Mental Health Services in Europe
Provision and practice

Edited by

NEIL BRIMBLECOMBE
Director of Nursing, Research and Development
South Staffordshire and Shropshire NHS Foundation Trust

and

PETER NOLAN
Visiting Professor in Mental Health Nursing
University of Birmingham
Emeritus Professor of Mental Health Care
Staffordshire University

Forewords by

DR MATT MUIJEN
Programme Manager, Mental Health and Degenerative Disorders
WHO Regional Office for Europe

DR PETER CARTER
General Secretary
Royal College of Nursing, London

IAN HULATT
Mental Health Adviser, Nursing Department
Royal College of Nursing, London

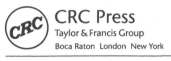

CRC Press
Taylor & Francis Group
Boca Raton London New York

CRC Press is an imprint of the
Taylor & Francis Group, an **informa** business

CRC Press
Taylor & Francis Group
6000 Broken Sound Parkway NW, Suite 300
Boca Raton, FL 33487-2742

ISBN- 13: 978-1-84619-436-8 (pbk)
ISBN- 13: 978-1-84619-827-4 (ebk)

Visit the Taylor & Francis Web site at
http://www.taylorandfrancis.com

and the CRC Press Web site at
http://www.crcpress.com

Contents

Contents

Contents

Foreword by Dr Matt Muijen

This is an important and timely book that illustrates some of the achievements of mental health reform in a range of European countries, but also recognises the long way we still have to go. Surprisingly, books systematically comparing mental health services in European countries are very rare. This book offers a wonderful opportunity to learn about the various service configurations and the challenges that countries face. The chapters also demonstrate the close connection between culture, wealth, health systems and mental health care, and the implications for the workforce and the quality of mental health care and the well-being of the population.

The thread of reforms unites this book. Some chapters describe the reform agenda and its implementation, others observe the lack of systematic reform in countries. This makes sense in the context of the last decade, in which nearly every country has drafted mental health strategies, policies or action plans. These strategies are remarkably similar, all aiming to close the large institutions, and to replace them with community-based mental health services, characterised by the strengthening of primary care, the creation of a range of community teams targeting different vulnerable groups, and the provision of beds in general hospitals. However, progress has been very variable, ranging from a comprehensive reorganisation of all components of the health system in countries such as the UK to countries in the eastern part of Europe which are still at the early stages. An attempt to explain this diversity is made in the conclusion and epilogue. One message that comes across strongly is that it is not simply about money. The political nature of mental health, including the human rights agenda, has to be acknowledged.

Another central message in this book, well summarised in the introduction and conclusions, is the broadening of the concept of what was formerly called psychiatry to mental health, as a consequence of the shift from narrow institutional care to a broad range of services in the community. This has meant that mental health promotion, the prevention and treatment of mental health problems, and the recovery and social inclusion of people have all come within the remit not only of mental health policy makers but also of the mental health workforce. That is a long way to travel in a short time, and no wonder many countries are struggling with its implications, let alone implementation. Reading this book offers a good understanding of the issues.

The challenge of reforming mental health services and creating community-based mental health care cascades to all aspects of the system. The evolution of nursing, centrally positioned in this book, exemplifies this. Whereas only 20 years ago the role of nursing would be largely similar in all the countries described in this book, i.e. caring for patients in hospitals, this has changed profoundly. Then, nurses could have moved from one country to another and taken up positions in hospitals that would have been practically identical. Now a nurse in one country works as a custodian in an institution, and after emigration can be expected to be an equal member in a multidisciplinary outreach team. Nurse training has evolved differentially between countries, following the changes of reform rather than leading it, and reinforcing the schism.

This book can be read in at least two different ways. One is to learn about the structure of mental health services and the challenges individual countries face. At this level, the book is highly informative. The other way of interpretation is to compare, to find similarities and differences and to identify the challenges across countries. One then realises how diverse Europe still is, how different the experience of service users and families must be and how complex it is to converge mental health care between countries. We can learn about mental health care from the variety of services in other countries, but we can also reflect on the diversity of societies in general, and the challenge to implement and sustain change in such different contexts. I have enjoyed reading this book a lot.

Dr Matt Muijen
Programme Manager, Mental Health and Degenerative Disorders
WHO Regional Office for Europe
January 2012

Foreword by Dr Peter Carter

I feel honoured to be able to provide a brief foreword to this excellent book. The editors have assembled a wide-ranging review of the state and shape of mental health services across Europe. There is of course variation in the journeys that have been made, but there is much in common. All of Europe has seen a concerted recognition that people fare better when treated and cared for at home (or at least close to it) and that large impersonal institutions are not a way to deliver services in the twenty-first century. All over Europe there are nurses engaged in the care and treatment of people who have mental health difficulties. Just as here in the UK, the changes sought and delivered will be carried forward on the energies and vision of those nurses. I am proud that we have achieved so very much in the transformation of mental health services here in the UK. Yet just as there have been changes in other areas of health care that nurses deliver, it is the vision of those nurses that things can be done in a better and more humane manner that has provided the necessary 'traction'. As the chief executive of the largest professional nursing organisation in Europe I know that it is the responsibility of all health care professionals and workers to not only engage in direct patient care, but also to become actively involved in influencing and shaping health policy.

Across Europe, as this book reveals, a range of mental health care professionals and carers are engaged in advocating on behalf of those they care for. I see it as an essential part of being a professional that one not only provides services, but ardently seeks to improve them. That surely is the intrinsic role of doctors, nurses, psychologists and many others involved in health care provision. Whilst we do have a duty to provide the best care for our clients, we also have a responsibility to influence those that determine how such services are provided. As mental health care professionals we can be a credible and respected voice in informing decision-makers how we believe services need to be provided. It can be seen across these chapters how the efforts of a range of disciplines, including academics, clinicians and other agencies across diverse cultures, are shaping, influencing and delivering the care and treatment that people need. United we can influence, we can shape policy, we can advocate for our clients, and we can do so together, confident that our vision will lead to the improvement of services and conditions for those who suffer various forms of mental health problems.

Dr Peter Carter
General Secretary
Royal College of Nursing, London
January 2012

Foreword by Ian Hulatt

This book is of real value in helping us understand more about approaches to mental health care provision across Europe. It provides overwhelming evidence that failure to recognise and support those at the cutting edge of service provision could result in untold damage to mental health services in the future. I was initially educated and trained in a small nursing school set in the grounds of a large rural psychiatric institution. There is now a generation of mental health nurses who have never worked in such a setting and indeed a generation of clients who will not have experienced such a care setting either. So much has changed and we have come to expect mental health services to be provided in settings that are modern, accessible and provided by people who have received the benefit of university-based education and training.

Yet, that is not the case over the (relatively) small continent of Europe. This book shows that mental health services are diverse in their structures and although countries may aspire to implement agreed policies, how they do so varies considerably depending on their systems, structures and cultures. There is not a race to a Utopian vision of mental health services, but clearly some countries are able to expend more resources upon these services than others. What they all share however is the determination of the nurses within them to shape not only the care provided to the clients and their carers, but also to exert influence within their respective organisations to improve the situation.

This book clearly demonstrates that the landscape is not only literally different across Europe, but also metaphorically with regard to the progress made. In the UK (for reasons still debated) we have largely eradicated large institutional settings for clients in which care and treatment were provided. Our progress to a community-focused system is an aspect of service provision we are rightly proud of. Yet models of institution-based care prevail in other parts of Europe. Our role here in the UK, informed by books such as this, is surely to offer support and a fraternal attitude of cooperation to our European nursing colleagues in their endeavours to progress.

Ian Hulatt
Mental Health Adviser, Nursing Department
Royal College of Nursing, London
January 2012

About the editors

Neil Brimblecombe, RN, PhD, is director of nursing, research and development for a mental health trust in central England and visiting professor at Nottingham University. He has worked in clinical, managerial and professional leadership roles, including director of mental health nursing for the English Department of Health. His research interests include crisis services, the history of mental health and international health issues.
neil.brimblecombe@sssft.nhs.uk

Peter Nolan, PhD, RMN, is professor of mental health care (emeritus) and has spent his working life in all aspects of mental health care – clinical, education and research. He has had a lifelong interest in the history of mental health services and has published widely in the area. His ambition is to see nurses get the recognition they deserve for the work they have done and are currently doing in continuing to improve services for those in the grip of mental health problems. He is currently visiting professor in mental health nursing to the University of Birmingham and emeritus professor of mental health care at Staffordshire University.
stallbrook@googlemail.com

List of contributors

Chapter 1
Ionela Petrea, PhD, is head of the Department of International Development, Mental Health at Trimbos-instituut in the Netherlands, a World Health Organization (WHO) collaborating centre for dissemination of good practices in mental health. Formerly technical officer with the Mental Health Programme at the WHO, she has published widely on European mental health services.
IPetrea@trimbos.nl

Chapter 2
Blanka Novotná, RN, started her career as a nurse in an acute psychiatric ward, later working for over 10 years as a psychotherapist and counsellor, and is currently deputy head nurse at the Bohnice Psychiatric Hospital in Prague. Novotná has completed long-term analytic psychotherapy training and studied in Belgium and the Netherlands. She lectures on communication courses for nurses and social workers, is vice-chairman of the Psychiatric Section of the Czech National Nurses Association and a board member of Horatio – European Psychiatric Nurses.
blanka.novotna@plbohnice.cz

Tomas Petr, MSc, BSc, RN, worked for over 8 years at the Bohnice Psychiatric Hospital in different positions – nurse, deputy head nurse, quality manager – and is currently head nurse in the acute psychiatric ward of the Central Military Hospital in Prague. Petr has extensive international experience, having worked in a private psychiatric hospital in the UK and attended various training programmes abroad. Chairman of the Psychiatric Section of the Czech National Nurses Association and member of Horatio – European Psychiatric Nurses, he has published and lectured widely on psychiatric nursing.

Chapter 3
Heikki Ellilä, RN, PhD, works as principal lecturer at Turku University of Applied Sciences. He is a member of the Mental Health Nursing expert group in the Finnish Nursing Association and a board member of Horatio – European Psychiatric Nurses. His main research interest is child and adolescent mental health.
Heikki.ellila@turkuamk.fi

Maritta Välimäki, RN, PhD, is professor in nursing science at the University of Turku and nursing director at the Southwest Hospital District. Her research area focuses on outcomes studies, patient-centred care and information technology in mental health services.

Lauri Kuosmanen graduated as a mental health nurse in 1992, MNSc in 2003 and PhD in 2009. His research interests include the use of seclusion and restraints in psychiatry, patients' rights, patient complaints, information technology in psychiatric care and primary care mental health.

Heli Hätönen, RN, PhD, works as a coordinator of preventive mental health services in the municipality of Imatra and as a researcher at the University of Turku. Her research and publications are focused on self-management and information technology in the field of mental health care.

Chapter 4
Michael Schulz, RN, PhD, is the first professor of psychiatric nursing in Germany and works at the Fachhochschule der Diakonie (University of Applied Sciences) in Bielefeld. He started his career as a psychiatric nurse in 1989. Schulz is a board member of Horatio – European Psychiatric Nurses, which seeks to link psychiatric nursing across Europe. He has researched and published on adherence, violence and stress in nursing.
Michael.Schulz@evkb.de

Chapter 5
Evmorfia Koukia, RN, MSc, PhD, is course leader and assistant professor at the University of Athens, School of Nursing, working with students at undergraduate and postgraduate level. She has previously worked in child, adult and mental health care, in both hospital and community settings, and has specific expertise in cognitive behavioural therapy and family psycho-education. Koukia is a member of the National Board of Nursing Development.
ekoukia@nurs.uoa.gr

Chapter 6
Ann J Sheridan, PhD, MEd, BNS, RPN, RGN, RNT, is a lecturer and researcher at UCD School of Nursing, Midwifery & Health Systems, Dublin. She has extensive experience in education and mental health, and her current areas of focus are collaborative learning with service users and nurses, and research on promoting and supporting recovery and social inclusion.
ann.sheridan@ucd.ie

Chapter 7
Claude Besenius was born in Luxembourg and obtained a BSc in psychology from the University of Leicester, followed by an MSc in health psychology from Stirling University. She recently completed her professional doctorate in health psychology at Staffordshire University whilst working for the Alcohol Community Team in Walsall, West Midlands. Claude's research interests include alcohol dependency, mental health promotion and services users' involvement in decision-making.
claude.besenius@gmail.com

Chapter 8
Roland van de Sande, RN, MScN, registered master's prepared psychiatric nurse, is working on a risk-management PhD thesis. Since 2002, he has been a senior lecturer at Utrecht University of Applied Science (NL) and academic nurse in the largest mental health trust in Holland, and since 2008 secretary general of Horatio – European Psychiatric Nurses.
roland.vandesande@hu.nl

Edwin Hellendoorn, RN, MA, is a clinical nurse specialist and project leader of a coercion reduction taskforce group, currently coordinating risk-management practice development projects on acute psychiatric wards and medium-stay locked psychiatric wards. Over the past years, Hellendoorn has provided clinical supervision, educational and research support in national coercion reduction programs (2006–11).

Chapter 9
José Carlos Pereira Santos is an adjunct professor at the Nursing School of Coimbra, a nurse specialist in mental health and psychiatric nursing, and holds an MSc in health socio-psychology and a PhD in mental health. Coordinator of several research projects about suicide prevention, he is president of the Portuguese Suicidology Society (2011–13) and has previously worked in intensive care, emergency and psychiatric wards.
jcsantos@esenfc.pt

Cândida Rosalinda Loureiro is an adjunct professor at the Nursing School of Coimbra (Department of MHNP). Having gained a master's in psychiatry and mental health in 2004, she is currently enrolled in a PhD in nursing sciences. As a nurse specialist in mental health nursing and psychiatry, Loureiro has been working with psychiatric patients in wards for acute and chronic patients for the last 10 years.

Aida Cruz Mendes is a coordinator professor at the Nursing School of Coimbra. A nurse specialist in mental health and psychiatric nursing, Mendes holds an MSc in occupational health and a PhD in psychology of education. She is also coordinator researcher of the 'Well-being, health and illness' section at the Health Science Research Unit: Nursing, as well as senior editor of the *Referência Journal of Nursing*.

Acknowledgements

We would like to express our gratitude to all who contributed to this book. In particular, we would like to mention their enthusiasm and readiness to respond to requests and the graciousness with which they accepted criticisms and suggestions. There are far too many colleagues to thank for various enlightening discussions we have had over the past two years and for which we are truly grateful. We owe a special debt of gratitude to Gillian Nineham, Jamie Etherington and Jessica Morofke of Radcliffe Publishing, who through gentle persuasion and focused questioning assisted considerably in bringing this book into existence. To all these people we extend our heartfelt thanks. Email addresses for main authors are provided.

Dedicated to the hope that services and conditions will continue to improve for all those who have suffered and continue to suffer with various forms of mental health problems throughout Europe.

Introduction

Neil Brimblecombe and Peter Nolan

In recent years, there has been a significant change in the language used to describe issues related to mental illness. The language of public pronouncements is powerful, argues Osbourne (2008): it provides definitions, offers directions and gives explanations; in addition, it seeks to alter our perception of reality and of how we relate to those around us. Recently, the language used in mental health care has increasingly reflected the cognitive dismantling associated with deinstitutionalisation, demedicalisation and deprofessionalisation of mental health services.

The World Health Organization (2010) has sought to recast mental illness in the context of the broader *mental health* domain, which it sees as the foundation for individual and community well-being. The claim that there is no health without mental health gives mental health a central position in the life of a community and its health services and increases recognition of the many factors that affect mental health either negatively or positively – factors such as rapid social change, stressful working conditions, gender discrimination, social exclusion, unhealthy lifestyles and human rights violations. This refocusing on mental health, rather than on mental illness, is both logical and timely; it challenges the stigmatising and pathologising frequently associated with institutionally based mental health care. It has also enabled the understanding that helping people to recover from mental health problems requires far more than the provision of services and treatments. There are many steps a person can take to enhance their own well-being, such as being physically active, connecting with family and neighbours, engaging in lifelong learning and volunteering in communities (The Foresight Project, 2009). Much has been learned from the voluntary sector about how people can look after themselves properly if supported and given appropriate information (Goddard, 2001). However, despite the WHO's recommendations for promoting mental health, for example by improving social support, stress management training, improved housing and reducing violence, the vast majority of countries approach mental health issues through a framework of treating mental *illness*

– particularly the more severe forms of mental illness, such as the psychoses and major affective disorders. The services they provide are typically referred to as 'mental *health* services', but in reality, they are mental *illness* services.

This book aims to explore the current arrangements for providing mental health services across Europe, how they have evolved, and plans for future development. It seeks to explore the broad question: Is there a common European approach to what mental health services should be and how they should be implemented? Lavikainen *et al.* (2000) point out that, even though there are EU policies stating what good mental health services should be, it is left to the discretion of individual countries to determine their preferred strategies for improving the mental health of their citizens. Whatever is devised has to be done within their capacities, capabilities and cultures.

The contributors were asked to focus specifically on nursing as a profession; its role, its relationships with other professions and the manner in which the profession had developed over time. There were a number of reasons to request a specific focus on this profession as opposed to others. Nursing is by far the largest profession working in mental health services across Europe, with a cursory glance at the figures in Chapter 1 suggesting over half a million in the EU alone. It is also one of the most flexible professions, with nurses working across health and social services. The history of modern mental health services is also, to a significant degree, the history of the development of nursing in the asylums and its subsequent stepping out into wider roles in different settings. The historical relationship between nursing and the medical profession, in the form of psychiatrists, reflects the implicit and explicit power of the psychiatric profession within mental health services. The majority of contributing authors to this book are from a mental health nursing background, which particularly equips them to describe and comment on nursing within their own countries.

In order to gauge the impact of these policies, in this book the mental health services of nine countries are explored. The authors were asked to address a number of themes (described below); although they have had considerable freedom to approach them in whatever way they chose. Additionally, in Chapter 1, Ionela Petrea sets the scene and provides an overview of comparative data and activity across Europe to allow a fuller contextualisation of the individual countries' contributions. The results from this and the subsequent chapters are discussed in a concluding chapter (Chapter 11), where commonalities and difference across Europe are highlighted. A brief epilogue then teases out key messages for the future.

The focus of this book is on mental health services, rather than the broader concept of mental health *care*. The differentiation here is based on a definition of *mental health services* as those that are specifically commissioned, normally by national or local governments, to provide specialist mental health interventions to people with mental illnesses. The reality is that in all countries, the majority of mental health *care* is not provided by such specialist services; rather, it comes in the form of informal care, provided by families, or non-specialist health or social care. Contributing to this, with varying degrees of skill, knowledge and enthusiasm, are health care workers, such as general practitioners and acute hospital staff, and a range of non-health care workers, including social care staff, priests, teachers and prison officers. A myriad charities and religious organisations are involved.

The particular countries contributing to this book were chosen for two main reasons; firstly, to reflect the distribution of countries across the European Union (EU), both in terms of size and geography. The reader will rightly note that large gaps are inevitably left unexplored in the European landscape. Secondly, countries were identified where authors were available who were in a position to comment in detail on their own countries' mental health services (in English), not just from a theoretical, research or policy perspective, but from their practical experience of delivering services. The authors were also deliberately chosen excluding those with medical backgrounds, so as to avoid descriptions provided by individuals specifically trained and acculturated in contemporary medical/psychiatric framings of mental health care. It is left to the reader to discern the benefits of taking a non-medical approach to the examination of European mental health services. Of course, just because a health professional is not a medical doctor does not mean that their understanding of mental health and illness, and the role of mental health services is not a *medicalised* one, i.e. consciously or unconsciously shaped by medical understandings, diagnostics, therapeutics and ways of seeing people and their problems. The possibility of seeking people who had used services to contribute to this book was considered, but decided against on the grounds that few countries appear to have well-established networks of experienced and confident service users who might help readers/professionals assess the strengths and weaknesses of different approaches and structures.

Terminology in this book reflects the differences in usage across Europe, and even within countries and between professions. The key variant is the word/s used to describe those people who use mental health services. The editors of this book use the phrase 'service users' in their specific contributions. The word 'patient' remains the more usual usage across Europe. The term *service user* is largely the result of the editors' acculturation within United Kingdom health care settings (as well as being an active philosophical choice). The term has arisen in the UK from a conscious attempt to avoid the use of the term *patient*, with its connotations of the person being a passive recipient of a health care intervention, to be replaced by a more neutral one. Such a distinction is still debated in the United Kingdom, but significantly, *service user* is now the official language of government, when referring to people who receive mental health services. The significance, or otherwise, of the fact that such a change does not yet seem to have a similar impact in many other countries is an issue that has yet to be explored in depth.

The chapters in this book can all be read individually. Individual descriptions of the arrangements in separate countries will provide sufficient detail to give a general sense of the needs, development and current issues in those countries. However, the editors believe that the real value in this book comes from noting that there is not only one way of providing mental health services and that the differences between countries may be as illuminating as those things that they have in common. The book provides a rich source for reflection on the many tensions within mental health services, the many attempts being made to reduce them and the considerable number of people who still do not have ready access to services.

Europe

In 2009, the population of the 27 countries of the European Union was close to 500 million (Eurostat, 2009). These countries are marked by huge diversity in size, population, wealth, health spend, history, geographical features and ethnicity. Yet on the surface, there seems to be much in common in terms of mental health services. All countries at least appear to be committed to a model of care that is based on the principles of the World Health Organization (see below). The histories of their mental health services all seem to include the establishment of asylums in the nineteenth century, followed by a stated aim to decrease reliance on institutional care late in the twentieth century (Priebe, 2004). The official framing of mental health problems across Europe is largely a medical one, based on international diagnostic categories, as diagnosed by medically trained staff. The fact that there exists two classification sytems for diagnosing mental health problems, i.e. ICD-10 and DSM-5, has added to the occasional confusion around definition and diagnosis. These are distinct approaches to problem identification, and it is not infrequent that clinical personnel who use different diagnostic critera encounter problems when seeking to ascertain what the nature of a problem is and what constitutes clinical evidence. This difficulty has come to light most notably in courts of law, when it appears that psychiatrists appear to be contradicting each other, when in fact they are appealing to different classificatory systems. Services are typically led (although in different ways) by medical staff specialising in psychiatric or neurological conditions. This book attempts to look beyond these generalities and to understand whether there really is a common understanding of what constitutes good mental health services and how near countries are to providing them.

Chapter structures
•••••••••••••••••••••••••••

The contributing chapters to this book are loosely divided into the sections laid out below. A raft of documents produced by the World Health Organization in the last 10 years has potentially set an agenda for mental health services in Europe (certainly representatives from many individual countries are amongst the signatories for many WHO proclamations and guidance documents) and these statements have helped raise issues that are explored in the chapters.

National profile and context

In describing features of the population, such as religion, wealth and ethnicity, the authors are contextualising the provision of their mental health services. Certain features of a population and their lifestyles may have a direct relevance to both mental health need and the manner in which that need may be met. An ageing population will produce an increasing number of mental health problems that are associated with old age, particularly dementia and depression, the latter being strongly linked with social isolation. Religion may tell us something about attitudes to life, living, illness and death. The historical role of the Catholic church in particular is interesting to consider, with its long history of providing care to people with mental health problems, and in some cases influencing aspects of the development of psychiatry itself.

The issue of ethnicity is one that was brought sharply to the attention of Europe in the 1990s, with the horrific sequelae of ethnic tensions being played out in the Balkans. For a country with a significant ethnic mix, a number of mental health issues can result. In the most extreme example, victims or survivors of ethnic violence and intimidation may be shocked and traumatised and require treatment for symptoms. Otherwise, different means of expressing emotions and distress are often confounders in a mental health system, with the dominant culture's modes of expression being recognised as more 'normal' than other ways of being. Labelling and misdiagnosing are always risks in such a situation. More fundamentally, issues of language and communication can make the practical delivery of mental health care challenging.

Else (2011) states that many of the causes of health problems are not to be found in individuals, but in how a society is structured. The bigger the gap, he argues, between the rich and the poor, the more it affects life expectancy, general health, levels of crime and violence, and mental illness. Being confined within the poverty trap can exacerbate the emotional pain associated with divorce, ill health and loneliness. However, in terms of wealth, there actually appears little evidence of direct impact of social class on the likelihood of developing schizophrenia (Mulvany *et al.*, 2001). Conversely, the effect of social circumstances on more common mental disorders is clear, with life stressors potentially contributing to the genesis of both anxiety and depression (Muscatell *et al.*, 2009). Unemployment has been strongly linked with psychological distress and, in some countries, an increased risk of suicide (Stuckler *et al.*, 2009). Financial status may also be a significant factor within health care systems where a direct payment is required for services, as this may directly deter individuals seeking treatment for their distress. The question of whether the disadvantaged in society, for example the unemployed, are disadvantaged in health systems is considered by several contributors, who describe features of their health cover and insurance systems.

The historical development of mental health services

In order to understand the current challenges of, and issues in, delivering mental health services across Europe, it is essential to understand the historical context. The way that services have been provided in the past and the manner and timing of changes to those services impacts on attitudes to mental health issues today. Attitudes are particularly important in shaping the 'culture' of mental health organisations. Here, 'culture' particularly refers to the way that mental health issues, the roles of staff and the relationships between staff and service users are perceived and understood, by staff, service users and others. There is existing evidence of considerable variation in the details of historical culture and practice in different countries' mental health systems (see, for example, Goldstein, 1987; Nolan, 1993; Goldberg, 1999; Boschma, 2003). The explorations provided within this book, from the nine contributing countries, paint pictures that have both similarities and differences between countries, but also make the important link with what has gone on before, what exists today and what may happen in the future.

Current national policy and priorities

The World Health Organization has put much store in the existence of national policies on mental health, carefully noticing who has and who does not have such policies. The report by Lavikainen *et al.* (2000) entitled *Public Health Approach on Mental Health in Europe* went much further than previous EU documents in voicing grave concerns about the consequences for the public good of ignoring mental health care. The report opens with an emphatic statement that:

> There is no health without mental health and it must be regarded as an indivisible part of public health.

It progresses by pointing out that mental health problems cause a heavy and increasing burden that contributes a high cost to our societies, long-lasting disabilities, increased mortality and enormous human suffering. Moreover, without the means of identifying the extent of these problems and strategies for effectively addressing them, mental health problems are set to become an even greater problem than they currently are. An action plan for the EU and its component countries has identified the following recommendations:

- Nation states should endeavor to promote positive mental health and tackle mental health problems utilising effective evidence-based measures.
- Each nation state should develop its own mental health strategy as an integral part of a comprehensive public health policy, taking account of the prevailing social and cultural circumstances.
- Mental health should be included in all policies at all levels and across all sectors of national and local governments.
- Closer collaboration between European states and the rest of the world is desirable as it promises substantial added value in the field of mental health promotion.

The Helsinki Agreement (WHO, 2005) affirmed the commitment of all EU member states to improved mental health care. It recognised the need for comprehensive, evidence-based mental health policies and sustainable means of implementing them. The following priority areas were identified:

- promoting individual and societal mental well-being
- tackling stigma, discrimination and social exclusion
- preventing the causes of mental health problems
- providing comprehensive and effective interventions for people with mental health problems whilst offering involvement and choice
- rehabilitating and including in society people who have experienced serious mental health problems.

As with previous policy statements, the Helsinki Agreement aimed to improve the general mental health and well-being of individuals, families and local communities. Mental health services should aim to enhance the well-being of people, build up their resourcefulness and resilience and enable them to enjoy a meaningful and productive life (WHO, 2005). Priebe (2006) comments that although ultimately the work of the conference may not be seen as seminal, it does illustrate important challenges to mental health care at the beginning of the twenty-first century and highlights important issues that might change the direction in the future. As later chapters in this book illustrate, some improvements have resulted from it, but in many areas only modest progress has been observed.

Some commentators (Dowding, 1995; Marmot, 2005) are critical of adopting a policy-first approach, which they consider naïve in that it fails to take account of the different health systems and infrastructures within the EU. There is no recognition of the circumstances – political, economic and social – that have given rise to gross health inequalities within and between European countries.

Without an understanding of these, health care policy may be little more than a cosmetic exercise. Without an understanding of the social determinants of poor health and a plan for addressing them, Marmot (2005) argues that public pronouncements on health are ineffective when endeavouring to activate political action. As described above, although there is clear evidence of links between social circumstance and many common mental disorders, such as anxiety and depression, the relative distribution of severe mental health problems, particularly psychotic disorders, is harder to understand in this way. Furthermore, one of the most significant mental health challenges across Europe, both now and in the future, is dementia, a disease whose growth is largely attributable to better living conditions and health care, resulting in longer lifespans. Dementia is becoming a huge social problem, but not one that arises from poor social conditions.

It is certainly a reasonable assumption to make that without a clear policy or strategy, systemic change and development is unlikely to happen. In the UK, the development of services able to respond to crises only became a routine part of what could be expected from services when it was ordained by a national strategy (DoH, 1999). The strategy was backed up by detailed guidance regarding the composition and aims of such services, and individual mental health-providing organisations were measured and held to account for delivering this. Prior to this time, the development of such services was localised and usually arose from the particular clinical interest and enthusiasm of charismatic clinical leaders, normally psychiatrists (Brimblecombe, 2001).

Staff and patients

The Helsinki Conference (WHO, 2005) acknowledged that although policies and legislation are important, of equal if not greater importance is having appropriately trained personnel to deliver them. Ionela Petrea (Chapter 1) clearly illustrates the wide variation between countries in the availability of different types of professional staff; for example, Finland has 163 nurses per 100 000 population, while Greece has only 3 nurses per 100 000. Whilst it is tempting to assume a simplistic relationship between more staff and proportionately better service, little evidence exists to actually prove that. However, it would be logical to assume that if the interventions required to make a positive difference to people with mental health problems are skilled activities that require training, then the presence of fewer staff capable of delivering them means less potential therapeutic benefit. The 'treatment gap' (that is, the difference between those who need a service and those who receive a service), must be influenced by such numerical differences. Generally, those services with more professionals available, for example, the health care systems of England, Finland and the Netherlands, tend to be more developed in terms of having a range of community services available. However, numbers provide no guarantee of comprehensiveness, as Ellilä and colleagues (Chapter 3), for example, point out the limitations in provision that still exist in Finland.

Conversely, it is clear that much of what makes a positive difference to people with mental health problems does not require psychiatrists, nurses or psychologists. Other factors are equally important, if not more so; employment, good housing and strong social relationships all have a positive effect (Office of the Deputy Prime Minister, 2004). Typically, there is a line, of varying rigidity, between mental health services that focus on *health* or *illness* issues, and social services and familial support which respond to *social* needs. This contentious boundary does appear to be perpetuated, to differing degrees, in the countries providing chapters here.

The World Health Organization (2003a) singled out mental health nurses as a primary means of combating psychiatric morbidity, and 3 years earlier the Munich Declaration (WHO, 2000) had advised that nurses should be central to mental health services because they could tackle public health challenges and were manifestly cost-effective. Nonetheless, despite the attention of the WHO, the chapters in this book illustrate that in most of Europe, the potential of mental health nursing remains largely untapped. Nursing remains bound by restricted roles and rules and by a subordinate relationship to medicine, sometimes enshrined in law. Other factors restrain the potential of nursing. In much of Europe, despite the profession increasingly becoming all graduate, the amount of specialist mental health training for nurses is limited, with only a handful of countries having specialist training at the level of initial qualification, while others provide only limited access to post-registration courses.

Mental health need

The established view is that mental health problems constitute a large and growing burden across Europe (WHO, 2005), yet mental health issues have received little governmental attention in proportion to the size of the challenge presented. The challenge with identifying need is deciding what should be done to alleviate it and this will undoubtedly become an even greater concern in the future. It is agreed that accurate data is hard to find, but the data that currently exists does call for much greater urgency in how these problems are dealt with. The individual chapters describe current evidence of need and consider whether provision is in line with that evidence. There is some doubt raised as to how reliable such data is, especially that comparing need between countries. It also appears that evidence of need sometimes does little to shape services in direct ways, with a number of countries noting inequality in provision, typically between cities and more isolated areas. The more general issue regarding the meaning and validity of psychiatric diagnostics, at both a practical and philosophical level, is considered in 'Conclusions' (Chapter 11).

Expenditure on mental health

To provide mental health services requires adequate and consistent funding. Different countries approach this necessity in different ways. The manner in which services are funded varies, with a range from individuals joining individual insurance schemes to services funded by central taxation. The level to which services are funded also shows great variation, with up to a sevenfold difference in the proportion of total health spend that actually goes on mental health (Chapter 1). Even taking into account the challenges of producing reliable figures on these matters, the differences are such that there are clearly major differences in the ability of countries to provide comprehensive mental health services and for individuals within each country to be able to access them.

The services

The structure and focus of services within a country are determined by political, cultural, professional and financial factors. Services can be categorised and judged in many ways, for example, comprehensiveness of response to a wide range of needs according to diagnosis or in terms of clinical pathway, such as crisis care and long-term rehabilitation. Politics may be influential at a national or international level, with countries signing up, at least theoretically, to the ambitions of the World Health Organization and the European Union. Cultural influence on services may be expressed through the attitudes of the population, politicians and professionals, and may result, for example, in resistance to the resettlement of long-stay patients into community-based settings. As above, the finances available are directly related to the potential extent of services, although as illustrated in some countries, such as Luxembourg, structural challenges may then prevent investment being as effective as possible.

Quality monitoring of mental health services

There are a number of approaches that can be taken to measure the quality of mental health services. The World Health Organization (WHO, 2003b) reasonably advises that 'A focus on quality helps to ensure that scarce resources are used in an efficient and effective way. Without quality there will be no trust in the effectiveness of the system.' Approaches that can be taken to measure quality can include gathering the experience of service users, comparing clinical outcomes between services through benchmarking processes, and evaluating as to whether the care provided is based on established best practice, derived from research evidence.

The particular approach to quality measurement taken in any given country is correspondingly likely to be influenced by attitudes to the role of service users in mental health services and the value attributed to their opinions, a willingness and means to self-assess, and access to suitable research and guidance on what actually constitutes best practice. Certainly, engagement with the research agenda seems to vary hugely across Europe, with the United Kingdom producing significantly more than other countries (with 10% of the total world publications, followed by Germany at 7% and other countries at 3% or less (Saxena *et al.*, 2006). There is, however, no evidence of a direct correlation between level of research output and quality of services provided. The reality is that there may be a different and simpler explanation for why some countries do not focus on quality measurement. 'In a context where resources are inadequate and mental health is emerging as a newfound priority, a concern for quality seems premature if not a luxury.' (WHO, 2003, p. 2).

The individual countries' contributions in this book appear to generally show a lack of well-established broad methodological processes to measuring quality in mental health services; a major issue for the well-being of the people they serve and a challenge to those who commission such services, for example, individual governments.

Mental health legislation

Mental health law is a point where the dilemmas and ambiguities inherent in mental health care come to the fore. The need to protect individuals and society from those with disordered minds has been recognised in Europe for many years, although the timing of the development of legislation to reflect this has varied widely. The history of mental health law and services demonstrates a dynamic interplay between the state's wishes to care and control, with the balance between the two impulses moving back and forth at different times and in different settings. In mental health services, the balance of protecting the individual's right to liberty has to be balanced on a daily basis with the state's right and duty to protect that person and others from harm.

Mental health is an arena in which the dynamic between state protection and individual liberty is played out within a medicalised framework which defines mental health problems. However, the existence of a mental health law (or other laws that perform a similar function) is not in itself a guarantee against human rights violations (WHO, 2005). In exploring the manner in which mental health law is applied in various states, a picture is built up of the range of approaches taken, in particular the balance held between legal and judicial power. It also shows the extent to which individuals are seen as being capable of making certain fundamental choices, even in the presence of significant mental health problems.

Attitudes to mental health problems

Attitudes to mental health problems in the general population and in health professionals have a tremendous impact on the lives of those with mental health problems, their families and those who work in mental health services. In addition to personal humiliation and rejection, negative attitudes can affect employment, housing, social relationships and personal safety (Office of the Deputy Prime Minister, 2004). The development of less institutionally based policies can be stymied by local resistance. Negative attitudes and stereotypes have been well documented through studies of public attitudes and media portrayals. The contributors to this book reveal the extent to which negative attitudes still exist. The Helsinki Agreement (WHO, 2005) made a specific pledge to tackle stigma, discrimination and social exclusion, and examples are provided of projects that are trying to face this huge problem across Europe.

Case scenario

A short case scenario has been provided to each of the national contributors to this book. They have provided a response to their view of the likely process that would be followed should the case described happen in their country. The case is a difficult one where an individual is described who may be threatening and whose initial actions suggest the possible presence of a serious mental illness. The situation where an individual is not willing to engage with mental health services is a challenging one everywhere, and the stories told by contributors suggest that many countries struggle to find an appropriate response at this point. The contributors then go on to describe likely interventions once the individual is in hospital, the reality being that across Europe, the inpatient context remains the central feature of mental health care. Finally, the case scenario describes the follow-up available after discharge, and this brings into sharp relief the differences in community resources available.

References

Alonso J, Codony M, Kovess V, et al. Population level of unmet need for mental healthcare in Europe. *Br J Psychiatry*. 2007; **190**: 299–306.

Becker T, Vazquesz-Barquero JL. The European perspective of psychiatric reform. *Acta Psychiatr Scand*. 2001; **104**: 8–14.

Boschma G. *The Rise of Mental Health Nursing: a history of psychiatric care in Dutch asylums, 1890–1920*. Amsterdam: University Press; 2003.

Bowers L, Douzenis A, Galeazzi GM, et al. Disruptive and dangerous behaviour by patients on acute psychiatric wards in three European centres. *Soc Psychiatry Psychiatr Epidemiol*. 2005; **40**(10): 822–8.

Brimblecombe N. Community care and the development of intensive home treatment services. In: Brimblecombe N, editor. *Acute Mental Health Care in the Community: intensive home treatment*. London: Whurr; 2001.

Department of Health. Mental Health Nursing: addressing acute concerns. *Report of the Standing Nursing and Midwifery Advisory Committee*. London: The Stationery Office; 1999.

Dowding K. *The Civil Service.* London: Routledge; 1995.

Else L. The happiness agenda. *New Scientist.* 2011; 16 April: 46–7.

Eurostat. *Total Population.* Luxembourg; 2009. Available at: http://epp.eurostat.ec.europa.eu/tgm/table. do?tab=table&language=en&pcode=tps00001&tableSelection=1&footnotes=yes&labeling =labels&plugin=1 (accessed 15 December 2009).

Foresight Project on Mental Capital and Wellbeing. *Mental Capital and Wellbeing: making the most of ourselves in the 21st century – final project report.* London: Government Office for Science; 2009.

Goddard M. Equity of access to health care services: theory and evidence from the UK. *Soc Sci Med.* 2001; **53**: 1149–62.

Goldberg A. *Sex, Religion and the Making of Modern Madness: the Eberbach Asylum and German society 1815–1849.* Oxford: Oxford University Press; 1999.

Goldstein J. *Console and Classify: the French psychiatric profession in the nineteenth century.* Cambridge: Cambridge University Press; 1987.

Healy J, Victor C, Thomas A, *et al.* Professionals and post hospital care for older people. *J Interprof Care.* 2002; **16**(1): 19–29.

Jones D. The free will delusion. *New Scientist.* 2011; 16 April: 32–5.

Lavikainen J, Lahtinen E, Lehtinen V, editors. *Public Health Approach on Mental Health in Europe.* Helsinki: National Research and Developmental Centre for Welfare and Health (STAKES); 2000.

Marmot M. Social determinants of health inequalities. *The Lancet.* 2005; **365**: 1099–104.

Marwaha S, Johnson S, Bebbington P, *et al.* Rates and correlates of employment in people with schizophrenia in the UK, France and Germany. *Br J Psychiatry.* 2007; **191**: 30–7.

Mossialos E, Murthy A, McDaid D. European Union enlargement: will mental health be forgotten again? *Eur J Public Health.* 2003; **13**(1): 2–3.

Mulvany M, O'Callaghan E, Takei N, *et al.* Effect of social class at birth on risk and presentation of schizophrenia: case-control study. *BMJ.* 2001; **323**: 1398–1401.

Muscatell KA, Slavich GM, Monroe SM, *et al.* Stressful life events, chronic difficulties, and the symptoms of clinical depression. *J Nerv Men Dis.* 2009; **197**(3): 154–60.

Nolan P. *A History of Mental Health Nursing.* London: Chapman Hall; 1993.

Office of the Deputy Prime Minister. *Mental Health and Social Exclusion. Social Exclusion Unit Report.* London: HMSO; 2004.

Osbourne T. *The Structure of Modern Cultural Theory.* Manchester: Manchester University Press; 2008.

Priebe S. Psychiatry in the future: where is mental health going? A European perspective. *Psychiatr Bull.* 2004; **28**: 315–6.

Priebe S. Sign of progress or confusion? A commentary on the European Commission Green Paper on mental health. *Psychiatr Bull.* 2006; **30**: 281–2.

Saxena S, Paraje G, Sharan P, *et al.* The 10/90 divide in mental health research: trends over a 10-year period. *Br J Psychiatry.* 2006; **188**(1): 81–2.

Stuckler D, Basu S, Suhrcke M, *et al.* The public health effect of economic crises and alternative policy responses in Europe: an empirical analysis. *Lancet.* 2009; **374**(9686): 315–23.

Wittchen H, Jacobi F. Size and burden of mental disorders in Europe – a critical review and appraisal of 27 studies. *Eur Neuropsychopharmacol.* 2005; **15**(4): 357–76.

World Health Organization. *Munich Declaration: nurses and midwives – a force for health.* Geneva: WHO; 2000.

World Health Organization, WHO Europe Mental Health Nursing Curriculum. *WHO European Strategy for Continuing Education for Nurses and Midwives.* Copenagen: WHO; 2003a.

World Health Organization. *Quality Improvement for Mental Health.* Geneva: 2003b. Available at: www.who.int/mental_health/resources/en/Quality.pdf (accessed 16 April 2011).

Mental health services in Europe

World Health Organization. *Report on the European Ministerial Conference on Mental Health*. Helsinki: WHO; 2005.

World Health Organization. *Mental Health: strengthening our response*. Geneva: 2010. Available at: www.who.int/mediacentre/factsheets/fs220/en/ (accessed 10 April 2011).

Mental health need in Europe

Ionela Petrea

Burden of disease

Mental health problems are one of the top public health challenges in Europe and represent a high burden of disease for the European population. It is estimated that 27% of the adult population (aged 18–65) in the European Union (EU), Iceland, Norway and Switzerland have experienced at least one mental disorder within a 12-month period, ranging from somatoform disorders, depression, anxiety and psychosis, to substance use or eating disorders. Women were more commonly affected than men (Wittchen and Jacobi, 2005). These figures represent an enormous human toll of ill health, with an estimated 83 million people affected. Yet even these figures are likely to underestimate the scale of the problem, as only a limited number of mental disorders were included in this meta-analysis. Additionally, this study did not collect data on those aged over 65, a group at a particularly elevated risk of mental health problems. These figures also fail to capture the complexity of the problems many people with mental disorders face. Indeed, 32% of those affected had one additional mental disorder, while 18% had two and 14% three or more.

The burden of mental health problems can also be reported as lost years of 'healthy' life, by measuring the gap between current health status and an ideal situation where everyone lives into old age free of disease and disability. This conventional health-gap measure, called disability-adjusted life years (DALYs), introduced by the World Health Organization (WHO, 2008a) in its Global Burden of Disease project, is particularly relevant to mental health. This is because it extends the concept of potential years of life lost to premature death to include equivalent years of 'healthy' life lost to states of 'less than full health', broadly termed 'disability'.

The most recent available data shows that neuropsychiatric disorders are

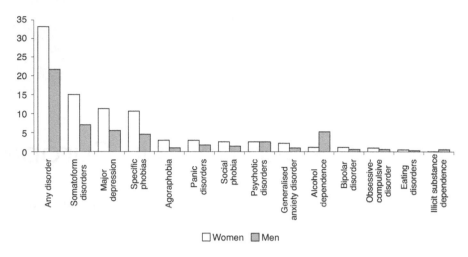

FIGURE 1.1 12-month prevalence rates by disorder among men and women (source: Wittchen and Jacobi, 2005)

the second-largest cause of DALYs in Europe[1] and account for 19%, only 4% less than the leading cause, cardiovascular disorders (*see* Figure 1.2). Mental disorders are among the top 10 conditions in all European countries, typically ranking 1 or 2 in EU countries, 3 or 4 in southeastern European countries and 5–6 in the Commonwealth of Independent States[2] (WHO Regional Office for Europe, 2005). The age group 15–29 is the most affected, with a burden twice as high as that of other groups, and with a pattern consistent across the European sub-regions.

Four of the top 15 diseases responsible for lost years of 'healthy' life are mental health disorders: unipolar depressive disorders are the third-leading cause of lost years of 'healthy' life (5.6% of all DALYs); alcohol use disorders rank sixth, accounting for 3.3% of all DALYs; self-inflicted injuries are the 11th-leading cause of DALYs (2% of all DALYs); and Alzheimer's and other dementias are the 14th-leading cause of DALYs (2% of all DALYs).

Another useful indicator calculates the burden of long-term conditions, including mental health problems, which place high demands on health systems. This is measured by years lived with disability (YLDs). Mental disorders are by far the most significant of the chronic conditions afflicting the population of Europe, accounting for 39.7% of the total burden of chronic conditions (*see* Figure 1.3).

---

1 Europe as defined in the UN system, with 53 member states.
2 The Commonwealth of Independent States (CIS) is a partnership on the basis of sovereign equality between 12 of the former Soviet Union republics (Armenia, Azerbaijan, Belarus, Georgia, Kazakhstan, Kyrgyzstan, Republic of Moldova, Russian Federation, Tajikistan, Turkmenistan, Ukraine and Uzbekistan) formed in December 1991 (source: www.cisstat.com/eng/cis.htm).

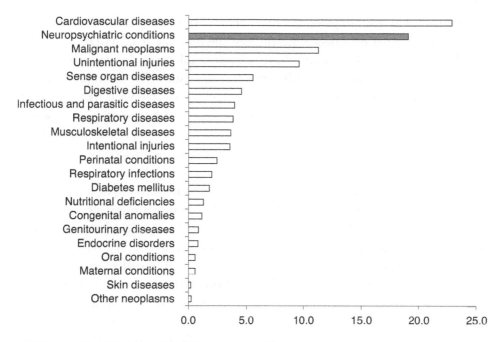

FIGURE 1.2 Disability-adjusted life years in the WHO European Region (source: WHO, 2008a)

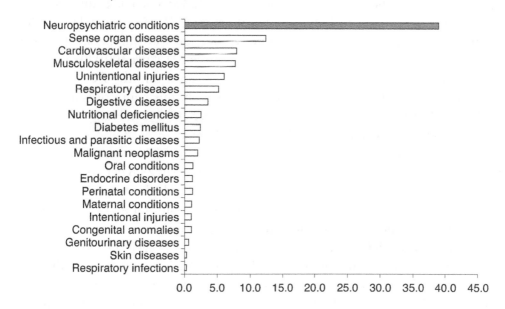

FIGURE 1.3 Years lived with disability in the WHO European Region (source: WHO, 2008a)

Unipolar depressive disorder alone contributes 13.7% of all YLDs, making it the leading chronic condition in Europe. This is followed closely by alcohol-related disorders, accounting for 6.23% of the total. Alzheimer's and other dementias are in seventh place, accounting for 3.8% of the total, ahead of schizophrenia and bipolar disorders, each responsible for 2.3% of all YLDs.

Ideally, policy-makers would have access to adequate information on the scale and nature of mental health problems, to ensure that the representation of mental health on the political agenda is commensurate with its magnitude, and to promote sufficient investment in strategies and interventions to address mental ill health. Ideally, one would seek data from national household surveys; nationally representative samples; internationally standardised data collection methods; a common set of indicators based on agreed definitions; and diagnostic instruments, and further would ensure effective monitoring of the quality of survey implementation that would be repeated at frequent intervals.

However, in terms of epidemiological data available to policy-makers, the situation in which European countries find themselves today is far from ideal. This is due to conceptual and technical obstacles involved in collecting data, some of which are not unique to mental health. Europe does not have a tradition of standardised surveys for mental health on a regional level. Findings presented above rely heavily on extrapolations from findings in a limited number of countries where epidemiological studies are carried out. While a far from perfect measure, one source of information that is always available is the suicide rate.

According to the most recent available data, 123 853 people commit suicide every year in Europe, of whom almost 80% are men (WHO Regional Office for Europe, 2010). The average suicide prevalence rates in Europe are 13.9 per 100 000, with the highest rates in the CIS countries (21.4 per 100 000), followed by the new EU countries (13.8 per 100 000). Even within the EU, where the overall average rate is 10.1 per 100 000 population, this figure rises as high as 30.7 per 100 000 population in Lithuania, 21.5 per 100 000 in Hungary, 18.5 per 100 000 in Finland and 18.4 per 100 000 in Slovenia.

Men are almost five times more likely to commit suicide than women in all countries of the European region (with an average rate of 23.8 per 100 000 population for men versus 5.2 per 100 000 for women). The highest male/female ratio occurs in CIS countries and the new EU member states (at a rate of 6 and 5.3 times more frequently in men than women, respectively).

The highest suicide rates are reported among people aged 65 and over (21.9 per 100 000 population) and 45–59 (21.5 per 100 000 population); both rates are around 1.5 higher than the European average. Among the age group 15–29, the highest rates are in CIS countries (21.9 per 100 000 population), 1.6 times higher than the European average.

In spite of the many methodological difficulties involved in data collection, the resultant limitations of available data and the type of indicator used, mental health problems are a leading health concern in Europe. Yet mental health problems remain largely untreated, as reflected by the substantial treatment gap. There is an obvious mismatch between the recognised needs of people with mental health problems and the actual evidence-based services available to them. It is estimated that even in countries with well-developed mental health systems, over 90% of people suffering alcohol abuse and dependence receive no effective treatment; nor do around 60% of those with anxiety disorders, almost 50% of those with panic disorders, 45% of those with major depression, 40% of those with bipolar affective disorder, 25% of those with obsessive compulsive disorder and 18% of those with schizophrenia and non-affective psychosis (Kohn *et al.*, 2004). However, limited availability of mental health services is responsible for only part of the treatment gap. Studies show that even when services are available, many of those who suffer from mental health problems avoid or delay treatment and choose not to engage or maintain contact with mental health services and adhere to treatment.

Political commitments to mental health care

Progressively, European governments have displayed their recognition of the scale and complexity of the challenges posed by mental ill health. Governments have committed themselves to protecting the rights of people with mental health problems, tackling discrimination against mental health service users and ensuring appropriate treatment and care. These commitments have been made in various fora, as member states of the United Nations (UN) and its specialised agency, the World Health Organization, as well as in the Council of Europe and the European Commission (EC).

United Nations

There are many United Nations documents endorsed by European member states that address the issue of equal rights to care and protection against discrimination. Some of these refer specifically to people with mental health problems.

The most recent is the Convention on the Rights of Persons with Disabilities, adopted by the United Nations General Assembly in 2006 and entered into force in 2008 (United Nations, 2006). This convention sets out the legal obligations of states to promote and protect the rights of persons with disabilities, including those with mental health problems.

The convention builds on previous documents, such as:

1. The 1975 UN Declaration on the Rights of Disabled Persons, which documented the rights of persons with disabilities (United Nations, 1975). This includes the right to receive special treatment for special needs, the right to medical and psychological treatment and the right to living conditions as close as possible to healthy people of their age.

2. The 1993 UN Standard Rules on the Equalization of Opportunities for Persons with Disabilities (United Nations, 1993). These rules require governments to guarantee persons with disabilities (including mental disabilities) the same level of medical care within the same system as other members of society and to develop national programmes for all groups of persons with disabilities, based on the actual needs of the persons with disabilities and on the principle of full participation and equality.

What is different about the 2006 convention is the way in which persons with disabilities are viewed. The 2006 convention conceptualises persons with disabilities as 'subjects' with rights, who are entitled to their 'physical and mental integrity on an equal basis with others' (Article 17) and are capable of making decisions for their lives based on their free and informed consent. They are not, as previously held, 'objects' of charity, medical treatment and social protection. Governments are required to ensure that people with disabilities, including those with mental health problems, have 'access to a range of in-home, residential and other community support services, including personal assistance necessary to support living and inclusion in the community and to prevent isolation or segregation from the community' (Article 19b, United Nations, 1993).

The convention confirms a number of civil rights, such as freedom to choose place of residence and nationality as well as rights to personal mobility, to property, to enter into contracts, to manage one's own financial affairs, to marry, work and retain custody of one's children, and to participate in political and public life. It prohibits discrimination against people with disabilities in health insurance, employment and education, and requires member states to prevent discriminatory practices in the delivery of health care.

Another key document adopted by the UN General Assembly is the 1991 Resolution on the Principles for the Protection of Persons with Mental Illness and the Improvement of Mental Health Care (MI Principles), which remains, to this day, a reference document for national mental health legislation (United Nations, 1991). The rights to which service users are entitled, according to the MI Principles, include the right to access mental health facilities equivalent to the access provided to any other health facility for any other illness, the right to treatment and care that meet the same standards as for people with other illnesses and the right of persons admitted to mental health facilities to the same level of resources as in any other health establishment. Though the document is not legally binding, it is stated within it that member states are expected to implement these principles fully.

World Health Organization

In 2001, the WHO took the initiative of dedicating, for the first time, the World Health Report, the technical discussions at the World Health Assembly and World Health Day to mental health. In the report, entitled *Mental Health: New Understanding, New Hope*, member states were urged to improve care for people with mental health problems, stressing that 'Effective solutions for mental disorders are available' (WHO, 2001, p. 109). The document states that governments are as responsible for the mental health as for the physical health of their citizens and should ensure that mental health policies are developed and implemented. The report calls for member countries to provide universal access to appropriate and cost-effective services for people with mental health problems, the provision of adequate care for service users and the protection of human rights for people with mental health problems. While acknowledging that the care required by people with severe and persistent mental health problems is similar to that of people with chronic physical problems, the document denounces the significantly poorer conditions in psychiatric hospitals as compared with other hospitals. It is recommended that ministries of health are 'to trade some efficiency gains to reallocate resources in the pursuit of equity' when developing their mental health strategies. The report formulates recommendations for member states to address the challenges faced in various areas of mental health. The 10 recommendations are:

1. Provide treatment in primary care.
2. Make psychotropic drugs available.
3. Give care in the community.
4. Educate the public.
5. Involve communities, families and consumers.
6. Establish national policies, programmes and legislation.
7. Develop human resources.
8. Link with other sectors.
9. Monitor community mental health.
10. Support more research.

By adopting the report, governments committed themselves to implementing its recommendations, based on the resources available in each country.

Pledges made at the global level have been tailored to the regional context in the form of regional or sub-regional commitments. The most important WHO European policy documents are the Mental Health Declaration and the Action Plan for Europe (WHO Regional Office for Europe, 2005a). Both of these instruments were endorsed by European health ministers in January 2005, at the first Ministerial Conference on Mental Health[3] in the region. Hosted by Finland, the

---

3   According to WHO regulations, the purpose of ministerial conferences is 'to transmit new

Helsinki Conference generated the political commitment to move from general agreement to detailed policy decisions within countries. Other key stakeholders, such as organisations representing users, carers and mental health professionals, also contributed to the preparation of these two documents that set the priorities for the next 7 years[4], as follows:

1. Foster awareness of the importance of mental well-being.
2. Collectively tackle stigma, discrimination and inequality, and empower and support people with mental health problems and their families to be actively engaged in this process.
3. Design and implement comprehensive, integrated and efficient mental health systems that cover promotion, prevention, treatment and rehabilitation, care and recovery.
4. Address the need for a competent workforce, effective in all these areas.
5. Recognise the experience and knowledge of service users and carers as an important basis for planning and developing services.

Health ministers who attended the Helsinki Conference committed themselves 'to recognising the need for comprehensive evidence-based mental health policies and to considering ways and means of developing, implementing and reinforcing such policies' in 12 priority areas for action. The Action Plan set out in detail the responsibilities of both the WHO and member states. These include reductions in stigma and discrimination, access to good primary health care, effective care in the community, partnerships across sectors, a competent workforce and adequate and fair funding.

A few sub-regional commitments are worth mentioning; a couple of which preceded the Helsinki Conference, and actually led to it. For instance, in June 2001, mental health professionals linked to national governments and mental health organisations in southern and southeastern Europe signed the Athens Declaration on Mental Health and Man-Made Disasters, Stigma and Community Care (WHO Regional Office for Europe, 2001), subsequently endorsed by a resolution of the Regional Committee for Europe at its 51st session. In the document, governments were requested to implement programmes aimed at reducing stigma and discrimination and to uphold the principle of equity in their mental health policies, programmes and services, and to accelerate the transfer

---

knowledge or review and discuss new policies and principles of interest to Member States. They bring together representatives of Member States, normally at ministerial level, to review broad strategic approaches to problems and seek a measure of agreement on important elements of particular problems, to further the application of the most recent knowledge and to foster common action on priority issues. They can also "round up" activities in a particular field to provide a springboard for practical application of the knowledge gained.'
4   A new WHO European Strategy for Mental Health is expected to be adopted in 2012.

of mental health care into the community. They were also asked to vigorously and systematically pursue the process of de-stigmatisation and the development of community mental health services. This, it was argued, would guarantee the civil and human rights of patients in receiving appropriate mental health services, education, housing and employment, so that their integration into society is based on solidarity and humanity as well as on pragmatic grounds.

The same year, health ministers from eight southeastern European countries signed the Dubrovnik Pledge: Meeting the Health Needs of Vulnerable Populations in South East Europe (WHO Regional Office for Europe and Council of Europe, 2001). This instrument expresses a strong political commitment by the respective countries to working in partnership so as to ensure equity of health care provision, increased access to appropriate, affordable and high-quality health care services, to address inequalities in health infrastructure and work on improving the balance between primary and secondary services in six health areas, including mental health. This event took place within the framework of the Stability Pact project for southeastern Europe, developed in partnership with the Council of Europe and the governments of other European countries (e.g. Greece, Italy and Sweden).

Finally, in 2008, WHO national counterparts from eight CIS countries signed the Merano Declaration on Mental Health in CIS countries (WHO Regional Office for Europe, 2008). On the basis of similarities in historical organisation of mental health services and the provision of mental health treatment and care in their countries, this document acknowledges a number of common challenges. These challenges are related to implementation of national policies and legislation, availability of mental health care in primary care settings, poor conditions in mental health institutions, which remain the main provider of mental health services in these countries, limited availability of specialist mental health staff and poor funding. The document sets a common work agenda around these areas and asks WHO Europe to support these countries and further the improvement of this work.

European Commission

The main EC policy initiatives with regard to mental health are the Green Paper on Improving the Mental Health of the Population and the European Pact for Mental Health and Well-Being (European Commission, 2005, 2008).

The green paper was launched in 2005, shortly after the WHO conference in Helsinki, and sought to initiate a public consultation on how better to tackle mental illness and promote mental well-being in the EU and to examine how best to develop a comprehensive EU strategy on mental health. The green paper identifies four areas of priority for a potential EU strategy:
1. Promote the mental health of all.

2. Address mental ill health through preventive action.
3. Improve the quality of life of people with mental ill health or disability through social inclusion and the protection of their rights and dignity.
4. Develop a mental health information, research and knowledge system for the EU.

Key stakeholders had the opportunity to comment on the green paper and give feedback to the commission. The report at the end of the consultation process concluded that there is indeed a need for an EU strategy in the area of mental health. However, instead of a strategy, the EC launched a European pact. This pact occurred by way of a high-level meeting organised in June 2008 and highlighted five areas of action, namely:
1. prevention of depression and suicide
2. mental health in youth and education
3. mental health in workplace settings
4. mental health of older people
5. combating stigma and social exclusion.

The recommendations contained within the pact were further endorsed by a European Parliament resolution on mental health in 2009.

Council of Europe

As with the UN, a number of key resolutions and recommendations of the Council of Europe are not aimed specifically at mental health, but nevertheless address issues relevant to the treatment and care of psychiatric patients. These include the Convention on Human Rights, the European Convention for the Prevention of Torture and Inhuman or Degrading Treatment or Punishment, which established a monitoring committee, the Revised European Social Charter and the Convention on Human Rights and Biomedicine (Council of Europe, 1950, 1987, 1996, 1997).

In 1994, the Parliamentary Assembly of the Council of Europe adopted Recommendation 1235 on Psychiatry and Human Rights. This recommendation is aimed at providing member states with an instrument for promoting legal measures guaranteeing respect for the human rights of psychiatric patients (Council of Europe, 1994).

Complementing the documents that seek to protect general human rights, including the right to health care, the 2004 Council of Europe Recommendation 10, concerning the protection of the human rights and dignity of persons with mental disorder, aims to enhance the protection of the dignity, human rights and fundamental freedoms of persons with mental disorders, in particular those who are subject to involuntary placement or treatment (Council of Europe, 2004). The explanatory memorandum attached to the recommendation elaborates on this, noting that 'Discrimination may also arise within health services themselves, for example by patients with mental disorders being given a lower priority for treatment of their physical illness'. On a wider scale, whether the allocation of personnel and financial resources to mental health services is fair in comparison to the allocation made to physical health services warrants consideration.

The strength of different international commitments

The impact at a national level of these instruments by international organisations is relative to their status and mandate, political influence and financial power. The United Nations, its specialised health agency (i.e. the World Health Organization) and the Council of Europe are all intergovernmental membership organisations aiming to promote cooperation between countries. The United Nations and the World Health Organization have 193 member states across all continents, while the Council of Europe has 47 member states entirely from the European region. In contrast, the European Union is an economic and political partnership between 27 European countries and the European Commission is the EU's executive arm.

The financial power of the UN, WHO and Council of Europe is limited to the extent that they are funded by their member states through membership fees. The WHO also receives further donations primarily from its member states, which account for up to 75% of its working budget. These donations can vary significantly (Kohn *et al.*, 2004). While this allows the WHO to implement a wider range of activities, it also makes it dependent on voluntary donors to implement its planned work. In contrast, the main source of revenue of the EU, accounting for about 75% of its total budget, is payment by each EU member state consisting of a uniform percentage rate applied to gross national income (GNI). Alongside other funding resources, such as the value added tax (VAT) or traditionally held resources, this allows the EC to implement and indeed fund a wide range of activities, making it a significant financial power.

All of these organisations are mandated by their respective member states to instigate adoption of policies and legislation. However, the scope of these international instruments differs from one organisation to another, depending on their mandate and sphere of influence. Thus, the WHO focuses on health-related policies, the Council of Europe on human rights and democratic practices, while the EC focuses on its established areas of competence; namely, types of services, key personnel and effective treatments.

The World Health Organization has been given the broadest mandate by its constitution to support member states in all areas of health, including mental health (WHO, 1948). One of its main roles is to bring countries together to address critical issues in health. Although it has done so several times since the

1950s, the WHO was relatively limited in its role with respect to mental health until the late 1990s and the turn of the century, when its role in this field is compared with its role in addressing other public health issues, such as tobacco control. Still, over the last 10 years it has adopted a number of influential policy documents, as noted above, that have steered policy-making on mental health in European countries. Although none of these documents are legally binding, they typically include a requirement from member states for the WHO to monitor their implementation. Different monitoring mechanisms, ranging from regional data collection to country-based national assessments, have been used to instigate policy development and implementation at the national level.

Unlike the WHO, the competence of the European Commission is limited in mental health, as hospitals and the health service remain the sole responsibility of the national state. The EC was not very active, either in the area of mental health or indeed in any area of health, until the late 1990s. It was only in 1992 that the EU received a mandate to work in the area of public health, with the advent of the Maastricht Treaty. The priority areas identified in the green paper and the mental health pact reflect the scope of the EC mandate in health. In addition, the current EC mental health policy documents remain at the level of consultation papers or loose agreements, with no binding commitments from the EU member states (Petrea and Muijen, 2008). Despite these limitations, the EC can still influence policy-making in mental health and support changes in countries, as it has done in some cases, by the use of some of its other mandates in protection of civil and social rights for the EU citizen, including the right to health care.

The only legally binding international agreements relevant to mental health have been adopted in the framework of the United Nations and the Council of Europe. The UN conventions have been influential, particularly in the area of disability. The Council of Europe played a special role in promoting fair mental health legislation and made an important contribution to addressing the treatment and care of persons with mental health problems from a human rights perspective. However, none of the Council of Europe documents that specifically address mental health (as referred to above) are legally binding, and their implementation is not easy to monitor.

National versus international policies

International policies can play an important role in driving change at the national level for those countries which endorse them. This is true even if the international instrument is not legally binding. Most of the time, international policies are the outcome of long-term processes involving international exchanges of good practices which are supported by a substantial base of evidence for their efficiency and/or effectiveness. They are generally adopted when the particular issue they address manages to capture sufficient attention from decision-makers and is raised on their political agenda. International agencies typically initiate negotiations on such policies when there is broad agreement on good practice in countries that have managed to achieve notable progress. Simultaneously, this is matched with the aspirations of champions for good practice (be they health professionals, decision-makers or beneficiaries) from countries where such practices have not been implemented at all or have not yet reached the mainstream.

Typically, countries with more advanced health care systems are at the forefront of promoting and developing international policies. Countries with less advanced policies and practices also endorse these international policies. On endorsement, all countries are expected to reflect on how the international policy will impact the national policy. As a result, countries with less advanced mental health policies need to make more significant changes to align themselves with the commitments within international policy.

International organisations mandated to monitor the implementation of international policies apply pressure on governments to adopt national policies which reflect the commitments made within these policies. These organisations, such as the WHO, provide technical support to the process of drafting national policies. However, in practice, policies are not the drivers of change in these countries and their adoption is not a valid indicator of a genuine willingness to induce change. The adoption of policies emerging primarily due to international pressure and for the purposes of public relations and convenience are often fairly meaningless and inconsequential in practice.

Policy-makers from countries with less advanced mental health policies and practices often have incentives to formally meet these expectations, even if the adoption of national policies is not the result of acknowledged needs at the national level. However, these national policies are not rooted in local processes and subsequently have insufficient ownership from key stakeholders and decision-makers. Internationally, adoption of legislation that complies with international requirements brings about financial support in the form of international funding for these countries, as well as political support and potential inclusion in different 'clubs' of countries (e.g. the European Union). Moreover, adoption of internationally sound and acceptable national policies also brings benefits nationally. Governments can use the adoption of these policies as a means of formally satisfying vocal requests for action from national champions, even if they have no intention to pursue their implementation.

National and international policies are generally complementary. Their comparative impact depends on the value attached to policies in a given country. At the national level, countries differ in the way in which policy-makers undertake the development and implementation of policy. This is because countries have dissimilar governing cultures and, from country to country, policy-makers develop policies with quite different mindsets and expectations for their implementation and accountability.

National policies have a decidedly stronger impact in countries where adoption of policy documents results in unambiguous expectations that commitments will be made and targets and milestones that have been set will be met. An additional precondition for the success of national policies is that decision-makers and relevant stakeholders are held accountable for the progress achieved during the time frame allocated for the implementation of that policy.

Measuring the impact of international policies at the national level is not straightforward. For national champions of such approaches, these policies can be key tools used to lobby for changes at the national level. They can also be used to give legitimacy to cross-country comparisons of practices, based on international monitoring of the implementation of commitments made by governments that have signed these international policies. Examples of areas in which cross-country comparisons have yielded improved services include early intervention, integrated health and social care, and various approaches to mental health promotion. While these comparisons are often disliked by politicians because of the ranking of countries they imply, they do tend to be powerful tools for instigating change, often for the same reason.

From international commitments to local action

As described above, international commitment has often been used as a means of putting pressure on governments to increase national action in the area of mental health. Most countries currently undergoing early-stage reform of their mental health systems have developed national mental health policies and legislation, often using international policies and recommendations as a guide. As such, national documents frequently set ambitious goals and cover a wide range of areas, from mental health promotion to deinstitutionalisation and human rights. What they often miss, however, are specific targets to be achieved within a determined time frame (the means by which any progress towards these targets will be measured), clearly established funding mechanisms and funding sources for the implementation of policy and achievement targets. In their absence, the goals set remain aspirational.

Although there has been an indisputable increase in awareness about mental health among governments in Europe, the impact of different political commitments is not always evident. However tempting it might be to simply blame decision-makers for not doing enough, one must acknowledge the challenges of translating political commitments into practical services and structures. Unlike other health areas, in which improvements can be linked to, for example, acquisition of high-quality equipment, linear correlations cannot be simplistically drawn in relation to improvements in mental health. While investments and commitment similar to other health areas are and should be a prerequisite, they are not sufficient in and of themselves. The interface between employment, social welfare, education, as well as the still-prevalent stigma and prejudices in society, impact significantly on mental health outcomes. Solutions to improving mental health remain complex.

Ongoing reforms in Eastern Europe illustrate these challenges well. The initial phase of reform is marked by high expectation for rapid change among some stakeholders contrasting with low priority given to mental health reform, as demonstrated by low budgets allocated and negligible investments in mental health. Mental health services in this phase are mainly based within large institutions, many with up to 2000 beds. Inpatient care is characterised by tough living conditions, where treatment is reduced to medication and patients often spend their lives dressed in pyjamas, engaged in few or no purposeful activities. The main achievement during this phase is the development of national mental health policies and legislation. But implementation strategies are not yet defined and commitment to the mental health agenda continues to be uncertain.

Political commitment is often stimulated by international pressure due to reports of human rights violations. Considerable funds are generally allocated to kick off the implementation of reform measures. Financial investment leads to improvements in mental health facilities, to increased infrastructure of mental hospitals and the setting up of pilot community services. However, the overall form and content of services remains largely unchanged. Most specialists are not yet fully behind the reform process in that they continue to provide individual services in the way they have always done. Where services have been radically transformed, it has taken local proponents, often working together with non-governmental organisations, to demonstrate how new collaborative arrangements can occur. Where effective innovation has taken place, training curricula for different staff groups have been developed and are in the process of being integrated into the curricula of faculties or centres for continuous education. While training courses are offered on a pilot basis to staff in affluent areas, they do not, however, reach remote, less developed areas. Some countries start building the capacity of primary health care to identify and treat people with mental health problems in an effort to both compensate for a shortage of specialist staff and to bring mental health services closer to the communities.

A turning point in the reform process typically takes place when, having benefited from investments over a sustained period of time, a critical number of services are modernised, living conditions in mental hospitals become decent and human rights violations are contained. Though not mainstream, modern evidence-based practices are accepted and endorsed by an influential proportion of the mental health staff, while leaders in mental health take ownership over mental health reform. The focus, now, is on how to ensure sustainability of successful initiatives, standardise good practices and learn from experiences and mistakes. Further challenges remain: introducing client-focused approaches to treatment, facilitating multidisciplinary team work and operational partnerships with other sectors, and integrating people with mental health problems into society and the workforce. Of major concern is how to protect the investments made in specialist staff; these professionals are usually the first to emigrate. Quality control becomes relevant, although setting up monitoring mechanisms will still take time and further investment.

A WHO study monitoring the mental health status in 42 countries, as compared to commitments made in the Helsinki documents, shows that while quality and provision of mental health care varies greatly across Europe, the vast majority of countries have made significant progress over recent years (Petrea and Muijen, 2008). Indeed, Europe now boasts several of the world's leading national processes in such areas as mental health promotion, mental disorder prevention activities, service reform and human rights.

Within the framework of mental health reform, the greatest need is to increase availability of community-based services, such as crisis care, home treatment, assertive outreach and early intervention. Many countries report that these services are available only to a small proportion of the population. Only Germany, Luxembourg and the United Kingdom (England and Wales) report that all or almost all people with mental disorders have access to home treatment and early intervention. In eight countries, home treatment is unavailable, while 11 countries report that early intervention services are virtually absent. Only the United Kingdom (England and Wales) reports that all or almost all people with mental disorders have access to assertive outreach. Conversely, 16 countries report that they do not provide these services at all.

There is large diversity in the models of care across Europe that includes some nations with well-established mental health systems and others that are still in an early stage of deinstitutionalisation. The pace of change, the improvements in treatment and care for people with mental health problems and the time frame and extent to which countries shift from institutional settings to person-centred community-based care varies from country to country.

Mental health resources – funding and workforce

Mental health funding

Funding for mental health remains small relative to the burden of disease. Data about mental health funding is available from 34 countries; however, the picture provided is not completely accurate, as mental health budgets are hard to define and are often subject to complex funding mechanisms (*see* Figure 1.4). In some countries, this budgetary information includes funds spent on mental health in primary care, in others not, while in still other countries they exclude time-bound investments in mental health reform.

While these figures are not perfect, they are indicative of the degree to which mental health is represented and prioritised by governments, and show the major differences between countries. These differences need to be interpreted in a broader societal context. One important observation is that wealthier countries, with a higher level of human development (as measured by the Human Development Index[5]), invest more money in general health and place a higher priority on mental health.

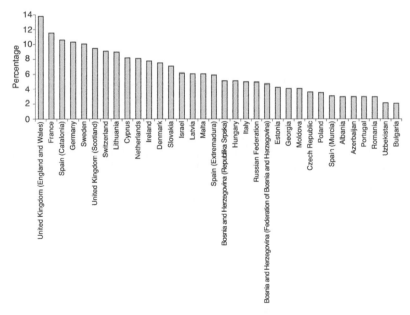

FIGURE 1.4 Mental health budget or expenditure as a proportion of the total health budget or expenditure (source: Petrea and Muijen, 2008, p. 118)

---

5   The Human Development Index (HDI) is a composite index that measures the average achievements in a country in three basic dimensions of human development: a long and healthy life; access to knowledge; and a decent standard of living (http://hdr.undp.org/en/media/HDR_20072008_EN_Complete.pdf).

Thus, mental health funding is correlated with GDP per capita such that more affluent countries spend more on mental health than do poorer countries within Europe (*see* Table 1.1). Looking beyond income, countries with higher achievements in different areas of human development also spend more on mental health. Furthermore, countries that give higher priority to health allocate a higher proportion of their health budgets to mental health. Mental health budgets are positively correlated with total expenditure on health as a proportion of GDP, as well as with per capita expenditure on health.

A high percentage of people that receive social welfare benefits or pensions because of disability have, as their primary condition, mental health problems. This indirectly increases the financial burden of mental health problems on a country. Data from countries where information is available shows that mental health problems account for as much as 44.4% of social welfare benefits or disability pensions in Denmark, 43% in Finland and in Scotland and 37% in Romania (*see* Figure 1.5). Even in Moldova, one of Europe's poorest countries, mental disabilities account for 25% of all social welfare benefits or disability pensions afforded by the government.

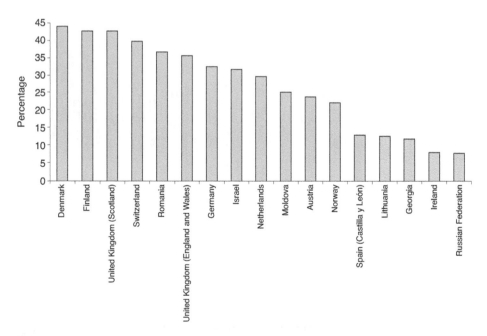

FIGURE 1.5 Proportion of people receiving social welfare benefits or pensions because of disability due to mental health problems (source: Petrea and Muijen, 2008, p. 127)

Considering the complex needs of people with mental health problems, integration of mental health service provision with other parts of the health sector and with other sectors is essential both to avoid double spending and to ensure better services for users. However, mechanisms for pooling of funds are rarely available. Even when strategies are developed jointly, they often lack specific targets and mechanisms to monitor and evaluate partnerships. At a practical level, human resources need to be allocated and trained for joint work in which mental health is part of the mainstream – yet another challenge.

Mental health workforce

People with mental health problems living in countries which invest more in mental health have significantly better access to mental health professionals. Higher investments in mental health are correlated with higher availability of psychiatrists and nurses working in mental health (*see* Table 1.1).

The availability of specialist mental health professionals (psychiatrists, nurses, psychologists) varies greatly across Europe (*see* Table 1.2). For instance, there are 30 times more psychiatrists per 100 000 population in Switzerland than in Turkey. This intercountry gap is even greater for nurses working in mental health. Finland has 163 nurses per 100 000 population, while Greece has only three nurses per 100 000 population. Psychologists are present in small numbers or are virtually non-existent in mental health services in many countries in the eastern part of the region, while in Austria there are 63 psychologists per 100 000 population, in Finland 47.2 per 100 000 population and in Norway 35 per 100 000 population. The availability of mental health professionals is highest in the EU countries that joined before 2004, and lowest in the CIS countries (*see* Table 1.3).

Mental health staffing differences between countries go beyond numbers. They are reflected in the quality of training and the roles and responsibilities assigned to different staff groups. Intercountry differences are just as diverse in these categories as in staff numbers. In some countries, people with mental health problems have access to multidisciplinary teams with clearly defined roles and responsibilities for each staff category. In others, they are confronted with psychiatrist-dominated care, where the impact of social workers, occupational therapists or psychologists is negligible. Even when they are present in these countries, their functions and status (revealed by substantially lower salary scales) undermine effective teamwork due to the diminished role and value attributed to these health professionals.

One striking difference across countries is the level of training, roles and responsibilities of nurses. A number of countries offer and require a period of specialised training to qualify as a mental health nurse, whereas others employ general nurses to work in mental health care and offer on-the-job training. In some countries, retraining courses have been established so that some qualified mental health nurses are entering the workforce. The priority given to workforce development can be judged by the proportion of training hours dedicated to mental health. This varies significantly, from 67% in Ireland and 49% in the United

TABLE 1.1 Correlations between GDP per capita, Human Development Index, expenditure on health and mental health, and numbers of mental health staff per 100000 population[6]

		GDP per capita, Int$	Human Development Index (value)	Total expenditure on health as % of GDP	Per capita total expenditure on health (PPP Int$)	Mental health budget or expenditure as a proportion of the total health budget or expenditure
Mental health budget or expenditure as a proportion of the total health budget or expenditure	Pearson correlation	0.673(**)	0.687(**)	0.487(**)	0.700(**)	1
	Sig. (2-tailed)	0.000	0.000	0.007	0.000	
	N	29	29	29	29	29
Number of psychiatrists per 100000 population	Pearson correlation	0.453(**)	0.638(**)	0.461(**)	0.532(**)	0.601(**)
	Sig. (2-tailed)	0.003	0.000	0,003	0,000	0,001
	N	40	40	40	40	29
Number of nurses working in mental health care per 100000 population	Pearson correlation	0.651(**)	0.576(**)	0.129	0.577(**)	0.553(**)
	Sig. (2-tailed)	0.000	0.001	0.490	0.001	0.004
	N	31	31	31	31	25
Number of psychologists working in mental health care per 100000 population	Pearson correlation	0.554(**)	0.673(**)	0.392(*)	0.612(**)	0.411
	Sig. (2-tailed)	0.002	0.000	0.039	0.001	0.072
	N	28	28	28	28	20

* Correlation is significant at the 0.05 level (2-tailed).

** Correlation is significant at the 0.01 level (2-tailed).

6 Author's calculations based on: 1) mental health data from: Petrea and Muijen (2008); 2) GDP per capita and health expenditure data obtained from WHO (2009); 3) Human Development Index from United Nations Development Programme (2007).

TABLE 1.2 Number of specialist mental health workers per 100 000 population in WHO European countries

Country	Psychiatrists	Nurses working in mental health care	Psychologists working in mental health care
Albania	3	7	0.5
Austria	13	37	63
Azerbaijan	5	8.4	0
Belgium	23	Information not available	Information not available
Bosnia and Herzegovina (Federation of Bosnia and Herzegovina)	7.4	10	0.5
Bosnia and Herzegovina (Republika Srpska)	5	4	3
Bulgaria	8.7	15.5	0.8
Croatia	8	Information not available	Information not available
Cyprus	6.5	52.5	6.7
Czech Republic	13.7	Information not available	Information not available
Denmark	11	9	10
Estonia	13	15	Information not available
Finland	26	163	47.2
France	22	Information not available	Information not available
Georgia	5.6	6.7	0.98
Germany	8.7	58	Information not available
Greece	15	3	14
Hungary	13.7	9.8	6
Ireland	7.3	126	Information not available
Israel	8.8	23.4	10.6
Italy	9.8	32.9	3.2
Latvia	11.3	38	1
Lithuania	18	39	7
Luxembourg	Information not available	Information not available	Information not available
Macedonia	9.5	24	2
Malta	4	109	6
Moldova	6	14	Information not available
Montenegro	6.4	Information not available	1.5
Netherlands	14.5	122	30
Norway	16	Information not available	35
Poland	5.5	16.4	4.9

(continued)

Country	Psychiatrists	Nurses working in mental health care	Psychologists working in mental health care
Portugal	6.7	13.2	2.3
Romania	4.7	22.4	Information not available
Russian Federation	10.9	49.7	2.4
Serbia	12	21	2
Slovakia	9	Information not available	3
Slovenia	5.4	5.8	1.7
Spain	6.1	9	4
Sweden	24	73	Information not available
Switzerland	30	Information not available	Information not available
Turkey	1	Information not available	Information not available
United Kingdom (England and Wales)	12.7	51.9	4.3
United Kingdom (Scotland)	10	122	3
Uzbekistan	4	9	1

Source: based on data from Petrea and Muijen, 2008, pp. 95, 96, 98

TABLE 1.3 Median rates of psychiatrists, nurses and psychologists per 100 000 population

WHO European region	Psychiatrists	Nurses	Psychologists
Europe (42 countries)	9	21.7	3.2
EU15	12.9	44.5	10
New EU countries since 2004	8.9	19	4.9
Southeastern Europe	8	15.5	1.5
CIS	5.6	9	1

Source: based on data from Petrea and Muijen, 2008, pp. 95, 96, 98

Kingdom (England and Wales) to only 2.9% in Lithuania and 3.3% in Bulgaria. Some hospitals in Eastern Europe have taken the initiative of offering training to their staff in priority areas (e.g. violence management, human rights, cognitive behavioural therapy, identification of mental disorders), utilising either internal or external training modules. However, one of the problems faced by managers in these countries is that returns from staff training are low as the best-trained staff are most likely to emigrate.

The roles and responsibilities of nurses remain limited in many countries in the central and eastern part of the region. On the one hand, nurses are not permitted to take on some of the tasks of psychiatrists, tasks which are usually delegated to nurses in countries with modern mental health services (e.g. care coordination, assessment of patient needs, consultation with other health professionals to establish and provide an individualised care plan, provision of high-level support to service users and their families). On the other hand, nurses working in inpatient units delegate to auxiliary staff many tasks that in other European countries would be considered core nursing tasks, e.g. carrying out assessments, administering medication and delivering psycho-educational programmes. The issue of distribution of tasks between nurses and auxiliary staff is rarely addressed. Auxiliary staff rarely have any training in providing care, nor experience in nursing people with mental health problems. However, these personnel can be preferred by hospital managers since auxiliary staff cost less than nurses, and they are readily available, as they are usually recruited from local communities in the surroundings of mental hospitals. Under these circumstances, the quality of nursing care received by service users is uncertain and sometimes substandard.

General practitioners and family doctors are increasingly asked to take more responsibilities in mental health care, since mental health resources are scarce and as a means of bringing mental health care to the community level. At the international level, political commitments and different initiatives directed towards low- and middle-income countries, such as the WHO Mental Health Gap Action Programme (mhGAP), are prioritising the shift towards making mental health care available in primary care settings (WHO, 2008b). In spite of its evident advantages, the feasibility of introducing mental health care into primary care is not a given, and it certainly is not a quick fix.

One concern is the degree to which GPs and family doctors have the capacity to provide mental health care, in terms of their training, time availability and motivation. In addition, the mandate of GPs and family doctors with respect to mental health is limited in many countries. In most European countries, GPs play an active role in the identification, diagnosis and referral of severe mental disorders. They are also regularly authorised to treat people with common mental disorders. However, for the most part, specialists are expected to give treatment for the majority of mental disorders, with GPs playing a supportive role. Only 52% of the European countries report that GPs diagnose severe mental disorders, and even fewer countries (40%) report that GPs give treatment. This figure includes no countries in southeastern Europe or CIS countries. In some CIS countries, GPs are not permitted by law to provide treatment for severe and enduring mental health problems.

Emigration of mental health staff across the European region

One of the biggest challenges faced by mental health services is to create incentives by which to retain existing mental health staff and stimulate the training and recruitment of new staff. There is currently a movement of specialised mental health staff from resource-limited countries to more affluent countries in the region (Pond and McPake, 2006). Most countries have no mechanism in place to monitor how many health workers leave the mental health system by emigrating to other countries. The low level of human-resource retention is particularly important in the context of governmental plans and commitment to increase the availability of community-based services, which require high numbers of competent staff. Under these circumstances, further staff cuts, linked to the recession, could make the situation critical.

In the few countries where such data is available, there is a vast difference in the rate of psychiatrists who emigrate abroad. This ranges from no emigration of psychiatrists in Malta and Spain (Murcia), to 1% in Albania, 2% in Estonia and Macedonia, and 4% in Georgia. In Moldova, this figure is 20%. Similarly, there is limited data available in countries of destination as to rates of professional immigration in the field of mental health. However, in Switzerland about 50% of the psychiatrists in clinics are non-Swiss citizens and in Spain (Murcia) 20% of new psychiatrists entering the mental health workforce are immigrants. In Luxembourg, immigrating psychiatrists account for only 3% of the psychiatric workforce.

The number of nurses emigrating is likely to be higher. Some local studies give an indication of the scale of the phenomenon for nurses in general, but little data is available on migration of mental health nurses specifically. For example, a 2007 study carried out in all hospitals in Romania showed that over 80% of health professionals who emigrated abroad were nurses (Rotila and Celmare, 2007).

Alongside retaining staff and preventing their emigration to other countries, another challenge is to attract mental health professionals to work in community-based settings. In some countries, legislation provides incentives for staff to choose employment in hospitals. Indeed, staff working in inpatient psychiatric services receive additional allowances of up to 75% of their salary (e.g. Romania, Serbia). Such allowances were well intentioned, so as to support the retention of staff in the most challenging services, but an unintended consequence has been that mental health staff are more inclined towards working in hospitals rather than in community services.

While staff shortages are a problem in most mental health services, the severity of the problem varies by geographical locality. Urban centres typically have a greater staff-to-patient ratio than rural or remote settings. The number of staff has reached critically low levels in some remote areas throughout Europe. This has resulted in an increased workload and overworking of the few remaining staff in these localities. The high volume of work, in combination with low salaries, leads to further demotivation of staff.

Conclusion

Since the situation in countries across Europe differs so dramatically, it is not possible to generalise and draw conclusions at the regional level. In many countries, there is a need for structural changes in the organisation of mental health systems, a redefinition of the packages of services to cover evidence-based community services (e.g. crisis care, home treatment and early intervention) and a restructuring of funding mechanisms. Equally, there is a need for a review and update of the roles and responsibilities of different staff groups and the pathways of care so as to limit duplication and improve efficiency. Many of the challenges to effective mental health service provision that have been described here have the largest impact on those most in need of long-term services. And we are still failing them.

Change takes time. Besides structural and organisational advancement, it requires first and foremost a change in societal attitudes towards people with mental health problems. This remains problematic even in countries with the most complex and advanced mental health systems. It is therefore essential to maintain a focus on the mental health agenda and monitor the implementation of various commitments made by decision-makers to ensure that further progress is being achieved.

References

Council of Europe. *European Convention on Human Rights and Its Five Protocols*. Rome; 1950. Available at: www.hri.org/docs/ECHR50.html (accessed 20 June 2010).

Council of Europe. *European Convention for the Prevention of Torture and Inhuman or Degrading Treatment or Punishment*. Strasbourg; 1987, as amended in 2002. Available at: www.cpt.coe.int/en/documents/ecpt.htm (accessed 20 June 2010).

Council of Europe. *Recommendation 1235 on Psychiatry and Human Rights*. Strasbourg; 1994. Available at: http://assembly.coe.int/Main.asp?link=http://assembly.coe.int/Documents/AdoptedText/ta94/erec1235.htm#1 (accessed 20 June 2010).

Council of Europe. *European Social Charter (revised)*. Strasbourg; 1996. Available at: http://conventions.coe.int/Treaty/EN/Treaties/Html/163.htm (accessed 20 June 2010).

Council of Europe. *Convention for the Protection of Human Rights and Dignity of the Human Being with Regard to the Application of Biology and Medicine: convention on human rights and biomedicine*. Oviedo; 1997. Available at: http://conventions.coe.int/treaty/en/treaties/html/164.htm (accessed 20 June 2010).

Council of Europe. *Recommendation 10 Concerning the Protection of the Human Rights and Dignity of Persons with Mental Disorder*. Strasbourg; 2004. Available at: https://wcd.coe.int/ViewDoc.jsp?id=775685&BackColorInternet=DBDCF2&BackColorIntranet=FDC864&BackColorLogged=FDC864 (accessed 20 June 2010).

European Commission. *Green Paper – Improving the mental health of the population: towards a strategy on mental health for the European Union*. Brussels; 2005. Available at: http://ec.europa.

eu/health/ph_determinants/life_style/mental/green_paper/mental_gp_en.pdf (accessed 20 June 2010).

European Commission. *European Pact for Mental Health and Well-Being*. Brussels; 2008. Available at: http://ec.europa.eu/health/ph_determinants/life_style/mental/docs/pact_en.pdf (accessed 20 June 2010).

Kohn R, Saxena S, Levav I, *et al.* The treatment gap in mental health care. *Bull World Health Organ.* 2004; **82**: 858–66.

Petrea I, Muijen M. *Policies and Practices for Mental Health in Europe – meeting the challenges.* Copenhagen: WHO Regional Office for Europe; 2008.

Pond B, McPake B. The health migration crisis: the role of four Organisation for Economic Cooperation and Development countries. *Lancet.* 2006; **367**: 1448–55.

Rotila V, Celmare L. Consequences of Romanian Health Care Workers Migration: the perspective of the managers from medical system. Analele Universitatii Dunarea de Jos, Galati, fasc. XX. *Sociologie.* 2007; **2**: 217–28.

United Nations. *Declaration on the Rights of Disabled Persons.* UN General Assembly (Resolution 3447); 1975. Available at: www.un.org/esa/socdev/enable/disdevelopmental.htm#_Toc35445325 (accessed 20 June 2010).

United Nations. *Principles for the Protection of Persons with Mental Illness and the Improvement of Mental Health Care.* UN General Assembly (Resolution 46/119); 1991. Available at: www2.ohchr.org/english/law/principles.htm (accessed 20 June 2010).

United Nations. *UN Standard Rules on the Equalizations of Opportunities for Persons with Disabilities.* UN General Assembly (Resolution 48/96); 1993. Available at: www.un.org/esa/socdev/enable/dissre00.htm (accessed 20 June 2010).

United Nations. *Convention on the Rights of Persons with Disabilities.* UN General Assembly; 2006. Available at: www.un.org/disabilities/default.asp?id=259 (accessed 20 June 2010).

United Nations Development Programme. Human Development Report 2007/2008. *Fighting Climate Change: human solidarity in a divided world.* UNDP; 2007. Available at: http://hdr.undp.org/en/media/HDR_20072008_EN_Complete.pdf (accessed 20 June 2010).

Wittchen HU, Jacobi F. Size and burden of mental disorders in Europe – a critical review and appraisal of 27 studies. *Eur Neuropsychopharmacol.* 2005; **1**: 357–76.

World Health Organization (WHO). *Constitution of the World Health Organization.* New York: International Health Conference; 1948.

World Health Organization. *Mental Health: new understanding, new hope.* Geneva: WHO; 2001. Available at: www.who.int/whr/2001/en/whr01_en.pdf (accessed 20 June 2010).

World Health Organization. *The Global Burden of Disease: 2004 update.* Geneva: WHO; 2008a. Available at: www.who.int/evidence/bod (accessed 20 June 2010).

World Health Organization (2008b). *mhGAP Mental Health Gap Action Programme: scaling up care for mental, neurological and substance use disorders.* Geneva: WHO; 2008b. Available at: www.who.int/mental_health/mhgap_final_english.pdf (accessed 20 June 2010).

World Health Organization. *National Health Accounts Series.* 2009. Available at: www.who.int/nha/country/en (accessed 20 May 2010).

WHO Regional Office for Europe, Council of Europe. Dubrovnik Pledge: *Meeting the Health Needs of Vulnerable Populations in South East Europe.* Health Ministers' Forum: *Health Development Action for South East Europe.* 2001. Available at: www.euro.who.int/__data/assets/pdf_file/0011/99749/E88512.pdf (accessed 20 June 2010).

WHO Regional Office for Europe. *Athens Declaration on Mental Health and Man-Made Disasters, Stigma and Community Care.* Madrid: Regional Committee 51 for Europe; 2001.

WHO Regional Office for Europe. *Mental Health Action Plan for Europe: facing the challenges, building solutions.* Copenhagen: WHO Regional Office for Europe; 2005a.

WHO Regional Office for Europe. *The European Health Report 2005: public health action for healthier children and populations*. Copenhagen: WHO Regional Office for Europe; 2005b.

WHO Regional Office for Europe. *Merano Declaration on Mental Health in CIS Countries*. 2008. Available at: http://test.cp.euro.who.int/document/mnh/merano_mtg.pdf (accessed 20 June 2010).

WHO Regional Office for Europe. *European Mortality Database (MDB)*. (Updated January 2010). Available at: http://data.euro.who.int/hfamdb (accessed 20 May 2010).

Mental health services in the Czech Republic

Blanka Novotná and Tomas Petr

Introduction

Among the many interesting topics addressed in this chapter is an account of the circumstances and challenges posed to mental health services when the political governance of a country shifts from that of communism to democracy; it is one of the first such accounts to be provided by those directly involved in service provision. The authors are well placed to describe where mental health services sit in relation to other public services and the level of support they attract from central government. The emergence of mental health services, how they are funded and the types of services provided are discussed, as are the roles of various personnel employed in the delivery of services. Of particular interest is nursing care and the preparation and educational and professional maintenance of mental health nurses.

National profile

Understanding the political, economic and demographic make-up of the Czech Republic provides the context in which to understand the factors influencing the shape of its mental health services and its approach to them.

The existence of the Czech Republic as an independent state started on 1 January 1993 with the break-up of Czechoslovakia into the Czech and Slovak republics. Many Czechs strongly identified themselves with the former state and perceived the separation as a loss and a political act performed, to a large extent, against the will of the citizens of both the new countries.

The Czech Republic became a member of the EU in 2004. The accession of the Czech Republic to the EU was supported in a referendum by 77% of those who voted; however, only 55% of voters participated in the referendum. The Czech Republic has also made a commitment to join the euro, but the original target date for the adoption was postponed and so far no exact date has been determined. As for their view of the EU, the Czechs are one of the more sceptical nations (together with the British, Hungarians and Latvians): for 46% of the population, membership in the EU is neither good nor bad. Nevertheless, 62% think EU membership has brought benefits to the country (Eurobarometer 72, Autumn 2009).

An important milestone in the recent history of the Czech Republic was the 'velvet revolution' of 1989, when the communist regime was overthrown and democratic principles started to be re-established in society. Forty years of communism was a burdensome legacy for the health care sector, and some of its effects can be seen to the present day. On the one hand, the health care system under directive management made some achievements primarily in the preventive and medical care of children; on the other hand, it suffered and still suffers from a chronic shortage of funds and financial management that continues to be very often ineffective. The communist propaganda also emphasised the idea that the state provided free health care to all people, resulting in the tendency today of people seeing the state as having ultimate responsibility for one's own health care. Upwards of 90% of the Czech population consider the health care sector to be highly problematic and inefficient, and view reformation of the system to be a necessity. Although improved services are called for, most of the population are unwilling to bear the costs of these reforms (Centrum pro výzkum veřejného mínění, 2006). The Czech people view with suspicion an invitation to participate in shaping health care due to the fact that historically individuals had no say in how welfare services were designed and provided; people were encouraged to see the state as having ultimate control over their well-being and that it should be regarded as a totalitarian, benign organisation which under no circumstances could be questioned.

Population and demographics

The population of the Czech Republic is some 10.5 million. Population density is approximately 133 people per square kilometre, which is a little higher than the European average (117 people/km^2). Some 71% of the population live in cities; 10% of all the people of the Czech Republic live in Prague. According to the data of the Czech Statistical Office, the population of the Czech Republic is growing very slowly (it was in decline between 1989 and 2006). The main reason is a very low birth rate, which, however, is partly compensated for by relatively high migration (the number of people in 2008 increased by some 15 000 due to natural reproduction and by more than 77 000 due to immigration).

In terms of ethnic composition, the Czech Republic is quite homogeneous, with more than 90% of people identifying themselves as Czechs (for details, *see* Table 2.1). Even though the dominant position of the Czech nationality has been preserved, there is a trend, which set in as a consequence of the post-1989 social changes, towards the decline in the proportion of the traditional ethnic minorities (Slovak, German, Polish, Hungarian) and the growth in the presence of other minorities, especially Vietnamese, Ukrainians and Russians (ČSÚ, 2003).

TABLE 2.1 Population of the Czech Republic by nationality in 2011

Nationality	% of total population
Czech	94.30
Slovak	1.89
Polish	0.51
German	0.38
Ukrainian	0.22
Vietnamese	0.17
Hungarian	0.14
Russian	0.12

Source: *CIA World Factbook*, 2011

A more varied situation is in the area of religious persuasion. Czech society is usually labelled as one of the most atheistic in the world; only 32% of people declare an affiliation with any religious denomination (for details, *see* Table 2.2). In a large-scale survey carried out by the Empirical Research Centre in 2007, the answer to the question 'Do you believe in God?' was 'yes' in the case of 28% of the respondents, while 48% said they did not believe in God and 24% answered 'I don't know'. However, a more in-depth analysis shows that rather than a lack of interest in spiritual values and faith, this hesitancy signals the existence of space, as it were, between atheism and a definitely declared faith or affiliation with any official church. Since 1989, society has continued to hold stable views on issues of religion and the proportion of people inclining to each belief variant remains rather unchanged (STEM, 2007).

The gross domestic product (GDP) per person in 2009 was CZK 345 727 (some €13,500); today's average gross salary amounts to CZK 25 752 per month (approximately €1,000). The long-lasting high unemployment rate in the north-west region of Bohemia and northern Moravia is related in the first place to industrial restructuring in these regions. On the contrary, Prague is definitely the most attractive region in terms of earnings as well as employment. The exclusive position of Prague is reflected in a wider supply of health care services as well, including services for mentally ill people.

TABLE 2.2 Composition of population by denomination

Denomination		%
Believers in total		**32.2**
Of which:	Roman Catholic Church	26.8
	Evangelical Church of Czech Brethren	1.1
	Czechoslovak Hussite Church	1.0
	Jehovah's Witnesses	0.2
	Orthodox Church of the Czech Lands	0.2
Non-denominational		**59.0**
Not identified		**8.8**

Source: www.czso.cz/csu/2001edicniplan.nsf/p/4101-01

General health care need

The adult population in the Czech Republic is most at risk of cardiovascular disease and malign tumours. There has been an increase in the occurrence of diabetes, allergies, psychic disorders and musculoskeletal disorders (ÚZIS, 2009). According to EHIS CR (2008), the percentage of people who suffered a chronic disease in the last 12 months was 57% in case of men and 69% in case of women. According to data provided by the same sources, the Czechs are ill for an average of 6–8 years throughout their lives, which is above the average of highly developed countries.

Similar to other EU countries, the Czech Republic is currently seeing the rise of an ageing population, with all the demands this makes on health and social welfare systems. People over 65 years of age make up some 15% of the population at present, but according to a forecast of the Czech Statistical Office (ČSÚ, 2011) this proportion is predicted to rise to 40% by 2040. The current average life expectancy is 74 years for men and 80 years for women. The elderly make up more than 80% of the clientele of physicians in outpatient care; the prevalence of chronic diseases in this group is higher than 90%. There is an increasingly high number of people in the age group of 65 years and above who, in connection with their illness, have difficulty coping with their normal daily lives and are becoming dependent on some form of assistance (45% of men and 66% women) (ČSÚ, 2010). Increasing life expectancy has inevitably led to an increase in the proportion of the population who are ill, disabled or both, thus requiring services which add considerably to health care costs. The ongoing debate consists of figuring out ways of funding expanding health services and assisting people in finding ways of accessing care other than that provided by the state. While an ageing population gives rise to many concerns, so also does the fact that those who provide the care – medical staff, physicians and nurses – are also ageing and not being replaced at a rate which replaces those who retire.

Health care services

Health care in the Czech Republic is financed by way of compulsory health insurance, which is subject to the Public Health Insurance Act of 1997. This law is based on the principle of solidarity in health care; that is, people contribute to the health insurance fund according to their capacities and use health care according to their needs.

The health insurance premium has been fixed at 13.5% of gross salary. Employees have 9% of this amount covered by the employer and their own contribution is 4.5%. The state covers the insurance premium for those who are not self-employed. This group includes children, students below 26, old-age pensioners, women on maternity leave, the unemployed, people in social need, prisoners and some other persons, such as asylum applicants.

There are nine private health insurance companies that oversee the collection and administration of insurance premiums and coverage of health care expenses to health care providers. The entire premium collected is distributed among the individual insurance companies based on the age structure of the insured clients. Všeobecná zdravotní pojišťovna ČR is the largest health insurance company (covering 65%–70% of the total insured population) and is the only health insurance company with a public guarantee, i.e. the government guarantees the company's solvency and fulfillment of its obligations towards the insured as well as health care providers (Figueras et al., 2002).

Since 2008, every insured person has been required to pay the health care providers 'regulatory fees' for the provision of health care. These fees have been set at CZK 30 per visit with a physician for clinical examination or treatment, CZK 60 per day spent in an inpatient facility and CZK 90 for use of emergency medical services (€1 equals approximately CZK 25). The main reason for the introduction of these fees was the attempt to eliminate inefficiencies and abuse of health care.

Most health care facilities in the Czech Republic are non-governmental; they have been established by regional governments, municipalities, churches and individuals (72% of non-governmental facilities are independent outpatient clinics with general practitioners and specialists). Governmental health care facilities make up less than 1% of all the health care facilities (these are typically university hospitals and medical treatment centres).

According to a survey carried out by CVVM, a public opinion research centre, in December 2009, one third of the Czech population is satisfied with the health care system (31%), one third is dissatisfied (34%) and 34% are indifferent. However, 73% of the Czech population stated that the biggest problem facing the public health care system is inadequate funding (CVVM, 2010). Respondents indicated that the source of this problem is not only the underfunding of health services but the ineffective use to which allocated resources are put. According to a study comparing the effectiveness of health care systems in Germany and the Czech Republic, the Czech health care system was found to be much less effective (MZ ČR, 2008).

So far, there have not been any standards of care defined which need to be achieved, nor is there any expectation that measurement of any kind should be conducted. Perhaps of even more concern is that there is no financial govern-ance system in place to ensure that money is spent efficiently and effectively (Figueras *et al.*, 2005).

Another serious problem of the Czech health care system is that people are poorly motivated to care for their own health. That is perhaps understandable given that the Czechs view health not as an individual issue, but as part of the public good to which individuals are entitled and which the state is obliged to pro-vide (Figueras *et al.*, 2005). In order to promote more individual responsibility for health care, people need to be able to have greater access to information, become aware of the types of services available and be able to make free choices. Despite this being the direction in which EU policy is taking EU countries, achieving it within the existing Czech system is impossible. The amount of relevant and understandable information available to people about health services and health education is grossly inadequate. While it appears that people have the freedom to choose an insurance company and a physician, in reality these companies cannot offer any degree of choice because they all provide the same services, which are defined by law and finance.

Other problems arise from the obsolescence of the health care structure and its inability to respond to individual need. The consequence is an unbalanced distribution of resources with much fewer services made available to those who live outside large conurbations. Lack of availability of services can have a pro-found effect on those with mental health problems and who may not be able to access care and treatment in the early stages of their illness, resulting in condi-tions deteriorating rapidly (Chytil *et al.*, 2008).

A major present-day problem which impacts, in the first place, on the elderly and chronically ill people is the division that exists between the management and financing of health and social services. Not only are they separate organisations, they have different cultures, different rules and regulations and different aims and objectives. Though most EU countries now recognise the importance of these two approaches to health care, in the Czech Republic they are managed by two discrete ministries which act independently of each other. As will be shown later, structural division like this can have disastrous consequences for mentally ill people whose recovery depends upon the close collaboration of health and social care.

The separation of health and social services can result in long-term, costly hospitalisations for those who have few financial resources and do not have a family on whom they can rely. Most of them need basic nursing care and, first and foremost, support in undertaking their everyday activities. The health care-oriented staff in health care facilities are not able to give these patients sufficient support to enable them to become self-sufficient; not only are they 'blocking' acute-care beds, as their numbers grow so does the cost to the nation. On the other hand, it appears that the quality of health care in residential social facilities is declining and consequently there are very strong tendencies to reduce the numbers of nurses and employ instead much less experienced and unqualified personnel (Gaskins and van Ginneken, 2009).

Although the quality of services may be under pressure, social care is defined by Act no. 108/2006 as 'an activity or a set of activities securing help and support to persons for the purposes of social integration or prevention of social exclusion'. These activities include help in coping with the common aspects of personal care, help in securing food, help in household maintenance, social consultancy, help in asserting rights, legitimate interests and arranging personal matters, phone emergency service, training in skills required for personal care, self-sufficiency and other activities leading to self-independence and social integration. Social services thus include, inter alia, protected living, homes for people with a chronic mental illness and services provided by community psychiatric nurses. While policy determines what the situation should be, there are many obstacles to making this a reality for all people.

Current profile of mental health need

According to an epidemiological study, 27% of the population of the Czech Republic have experienced mental illness at least once in their life (Scheffler and Potůček, 2008). The highest total prevalence of mental illnesses is in Prague, which is 78% higher than the total average for the Czech Republic (ÚZIS, 2009).

In 2009, there were 482 970 new patients seeking the help of a psychiatrist in the Czech Republic, which is an increase in comparison with 2008 (16 618 patients). Compared to 2000, the number of adult patients rose by more than one third (39%). The number of ill women is growing much faster than that of men and, as would be expected, they are seeking psychiatric help more often than men. Women account for some 60% of the total number of examinations and of initial examinations (ÚZIS, 2010). The most frequent psychiatric diagnoses for which patients are treated include neurotic disorders (44.5%) and affective disorders (14.9%). Other frequently diagnosed disorders are organic mental disorders and schizophrenia. In 2009, 41 419 patients were actively treated and received outpatient care for the abuse of psychoactive substances, which is almost 3% less than in 2008; 67% of these service users were men.

A comparison of the number of patients in the individual groups of psychiatric diagnoses classified by sex clearly shows that women more frequently suffer from affective, neurotic and organic mental disorders, making up 66% of the total number of patients. Men were considerably more frequently treated in connection with sexual disorders (deviations), disorders caused by alcohol and other psychoactive substances, and developmental disorders in childhood and adolescence (Dlouhý, 2004).

The most frequent diagnoses for children up to the age of 14 were developmental disorders in childhood and adolescence and neurotic disorders; in all, more than 85% of the patients in this age group were treated for these disorders (ÚZIS, 2010).

Care of mentally ill people in inpatient settings

In 2009, there were 18 454 patients hospitalised in psychiatric wards and 38 185 patients hospitalised in psychiatric sanatoria (the difference is explained below). This amounts to 550 hospitalisations per 100 000 people, an insignificant decrease of 1% compared to the previous year. The second-most-frequent group of diagnoses for which the patients were hospitalised were schizoaffective disorders. This group made up more than a quarter of the total number of hospitalisations. The most frequent reason for hospitalisation was for the the treatment of disorders related to alcohol abuse (ÚZIS, 2010).

The Czech Republic has an average rate of suicide among all European countries, currently occupying 22nd position with a rate of 13.7 suicides per 100 000 population. The CIDI/ICD-10 study (2000) revealed that one person in 10 considered suicide at some point during their lives, 5% acknowledged that they experienced suicidal thoughts at various times and 2% actually attempted to commit suicide. Men reported that they entertained suicidal thoughts less often than women. In 2008, there were 1,379 suicides committed in the Czech Republic.

Disability and incapacity due to mental illness

Of all those granted full disability pensions, 14.2% were given to those with a mental illness. For partial disability pensions, 9.5% were granted to those with psychiatric problems (Dlouhý, 2009). In 2009, the total number of partial disability pensions granted in the Czech Republic to people with mental health problems was 2840. Alomost two thirds of these were granted to women. Incapacity to work caused by a mental illness accounted for 3.3% of the total number of sick days in the Czech Republic in 2006. In 2009, there were 36 022 cases of incapacity to work due to a psychiatric diagnosis. The most frequent diagnoses in women were affective disorders, such as depression, anxiety, persistent tiredness and sleeplessness. Two other groups which were awarded disability pensions were those with schizophrenic illnesses and learning disabilities (ÚZIS, 2010).

Social views on mental health

Those with mental health problems are still strongly stigmatised in the Czech Republic, and despite several attempts to reduce the impact of this on individuals, it continues to pose a serious problem (Sartorius and Schulze, 2005). Suffering a mental illness is often viewed by the public as a failure that may largely disqualify a person from work, education and training, and various other aspects of social life. Another and probably even more important consideration is the low professional and social standing of psychiatrists and nurses in comparison to other professions. Research activity in the field of mental health care remains minimal, due to limited resources being available and few professionals being interested.

Surveys focusing on the prestige of the profession of psychiatrists and psychiatric nurses have yielded similar results. In a study by Janoušková (2004), 1248 respondents were invited to evaluate the prestige of various medical professions on a scale from 1 (lowest score) to 10 (highest prestige). Psychiatric nurses scored 5.8, placing 11th out of 17 nursing specialities. These results indicate how society at large, as well as other professionals, view those involved in caring for the mentally ill.

The World Psychiatric Association's programme 'Open the Doors, Open Your Hearts' (1996) sought to eliminate stigmatisation and discrimination of schizophrenic patients worldwide. The Czech Republic joined this programme in 2004. Later, a 3-year initiative called 'Change' was started, which focused especially on patients with schizophrenia, bipolar disorders and children's mental disorders (Scheffler and Potůček, 2008). As a result of this initiative, a survey involving 700 respondents was carried out in the Czech Republic in 2004 mapping the attitudes of the adult population to schizophrenia. The results showed that the level of knowledge about schizophrenia among the general population was very low and there existed widespread stereotypical views of patients' behaviour being highly dangerous and unpredictable. These results were not much different from those of similar surveys around the world, indicating that all countries have a considerable way to go to reduce the level of stigma that exists.

The attitudes of the Czech public towards mentally ill people ranges from seeing them as 'poor people', or 'ill people' to describing them as 'weirdoes, loonies or maniacs' (Scheffler and Potůček, 2008). General awareness of the nature and manifestations of schizophrenic disorder is low and the general public is ill informed with respect to what it is like to suffer from a mental illness. A more positive attitude to people with psychiatric problems is held by those members of the population who have some understanding of and are involved in relating to people with schizophrenia on an interpersonal level as a family member, as friends or at a workplace. Such people strongly disapprove of segregation and keeping the mentally ill in isolation, and tend to see all mental illnesses as curable. Where negative attitudes do exist, they mainly involve seeing mentally ill people as potentially aggressive, unpredictable and instilling fear in those they meet (Sartorious and Schulze, 2005).

Similar to other countries, the Czech health care facilities that provide care to mentally ill people have been found to have a strong stigmatising effect as well. Large psychiatric sanatoria on the outskirts of cities, where the conditions for the provision of health care are much worse than in the majority of hospital wards for patients with somatic illnesses, create a negative and frightening image in the public mind. No less important is the influence of the media and the impressions of the mentally ill they provide, particularly in relation to aggression and violence. Nawková (2010) reviewed 203 articles relating to the topic of mental ill health and demonstrated that 37% contained stigmatising statements relating to people with a mental illness. The predominant description was that mental illness was closely associated with aggression, fear and violence. Less than a fifth of the articles referred to the fact that mentally ill people were more likely to be victims of violent acts than the population at large.

The major goals outlined by the Change initiative included a systematic education of the public – families as well as professionals and civil servants – and transfer of the base of care from large psychiatric sanatoria to community facilities. One of the activities aimed at destigmatisation of mentally ill people was the launching of a specialised website, www.stopstigmapsychiatrie.cz, which offers online consultancy and a large volume of information and brochures to download. In 2009, this website was visited by 56 876 persons and the online consultancy service answered 909 inquiries (Wenigová, 2005).

A number of destigmatisation-related activities take place across the country, and are aimed at changing public attitudes towards mentally ill people. These include, for instance, the Week of Mental Health, which is an annual event to highlight the difficulties that people with poor mental health have to endure and what needs to be done about it. Various psychiatric organisations host musical and theatre festivals about aspects of mental illness and mental health and the public are invited to see what takes place within hospitals and organisations. Online consultancy services have sprung up to provide direct help to people in the form of education, advice and where various services can be located. While this is an honest attempt by sincere and enlightened individuals, it lacks governmental support, planned direction and evidence as to how to address negative public attitudes. Such activities unquestionably demonstrate that social education is required in order to improve mental health services and that there are people who are prepared to do it.

Expenditure on mental health care

Health care expenditure in the Czech Republic has oscillated around 7% of GDP in recent years (Scheffler and Potůček, 2008). Funding of services for people with a psychiatric illness is highly unsystematic and ill-conceived in the Czech Republic. The several stable sources of funding for these services include:

- **The Health Insurance Fund**, which covers health care services. The services covered are those offered by inpatient and outpatient psychiatric facilities, daily clinics and occasionally also other services (home care). The payments are made either as fixed lump sums (inpatient facilities) or on the basis of reported workload (outpatient services).
- **Subsidies of the Ministry of Labour and Social Affairs and the Ministry of Health to non-governmental non-profit organisations.** These sources are partially used (up to 70% maximum) to cover the costs of NNOs which primarily offer community services, i.e. social services, or services on the border of the social and health care sectors, not covered by health insurance.
- **Subsidies from the Ministry of Health to health care facilities.** These are mainly investment grants to hospitals within the government's responsibility, or regions or municipalities.
- **Direct payments by recipients of services/patients.** A direct payment system is employed mainly by private facilities in relation to above-standard services.
- **Grants** provided, for example, by foundations, sponsors, foreign donors, etc. These are grant programs for social and health services. In the majority of cases, these grants may be applied for by NNOs, private and municipal facilities. Though shown to be useful, these grants are generally aimed at time-limited projects and are generally less then €15 000.
- **Participation by providers.** Most of the providers cover part of their costs from their own resources, for instance, from the sale of their own services and products (CMHCD, 2003).

TABLE 2.3 Estimated mental health expenditure in 2006

Expenditure	Amount (CZK million)
Sickness benefits and costs of assistance in nursing a family member	944
Expenses on full disability pensions	5 281
Expenses on partial disability pensions	1 126
Expenses on health care for mentally ill people	8 032
Total expenditure on mental health	15 362
Of which: sickness benefits	6%
full disability pensions	34.4%
partial disability pensions	7.3%
health care	52.3%
Proportion of mental health expenditure in GDP	0.48%

Source: Dlouhý, 2009

Compared to other EU countries, mental health care in the Czech Republic is severely underfunded. Of the total volume of funds flowing to health care, only 3.5% is allocated to mental health (compared to 12% in the UK or 10% in Germany). Hence, the Czech Republic is one of the countries with the lowest volume of funds invested in mental health care (European Commission, 2005). Mental health expenditure is not connected with health care only, but includes sickness and pension benefits as well. Most of the money allocated to mentally ill patients is consumed in the inpatient sector (psychiatric sanatoria and psychiatric wards), which precludes the development of community services. The major difficulties in funding mental health care may be summarised as follows:

● In comparison with the highly developed EU countries, the volume of funds allocated to mental health care is insufficient. The Czech Republic is one of the countries with the least money spent on the care of mentally ill people.

● The existing formula for funding services results in an uneven distribution of resources across the Czech Republic. For instance, city-based facilities, teaching hospitals and university-linked services get considerably more funding than isolated or rural areas.

● A rigidly organised structure of services and their funding inhibit a flexible development of the services so as to reflect the needs of the patients. Finding ways to finance alternative services is highly difficult. The resources available are not used in line with the needs of the population. Psychiatric sanatoria use up most of the resources, which thus cannot be applied to building a community service network (Gaskins and Ginneken, 2009).

● Insufficient coordination of health and social services results in insufficient funding of the services on the border of health and social care (Gaskins and Ginneken, 2009).

- Funding of some services, particularly community services, is unstable. For community services, there is no basic certainty as to the availability of funding in future periods; moreover, the situation changes every year.
- No assessment is made of the effectiveness of the funds expended (David *et al.*, 2003).
- There is an urgent need to assess the amount of funding required to undertake a properly planned mental illness prevention and mental health education programme in primary care (Sartorius and Schulze, 2005). The need for primary prevention in the area of psychiatric care is indisputable as timely and appropriate care reduces the likelihood of long-term disability (Wenigová, 2005). Some educational approaches have been shown to assist patients to recover faster than they normally would have, and members of the public with negative attitudes have been shown to reduce their stigmatisation of mentally ill people (Scheffler and Potůček, 2008). However, the dependability of robust research upon which to make decisions and the availability of personnel available to do this falls short of that which exists elsewhere.

The volume of financial resources allocated to mental health may be regarded as an indicator of society's interest in mentally ill people. From this viewpoint, the Czech Republic is not doing very well in comparison with other European countries. International comparisons of mental health expenditure in health care sectors make the insufficient funding of mental health care in the Czech Republic more visible. According to a study on mental health care in Prague, the limited resources allocated to mental health are used to finance costly health and social inpatient facilities, rather than home and community care (Bašný *et al.*, 2003).

History of mental health care

The development of care for mentally ill people in the Czech Republic was similar to the situation in the rest of Europe. Virtually until the end of the eighteenth century, the standards of psychiatric care were comparable to those of the Middle Ages. The actual origins of care for the mentally ill in the Czech Republic date back to 1783, when Emperor Joseph II ordered the establishment of a ward for mentally ill priests in the Brothers of Mercy Hospital in Prague. Another of Emperor Joseph II's achievements was the establishment of the General Hospital on Charles Square in Prague in 1790, part of which was also a separate facility for mentally ill patients. The number of psychiatric beds in Prague further increased in later years (Šnajdr, 2004). In the 1840s, the Prague sanatorium with 500 beds had the reputation as one of the most modern facilities in the whole of Europe. At this time, Josef Riedel, the first professor of psychiatry, who held posts both in the university and the psychiatric hospital, started to devise courses and a series of lectures on the causes and treatments of 'insanity'.

Establishment of large psychiatric sanatoria

The period from 1860 to 1920 is characterised by the establishment of large facilities for mentally ill patients. The majority of these facilities were located outside of large cities, in a pleasant setting. For example, in 1870 a monastery in Kosmonosy was bought and after several modifications turned into a sanatorium where patients from Prague were moved. In 1880, a sanatorium in Dobřany was completed and ceremonially opened, with Arnold Pick, a prominent psychiatrist, as its first director (Vencovský, 1983). Building of other large sanatoria in various parts of the country followed.

The majority of these were large-capacity facilities outside large cities, many of which were overcrowded. Between 1919 and 1937, the number of psychiatric facilities rose from 11 to 15 and the number of beds increased from 9.4 to 13.9 per 10000 people. Also, the number of psychiatrists increased significantly, by as much as 40%. The average hospitalisation period was long – in 1937, it was 224 days. The major function of the psychiatric facilities was protection.

Post-war period

During the war, and until 1947, psychiatric care was on the decline due to lack of interest and funds. After the end of the war, Czechoslovakia found itself under the control of the Soviet Union, and was to remain so for 40 years. The health care system was nationalised and managed centrally. The development of alternative types of care, such as the foundation of self-help parent or patient associations or non-profit organisations, was suppressed. Next to the large psychiatric sanatoria, there were psychiatric wards opened as part of large general hospitals, especially in the post-war period. Psychiatric care was concentrated primarily in inpatient facilities.

Conditions at the large psychiatric sanatoria were sub-standard. Scant resources were channelled into what was then regarded as the insignificant field of psychiatry. Apart from being admitted, the mentally ill were not offered any other treatment options, such as home care, crisis intervention, protected homes or other types of community care. These extramural services did not begin to take shape until after the 1989 revolution. Little scholarship exists about how psychiatry was used for political purposes similar to that which took place in the Soviet Union and Czechoslovakia under communism. It is beginning to emerge that psychiatric practitioners were directed to extract information from those who were considered dissenters and in certain instances eliminate them. The implication of psychiatry in torture and cruelty is still closely associated in the minds of people old enough to remember the worst aspects of the communist regime. Baštecký (1997) has pointed out that in the past, people who were regarded as being against the system were labelled psychopaths or paranoiacs and were forcibly hospitalised for an indefinite period. During the communist regime (that is, before 1990), the ratio of forced admissions to voluntary admissions was 80 : 20 and after 1992, it markedly altered to 20 : 80. This change resulted from a revision of why people should be admitted. Under the new system, people were admitted solely to have their mental health problems addressed and not for punishment or interrogation. Prior to 1989, local governments were empowered to decide whether or not a person should be admitted, but after that time, responsibility to admit was the sole prerogative of the courts (Baudiš and Libiger, 2002).

Post-1989

Until 1989, psychiatry was largely isolated from other medical branches, but after that time, due to the major political and social changes occurring, the whole health care system, including psychiatry, was set to change. Mental health and psychiatric disorders became of interest to the public and these and related topics were frequently discussed in the media, indicating that a significant shift in attitude was beginning to take place in the public mind. Perhaps the greatest change to take place was that doctors and nurses were attempting to do their best to help people cope with their problems, while patients themselves talked freely about how they felt and what it was like to suffer from a mental health problem. This openness resulted in psychiatry moving closer to general medicine, in a reduction of the fear that once prevailed, and in mental health care personnel developing closer relationships with patients and their relatives.

Voices calling for the reform of psychiatric care leading to its deinstitutionalisation and development of community care were becoming more and more frequent. There was a slight decline in the number of beds in psychiatric sanatoria, and several centres were established around the Czech Republic offering community services for people with a mental illness. However, for the last 10 years this process has been at a standstill. Eighty-seven per cent of the care is still provided in psychiatric institutions built at the beginning of the twentieth century and no new alternative services have materialised to date.

Following the Czech Republic joining the EU in 2004, the vocational training of doctors and nurses was reviewed, harmonised with EU directives and generally improved. Doctors and nurses were encouraged to innovate and become involved in the management of services and a number of EU-initiated projects involving the Czech Republic. Although the education of health care staff improved and national studies commenced, the actual practice of psychiatry and what transpired within services remained unchanged. It became apparent that much more is required if society in general and patients in particular are to have a greater say in creating the types of services that are effective.

Types of services provided

The Czech Republic is one of the minority of EU countries that do not have a national programme for the provision of mental health care (Gaskins and Ginneken, 2009). The consequences of this are numerous, including an unsystematic approach to the location of psychiatric facilities, unevenly distributed outpatient services, obsolete inpatient facilities and a lack of appropriate community care facilities. Not surprisingly, availability of psychiatric care is therefore haphazard and unsatisfactory. However, in September 2010, the Czech Republic announced the creation of a national plan for those with Alzheimer's disease, although it was not fully operational in June 2011, when it was due to commence. This venture combines the efforts of five distinct ministries: Health, Labour, Social Affairs, Finance and Justice.

Psychiatric care is currently provided through a network of facilities offering a range of services to mentally ill patients. The basic elements of this network comprise psychiatric outpatient clinics, outpatient clinical psychology centres, inpatient facilities (psychiatric sanatoria, psychiatric wards in general hospitals and psychiatric clinics) and community care facilities which combine psychiatry and social services.

Psychiatric outpatient clinics

In 2009, there were 825 psychiatric outpatient facilities in the Czech Republic, with 1270 specialists, including 730 outpatient psychiatrists, 415 non-medical staff and 84 psychologists (ÚZIS, 2010). Various studies show that outpatient psychiatrists are overburdened with large numbers of people with long-term mental health problems, resulting in them not having enough time to devote to each patient or to collaborate with other service providers (Wenigová et al., 2009). Aside from psychiatric outpatient clinics, there are specialised outpatient clinics as well, e.g. paediatric, gerontopsychiatry, addiction treatment, psychotherapy and other specialised treatments.

Inpatient care

There are two types of inpatient psychiatric care – acute care and after-care. The general strategy in psychiatry requires that acute care should be provided in psychiatric wards at general hospitals and after-care at psychiatric sanatoria. However, the actual situation is different because of the lack of beds in psychiatric wards. In the Czech Republic, 80% of psychiatric beds are placed in psychiatric sanatoria. This is why acute care has been provided to a large extent at psychiatric sanatoria instead of psychiatric wards of general hospitals.

Psychiatric sanatoria

The task of psychiatric sanatoria is to provide long-term treatment and rehabilitation for people with a psychiatric illness for all age groups. At the same time, they fulfil the function of providing psychiatric inpatient care in regions where no psychiatric wards have been established so far, or where the accommodation capacity is insufficient. In the Czech Republic, there are 17 psychiatric sanatoria for adult patients, with a total accommodation capacity of 9207 beds, and three psychiatric sanatoria for children, with 260 beds. The average length of hospital stay is 83.8 days (ÚZIS, 2010).

Psychiatric wards

Usually, psychiatric wards are part of hospitals, but some exist as self-contained facilities as well. A special type of psychiatric ward is one attached to a university hospital, with the status of a clinic existing as part of a faculty of medicine. Apart from health services, these facilities provide education to university and postgraduate students, and are places where research is carried out. They also offer supervisory consultancy services and provide psychiatric care in especially complicated cases. There are 31 psychiatric wards with a total of 1383 beds in the Czech Republic. The average length of hospital stay is 20.6 days (ÚZIS, 2010).

Community care

Currently, there are 21 day clinics available in the health care sector for the treatment of mental disorders in the Czech Republic, roughly half of which exist as part of larger inpatient facilities and half as independent facilities. As for their geographic availability, daily clinics are often usually found in larger cities. New facilities were established during the 1990s, and after 2000 almost no new facilities were opened due to lack of resources. In the whole country, there are only three crisis centres providing 24-hour access to a psychiatrist, two in Prague and one in Brno.

The profession of community psychiatric nurses, who specialise in case management and individual rehabilitation of patients in their own homes, was introduced into the health care system in 2006. Currently, there are only three facilities offering this service (two in Prague, one in Ostrava).

During the two last decades, what is commonly referred to as 'psychiatric rehabilitation' has been firmly located within social services. At present, this activity is carried out by only 29 non-profit organisations, which in 2007 employed

470 social workers in direct care for some 4600 clients (Asociace komunitní péče – Community Care Association, 2007). These facilities are located mostly in larger cities in some regions (e.g. Karlovy Vary or Zlín), while in other areas they do not exist at all. The fact that the services of daily clinics, crisis centres and psychiatric rehabilitation services are only available to a very small group of patients is demonstrated by the data in the table below.

TABLE 2.4 Numbers of patients using community services in 2007

Daily clinics	7747
Crisis centres	10059
Psychiatric rehabilitation	4600
Psychiatric outpatient clinics	464836

Source: Institute of Health Information and Statistics, Community Care Association, Association of Daily Clinics and Crisis Centres, 2007

Legislation

Major changes in legislation came after 1989. These enabled the establishment of independent professional organisations and associations defending the interests of patients or parents. The formation of the Czech Republic in 1993 was followed by adoption of the Constitution, as the supreme law, and the Charter of Fundamental Rights and Freedoms.

Mental health care is regulated by general health care legislation. The Czech Republic has not adopted any special law on psychiatry, as is the case in some other European countries, and the question of the necessity of such a law is frequently discussed in professional circles. The care for mentally ill patients is regulated by several legal norms with different legal weight. On the constitutional level, it is the Charter of Fundamental Rights and Freedoms which guarantees fundamental rights and freedoms to psychiatric patients. As for international documents that have precedence over national law, an especially important piece of legislation is the Convention of Human Rights and Biomedicine.

On the statutory level, the details of the provision of health care are set forth in the Public Health Care Act of 1966, which has been amended several times. Issues concerning a patient's admission against his or her will are provided for in Act no. 99/1963 Coll., Civil Procedure Code, which lays down the procedural rules for the 'involuntary admission'. This act also determines time limits for decisions of courts (the whole procedure is described below). Other laws regulating psychiatric care are the Criminal Code, which deals with issues relating to compulsory treatment, and the Preventive Detention Act.

Important by-laws include the Methodological Measures of the Ministry of

Health, which, however, are only binding on institutions subordinated to the ministry. Since 1992, the National Program of Care for Mental Health has been in preparation in the Czech Republic. A conceptual plan for psychiatric care drawn up by the Psychiatric Medical Association was adopted by the Ministry of Health in 2002. The major goals of this plan are deinstitutionalisation and building a network of community services. Nevertheless, the effort to implement the plan for psychiatric care has failed, primarily because of rigid restrictions on health care funding.

Other important documents relating to patients' rights are codes of ethics. These rights are acknowledged by the Central Committee for Ethics of the Ministry of Health in 1992 (Haškovcová, 2002) and the Codes of Ethics of the Czech Medical Chamber adopted in 1996 (ČLK, 1996). Another agent playing an important role in defending the rights of patients is the office of the Public Defender of Rights of the Czech Republic, which performs regular inspections of psychiatric facilities.

Because of the effects of mental illness on the functioning of a person, they are some of the most vulnerable people in society and require the protection of effective legislation. A number of patient organisations have been established, and they have pointed to a number of problems within the services, e.g. lack of privacy, lack of relevant information, poor relationships with doctors, lack of freedom due to the lack of staff and an inability to explore other services that might be of use to them (Shaywitz and Ausiello, 2002). One of the sources of these problems, in their opinion, is the unavailability of specific legislation regulating the issues of involuntary hospitalisation and questions relating to insufficient decision-making capacity of patients.

Therefore, an important goal to be achieved by legislation would be either to modify the existing legal regulations or to draw up a specific law on psychiatry which would also set rules for regular and independent monitoring of the rights of mentally ill patients (Scheffler and Potůček, 2008).

Involuntary hospitalisation

Hospitalisation without the patient's consent is provided for by the following laws:
- Convention for the Protection of Human Rights and Dignity of the Human Being with Regard to the Application of Biology and Medicine no. 96/2001 Coll.
- Constitutional Act no. 23/1991 Coll. (Charter of Fundamental Rights and Freedoms).

Every patient is entitled to give or refuse consent to both the actual hospitalisation and anything concerned with diagnosing and treating. No consent is required in some issues which are clearly defined in law. These conditions include:

- when a person demonstrating signs of a mental illness or intoxication is a threat to herself or people or objects around her
- when it is impossible to request the patient's agreement due to his condition of health while providing urgent treatment which is required to save the patient's life or health.

The patient may, at any time, withdraw his or her consent. Hospitalisation without the patient's consent has the following stages:

1. If the patient does not give written consent to her hospitalisation on admission, the physician will assess her condition of health and either release the patient or decide on forced hospitalisation. If the psychiatrist decides to hospitalise the patient without his or her consent, the physician must give notice to a court within 24 hours after admitting the patient to the effect that he has detained the patient without their consent.

2. The court must determine within 7 days of the notice whether or not admission without the patient's consent was on legal grounds. Representatives of the court will appear on the ward to discuss the case with the patient and the physician.

3. The court decides that admission into institutional care has been done on legal grounds, and the process continues with a view to determining permissibility of further detention of the patient at the institution. The court will appoint an expert psychiatrist to verify the patient's condition (he or she cannot be a physician who works for the health care facility where the patient is hospitalised) and then decide on whether or not further detention of the patient is permitted and for how long (1 year maximum). This decision must be made within 3 months of the ruling whereby admission into the facility was permitted.

4. The patient is entitled to be heard by the court, choose his legal representative and appeal any decision of the court. If the patient does not himself select a legal representative, the court will appoint a legal representative from available attorneys. The government will pay legal representation costs in this case.

Role of mental health nurses

Up to the twentieth century, nursing care in facilities for the mentally ill was often in the hands of non-trained nurses. Psychiatric sanatoria themselves had to provide for the basic training of their staff. The first courses specialising in the care for the mentally ill were opened only after the Second World War. In 1960, the Institute for Further Education of Health Care Workers was opened, offering courses and specialised education, inter alia, in the field of care for mentally ill patients (Marková, 2005).

After 1989, there were lots of changes made in the education of psychiatric nurses. During 1992–96, there were three nursing schools in the Czech Republic offering a 1-year post-secondary education programme with specialisation in nursing care in psychiatry, which was open to the graduates of secondary nursing schools. In 1997, this programme was replaced with a new one called Certified Nurse for Psychiatry, which was open to all graduates who had completed an advanced level of secondary education. After 2004, this study programme was terminated completely (Marková, 2005).

Since 2004, in connection with the accession of the Czech Republic to the EU, many changes have been made that were required by European directives. These changes affected the education of nurses as well. At present, the qualification of a general nurse may only be achieved through study at higher nursing schools or universities in a bachelor's programme. Only then is field specialisation possible.

Since 2004, nurses have been able to register with the Ministry of Health to obtain a certificate authorising them to work as a health care professional without professional supervision (without the supervision of another qualified nurse). The prerequisites for this registration are a professional health care qualification, a minimum of 1 year of practical experience in a health care setting in the previous 6 years and evidence of involvement in lifelong learning programmes, resulting in the achievement of 40 credits. Registration is only valid for a period of 6 years, after which suitability to practice must be reassessed. Unregistered nurses may provide similar nursing care, but only under the supervision of a registered nurse. Even though this process looks thorough, in reality it does not function very well. Being qualified and registered is not a guarantee of one's ability to provide care of a high quality. Lifelong learning, which is cherished as evidence of academic ability, is frequently no more than a 'hunt for credits' rather than acquiring an in-depth understanding of the needs of patients. The term 'professional supervision' is very vague and remains largely undefined, resulting in any activity being called supervision. Hence, registration is just a means of counting the number of registered health care workers, not evidence of the quality of their work. Though this is not a position held by officials in the Ministry of Health, it is one firmly held by the authors.

The specialisation course Nursing Care for Mental Health may currently be studied at two educational centres attached to four accredited clinical facilities for undertaking the practical component of the programme. It is a 3-year study programme, and the practical part comprises 50% of the course. However, the programme is not run regularly, and on completion students may have to wait for a considerable period to be registered as a nurse. About 50 applicants were accepted for training in 2010, but twice that number were awaiting registration in order to be recognised as 'qualified nurses'.

Nevertheless, this specialisation is not necessary for working as a nurse in psychiatry. It is required only for undertaking managerial positions, such as ward and head nurses, and for the profession of community psychiatric nurse. The exact number of nurses who have obtained specialisation for work with mentally ill people cannot be determined at this moment. The number is estimated at some 30% of all nurses working in psychiatry. In 2009, there were 3335 nurses working in inpatient and outpatient facilities for mentally ill patients, of whom 2976 worked in psychiatric sanatoria (ÚZIS, 2009).

As in the other health care sectors, psychiatry is primarily the domain of female nurses. There is no exact data available on the numbers of women and men working in psychiatric nursing care. Nevertheless, the composition may be illustrated by looking at the nursing staff in one of the large psychiatric sanatoria. In 2010, there were 385 women (88%) and 53 men (12%) in the total of 438 nurses. The women-to-men ratio in other psychiatric facilities may be expected to be comparable. Most managerial and clinical positions are occupied by women as well. Information available on the websites of psychiatric sanatoria shows that in 2010 the jobs of the main nurses were performed by 12 women (80%) and two men (13%), and in one case a position was left unfilled. Further, it follows from the data available that the women-to-men ratio in lower managerial positions (head nurses and charge nurses) is similar.

As mentioned above, no specialised education in the area of nursing in psychiatry is required to work in a psychiatric facility, although it is an important factor when applying for senior positions. A nurse applying for a job must have the qualification of a general nurse, must be medically fit and without a criminal record (i.e. no final unsuspended sentence of imprisonment for a premeditated crime in connection with the provision of health care). The nurse is then trained on a psychiatric ward as usual in the given facility. Nurses may attend seminars, training courses and conferences organised by their home health care facility, educational agencies or the psychiatric section of the Czech Nurses Association. The competencies and the scope of working duties of nurses in psychiatry are thus identical to a large extent to those of general nurses. Nurses are usually able to provide somatic and practical care of a very high standard, but with respect to specialised psychiatric skills, these are acquired after they have started to work in a psychiatric facility. Though such skills would add credibility, there are instances where individuals do not acquire any, nor is there any obligation on them to do so. The specific skills of a psychiatric nurse and the required competencies are not defined; what is required of nurses is left entirely to those who manage various facilities.

Hence, the job of a nurse at an inpatient facility involves, primarily, basic nursing care, i.e. responsibility for patients' hygiene, nutrition and hydration, serving medication and food, supervising the behaviour and securing the safety of patients, and pacifying restless and aggressive patients. The degree to which nurses participate in specialised activities such as relaxation, psychotherapeutic and support groups or occupational therapy varies greatly between individual facilities. Nurses themselves often view these activities as falling within the exclusive competence of psychologists and psychiatrists.

With increasing specialisation in psychiatry, the competence of nurses is expanding, and roles may include education for acquiring the skills of providing supportive psychotherapy, relaxation techniques, training in cognitive functioning, crisis intervention and preparation of a patient for follow-up care following discharge. The fact that a nurse has obtained specialisation does not necessarily mean that his or her extended skills will be utilised. Specialised nurses usually have the same responsibilities as nurses without specialisation. The reason for this is that, first, not many posts for specialised nursing positions exist, and second, if they did, they would add considerably to the cost of providing the service.

The conditions for the provision of psychiatric nursing care are different depending on the type of inpatient facility. Psychiatric wards in hospitals tend to have fewer beds, larger numbers of staff and more up-to-date equipment. The composition of patients is more favourable because patients with behavioural problems and/or a negative prognosis are sent to psychiatric sanatoria. A typical ward has a linear structure, with the nurses' room in the middle part. Usually there are two- to four-bed rooms, sometimes with separate sanitary facilities; sometimes there are common toilets and a bathroom for the entire ward. Patients have a shared dining room which is often used as a common room.

All the psychiatric sanatoria were built in the first half of the twentieth century. These are very old buildings, the layout of which is the product of the organisation of care at the time of their establishment, which makes them rather unsuitable for the provision of acute psychiatric care in particular. The wards are usually chaotic; some patient rooms are accessible only through other patient rooms and it is difficult to secure patients' privacy. The size of the rooms varies depending on the spatial conditions. Some wards have two- to three-bed rooms, but even today one can find rooms with six, eight or ten beds. Modernisation of these facilities is extremely expensive.

The patient composition on individual wards is determined by age (children's wards, adult-patient wards and wards for the 65+ age group), health condition (acute care, after-care, resocialisation wards) or diagnosis (specialised wards for treatment of neuroses, affective disorders, addictions, eating disorders, compulsory treatment). Acute care wards are usually divided into male and female, while in after-care wards and psychotherapeutic wards men and women may be hospitalised together.

The treatment provided at inpatient facilities is mostly biological in nature. Czech patients can get virtually all the latest psychopharmaceuticals. Prescription of any medication is the exclusive domain of a physician. Principles of psychiatric rehabilitation are applied on a larger scale in after-care and to chronically ill patients; even then, however, it is sometimes viewed just as one of the possible ways to fill up free time during hospitalisation. Psychotherapy is applied on the largest scale on wards treating neuroses and addictions.

A higher proportion of non-biological therapy is found in outpatient facilities, such as crisis centres or daily clinics. Systematically applied are various forms of individual and group psychotherapy; art therapy is frequently used, for example. Daily clinics for persons with a psychotic illness give more space to psychiatric rehabilitation and resocialisation as well.

The average monthly salaries in health care in 2009 are stated in Table 2.5. Compared to 2008, the average salary increased by 7.6% in state facilities and by 6.8% in private facilities (ÚZIS, 2010). In view of the radical cuts in expenditure of the new government elected in May 2010, it is likely that salaries will decline further.

TABLE 2.5 Average salaries in health care

	Average salary			
	Facilities established by state and local authorities		Private facilities	
	CZK	EUR	CZK	EUR
Health care workers in total	26760	ca 1070	22840	ca 913
Nurses	**26261**	**ca 1050**	**22371**	**ca 894**
Medical professions	48723	ca 1950	47266	ca 1889

Source: ÚZIS, 2009

TABLE 2.6 Number of specialists in psychiatric sanatoria

Physicians, dentists and pharmacists	550
Nurses	2976
Occupational therapists	39
Social workers	99
Psychologists	120
Physiotherapists	60
Other specialists	147
Non-physicians under specialist supervision (orderlies in particular)	1763

Source: ÚZIS, 2010

TABLE 2.7 Number of specialists in outpatient facilities

Physicians	730
Nurses	415
Psychologists	84
Other	40

Source: ÚZIS, 2010

A typical team providing care at inpatient psychiatric facilities comprises psychiatrists, psychologists, nurses, social workers and care support workers. For illustration, this is the staff of a 40-bed psychiatric ward: four psychiatrists, twenty nurses, one psychologist, one social worker, and four care support workers. The following is a brief outline of the main activities of each employee category:

- A **psychiatrist** defines a therapy plan, does ward rounds every day, communicates with families, provides psychotherapy and organises subsequent care.
- **Nurses** complete psychiatrists' orders, define care plans based on patients' needs, and independently provide education to patients (for example about adherence with medication, physical health, addiction problems, etc.) and some psychotherapeutic activities (such as relaxation, art therapy and cognitive functions training).
- A **psychologist** performs psychological testing and psychotherapeutic interviews with patients, including group psychotherapy.
- **Care support workers** provide the basic nursing care – supporting hygiene, administration of food, patient supervision, escorts, disinfection and cleaning.

Future developments

In 2004, the Committee for Implementation of the Conceptual Plan in Psychiatry was set up as an advisory body to the Ministry of Health. It was composed of the representatives of the individual mental health care sectors, the Psychiatric Association of the Czech Medical Association, the Centre for Mental Health Care Development and the representatives of patients and relatives of psychiatric patients. The task of this committee was to formulate concrete proposals, systems and procedures that would allow the conceptual plan to be implemented in practice. Unfortunately, shortly after the commencement of this work, changes took place in the Ministry of Health which resulted in these plans being abandoned.

However, a more recent revised plan for psychiatry produced by the Psychiatric Association of the Czech Medical Association was approved by its board. This plan provides a detailed description of an adequate structure for individual services for patients with mental illnesses. It sets forth a new definition of primary psychiatric care at psychiatric outpatient clinics which should be systematically linked to other follow-up services; it defines psychiatric hospitals to which psychiatric sanatoria are to be converted; acute and after-care are defined as specialist care, and newly devised structures for community care are to be put in place. The revised plan contains chapters dealing separately with gerontopsychiatry, substance abuse, child and adolescent psychiatry and a programme of care for criminals with mental illness. The revising of structures and systems by a medical organisation could be seen as progressive in that in the past there existed the naïve belief by civil servants and politicians that the mere devising of policies equated with their being implemented. However, a problem still exists. Is there a political will to fund the proposed services, particularly at a time when the economic recession is affecting the provision of health care in other EU countries?

Conclusions

No major changes in psychiatry have occurred in the Czech Republic over the past 10 years. After 1989, initial efforts to develop community care began. However, activities of this kind have been more or less stagnant in recent years. The development of care for mentally ill people is currently ill-conceived and unsystematic (Bašný *et al.*, 2003).

To improve the current situation, the range of existing services needs to be extended, especially incorporating community services which aim to help clients in their natural surroundings. Improving the standard of education of health care professionals, especially nurses, is another important factor in improving service quality. More attention should be paid to increasing and protecting mental patients' rights. A significant role can be played here by self-help associations of patients and their families, which have been steadily emerging and whose voice has become increasingly strong.

Case scenario

A 23-year-old unemployed man is reported by his landlord as acting increasingly strangely. He has barricaded his room, and is talking about being spied upon by the CIA. He can be heard shouting within his room in an angry and incoherent way. He has not been seen by a psychiatrist in the past, although his mother has told the landlord that he has been isolating himself and acting increasingly oddly over the last couple of years.

If the young man consents to be examined by a physician, he can be examined by an outpatient psychiatrist or a psychiatrist at an inpatient facility based on, or without, his GP's referral. If the man does not consent to a medical examination, he can be escorted by the rescue service, including with the assistance of the police, to a local psychiatric facility to be examined by a psychiatrist in the event that he is a threat to himself or people or objects around him. The psychiatrist must decide on whether or not the patient is mentally ill and needs to be hospitalised. Hospitalisation is only possible without the patient's consent if the patient is mentally ill or intoxicated or a threat to himself or people or objects around him. If the physician decides to hospitalise the patient without his consent, the physician will inform the court within 24 hours after the patient was detained. No other approaches, such as mobile crisis teams and monitoring of patients by visiting them at home, have developed in the Czech Republic.

The patient would be admitted to a psychiatric facility – that is to say, a psychiatric sanatorium or, less probably, a psychiatric ward in his town. The patient's condition would be assessed during hospitalisation. The assessment includes a comprehensive psychiatric examination, a laboratory analysis, often a CT brain scan and a psychological examination. Treatment, which is predominantly biological during the first stage, would begin if a mental illness were diagnosed.

The main tasks of the nursing staff in this phase would be to observe the patient's behaviour and to interview the patient, administer medication, and ensure his safety and that his basic biological needs are met (for example, hydration, nutrition, hygiene, rest and sleep). In cooperation with social workers, nurses would help to contact the patient's relatives, provide appropriate clothing and assist in suggesting the use of various hygiene aids. Nurses record their observations and the information derived from interviews at least twice a day in order to elicit a good description of the patient's condition.

As his condition improves, the patient would be gradually involved in therapeutic activities (art therapy, music therapy, rehabilitation exercises and so on). He would also be permitted to visit his home during hospitalisation, accompanied by members of his family at first and later on his own. In regions with developed community care, the patient could be put in touch with community services, such as a day centre, after he had been released from hospital. However, he would be more likely to be referred to an outpatient psychiatrist, whom he would see for regular health checks.

References

Bašný Z, Fialová R, Herman E, *et al.*, 2003. *Koncepční východiska k systému péče o lidi s duševním onemocněním v Praze.* [*Conceptual Basis for System of Care for People with Mental Illness in Prague.*] Prague: CRPDZ. Available at: www.cmhcd.cz/dokumenty/koncepce-praha.pdf (accessed September 2009).

Baštecký J. *Psychiatrie, právo a společnost.* Prague: Galén; 1997.

Mental health services in Europe

Baudiš P, Libiger J. *Psychiatrie a etika*. Prague: Galén; 2002.

Central Intelligence Agency. *The World Factbook*. CIA; 2011.

Centrum pro výzkum veřejného mínění. *Reforma zdravotnictví: názory veřejnosti na problémy zdravotnictví*. Tisková zpráva; 2006. Available at: www.cvvm.cas.cz/upl/zpravy/100571s_oz60406.pdf (accessed 6 April 2006).

Centrum pro výzkum veřejného mínění. *Česká veřejnost o zdravotnictví*. Tisková zpráva; 2010. Available at: www.cvvm.cas.cz/upl/zpravy/100992s_oz100111.pdf (accessed 11 January 2010).

Česká lékařská komora. *Etický kodex České lékařské komory*.1996. Available at: www.lkcr.cz/dokumenty.php?item.id=285&do[load]=1&filterCategory.id=9 (accessed 11 January 2010).

Český statistický úřad. *Sčítání lidu, domů a bytů v roce 2001*. 2003. Available at: www.czso.cz/csu/2005edicniplan.nsf/p/4132-05 (accessed 26 October 2006).

Český statistický úřad. *Statistická ročenka České republiky 2010*. 2011. Available at: www.czso.cz/csu/2010edicniplan.nsf/publ/0001-10- (accessed 7 June 2011).

Chytil M, Roubal T, Voňková K, *et al. Zpráva o stavu, vývoji a výhledu zdravotnictví v ČR*. Prague: Ministerstvo zdravotnictví; 2008. Available at: www.kulatystul.cz/cs/node/236 (accessed 17 June 2008).

David I, Kebza V, Paclt I, *et al.* Mental health in the Czech Republic: current problems, trends and future developments. *J Public Ment Health*. 2003; **5**: 43–7.

Dlouhý M. Mental health care system and mental health expenditure in the Czech Republic. *J Ment Health Policy Econ*. 2004; **7**: 159–65.

Dlouhý M. Ekonomie péče o duševní zdraví v České republice. *Polit Ekon*. 2009; **6**: 797.

European Commission. *Green Paper – Improving mental health of the population: towards a strategy on mental health for the European Union*. Brussels: European Commission; 2005.

Figueras J, McKee M, Mossialos E, *et al. Funding Health Care: options for Europe*. Buckingham: Open University Press; 2002.

Figureas J, Robinson R, Jakubowski E. *Purchasing to Improve Health Systems Performance*. Maidenhead: Open University Press; 2005.

Gaskins M, van Ginneken E. Czech Republic health system review. *Health Syst Transit*. 2009; **11**: 1.

Haškovcová H. *Lékařská etika*. Prague: Galén; 2002.

Janoušková H. *Prestiž povolání sestry ve zdravotnictví*. Diplomová práce. 1. lékařská fakulta University Karlovy v Praze; 2004.

Marková E, Venglářová M, Babiaková M. *Psychiatrická ošetřovatelská péče*. Praha: Grada; 2005.

Ministerstvo zdravotnictví ČR. *Mýty a pověry ve zdravotnictví*. 2008. Available at: www.mzcr.cz/dokumenty/reseni-je-snadne-penize-vice-penez_3279_1380_1.html (accessed 30 September 2008).

Nawková, L. Obraz duševní nemoci v tisku. *Zdravotnické noviny*. 2010; **59**(22): 6.

Sartorious N, Schulze H. *Reducing the Stigma of Mental Illness: a report from a global programme of the World Psychiatric Association*. Cambridge: Cambridge University Press; 2005.

Scheffler R, Potůček M, editors. *Mental Health Care Reform in the Czech and Slovak Republics, 1989 to Present*. Prague: Karolinum; 2008.

Shaywitz DA, Ausiello DA. Global health: a chance for Western physicians to give – and receive. *Am J Med*. 2002; 113, 354–7.

Šnajdr B. *Návštěvní kniha*. Prague: Gasset; 2004.

Středisko empirických výzkumů (STEM). *Češi a víra v Boha*. [*The Czechs and Belief in God.*] Press release. Prague: Středisko empirických výzkumů; 16 March 2007. Available at: http://www.stem.cz/clanek/1516 (accessed 16 March 2007).

Ústav zdravotnických informací a statistiky ČR. *Zdravotnická ročenka ČR 2008*. 2009. Available at: www.uzis.cz/publikace/zdravotnicka-rocenka-ceske-republiky-2008 (accessed 16 December 2009).

Ústav zdravotnických informací a statistiky ČR. *Psychiatrická péče 2009*. 2010. Available at: www. uzis.cz/novinky-ustavu-zdravotnickych-informaci-statistiky-ceske-republiky-edition-5 (accessed 23 November 2010).

Ústav zdravotnických informací a statistiky ČR. *Evropské výběrové šetření o zdravotním stavu v ČR – EHIS CR (Duševní zdraví, vitalita, kognitivní schopnosti)*. Tisková zpráva; 2010. Available at: www.uzis.cz/rychle-informace/evropske-vyberove-setreni-zdravotnim-stavu-cr-ehis-cr-dusevni-zdravi-vitalita-kogni (accessed 19 May 2010).

Ústav zdravotnických informací a statistiky ČR. *Mzdy a platy ve zdravotnictví v roce 2009*. Tisková zpráva; 2010. Available at: www.uzis.cz/rychle-informace/mzdy-platy-zdravotnictvi-roce-2009 (accessed 2 July 2010).

Ústav zdravotnických informací a statistiky ČR. *Evropské výběrové šetření o zdraví v České republice EHIS 2008. [European Health Interview Survey in the Czech Republic EHIS 2008.]* Prague: Ústav zdravotnických informací a statistiky ČR; April 2011. Available at: www.uzis.cz/en/publica tions/european-health-interview-survey-czech-republic-ehis-2008 (accessed 02 March 2012).

Vencovský E. *Čtení o psychiatrii*. Prague: Avicenum; 1983.

Wenigová B. *Stigma a psychiatrie (napříč časem)*. Prague: Sanquis 38; 2005.

Wenigová B. *Pilotní model péče o duševně nemocné v Karlovarském kraji*. Prague: CRPDZ; 2009.

Zastoupení Evropské komise v ČR. *Národní zpráva Eurobarometr 72: podzim 2009. [Eurobarometer 72 National Report: Autumn 2009.]* Prague: Zastoupení Evropské komise v ČR; 2010. Available at: http://ec.europa.eu/ceskarepublika/news/100121_eurobarometr_72_cs.htm (accessed 21 January 2010).

3

Mental health services in Finland

*Heikki Ellilä, Maritta Välimäki, Lauri Kuosmanen
and Heli Hätönen*

Introduction

In this chapter, Finnish mental health services and their evolution are described, as are the current population and demographics of the country. An overview of the general health of the population is also provided, followed by a description of the general health care system. The state of public mental health and the Finnish system of mental health are discussed, including mental health legislation, public attitudes towards mental health and expenditure on mental health services. The current position of psychiatric nursing is examined, as is the future direction of mental health services in Finland.

Population and demographics

Finland is a parliamentary, democratic republic with a semi-presidential system. It joined the European Union together with Sweden and Austria at the beginning of 1995. The currency in Finland is the euro and the population is 5.35 million.

Except for a small highland region in the extreme northwest of Lapland, the country is lowland, less than 180 m above sea level. Off the southwest coast are the Swedish-populated Åland Islands (1505 km²), which have had an autonomous status since 1921. All together the population of Finland is spread over approximately 330 000 km². This makes Finland the most sparsely populated country in the European Union. There are two official languages: Finnish, which is spoken by 92% of the population, and Swedish, which is spoken by 5.5% of the inhabitants. The mean age in 2009 was 39.8 years for males and 42.7 for females (Statistics Finland, 2010a). Finland has an immigrant community consisting of only 1.99% of the population, which is small in comparison to other European countries. Approximately 40% of immigrants have moved from the former Soviet Union, Estonians being the biggest immigrant group. Regarding religion, over 83% of the population belong to the Evangelical Lutheran Church of Finland (Evangelical Lutheran Church of Finland, 2005).

Finnish people generally have a high standard of education. Young people, in particular, have been rated highly in international comparisons in the OECD Programme for International Student Assessment (PISA) surveys. In 2000 and 2003, Finnish educational success was seen as outstanding in reading assessment and has also fared quite well in mathematics and science (Ministry for Foreign Affairs of Finland, 2007; OECD, 2010). Sixty-five per cent of the population aged 15 and over have attained an educational qualification. Tertiary degrees are held by 24% of males and 30% of females (Statistics Finland, 2010c). According to the Adult Education Survey (Statistics Finland, 2010b), more than half the Finnish population aged 25 to 64 participate in some form of education or training annually in order to improve their skills and knowledge through informal learning. The level of education people have had is significantly, and consistently, associated with nearly all indicators of health and functional capacity. Educated and married persons tend to be significantly healthier than single, uneducated, cohabiting, divorced and widowed persons (Palosuo *et al.*, 2007). Additionally, regional variation in health and functional capacity has also been found to be significantly related to health status (Helakorpi, 2009). About 8%–10% of the population is living in marginal circumstances, suffering from a wide range of socio-economic, psychological and somatic problems, which adversely affect their health (Palosuo *et al.*, 2007).

There were 2 517 000 household-dwelling units in Finland at the end of 2009 and there has recently been an increase in the numbers of one and two-person household-dwelling units. In contrast, the number of larger household-dwelling units with at least three members decreased (Statistics Finland, 2010d). In 2008, the mean income per person was €24 696: €29 089 for men and €20 566 for women (Statistics Finland, 2010 e).

The current most important creators of employment are the electronics industry, forestry, business services, social and health services as well as trade. These branches of the employment sector are also growing fast, while jobs are still decreasing in the food and textile industries (Statistics Finland, 2007f).

According to Statistics Finland's Labour Force Survey, the unemployment rate in May 2010 was 10.5%, 0.3% lower than the previous year. Those employed are facing greater stress and more pressures than ever before. For example, the latest Quality of Work Life Survey (2008) describes the changes that have taken place in working conditions during the past 30 years. Positive changes include greater opportunities to engage in more on-the-job training in order to acquire more skills to meet the demands of changing working conditions. Negative developments include an increase in problems related to time pressure, insecurity of employment and social relationships. These developments have especially been observed in the public sector. Negative developments started to appear in the local government sector from about the time of the recession in the 1990s, but according to the latest survey, the 2000s have also seen an increase in work–life problems, especially in the central government sector (Statistics Finland, 2010f).

General health need

The general health status among the Finnish population has historically been relatively poor, especially in comparison with other Scandinavian countries (Koponen and Aromaa, 2005). Until 1970, Finland was a country with a high incidence of musculoskeletal diseases, and mortality due to cardiovascular diseases was among the highest in the world (Peltonen *et al.*, 2007). Poverty and other socio-economic problems among the population, accompanied with other risk factors such as smoking and unhealthy nutrition, were identified as the main reasons for the high incidence of general diseases and for short life expectancy (Statistics Finland, 2007).

The general health profile among the population has improved significantly over the past three decades and mortality from cardiovascular diseases has decreased by 80% in the middle-aged population (National Public Health Institute, 2008). The prevalence of many other common diseases, including musculoskeletal diseases and caries, has also decreased. Most of this decline can be explained by changes in relation to the main cardiovascular disease risk factors, such as decreased smoking and healthier eating habits (Peltonen *et al.*, 2007). According to the Finnish Cancer Registry (2009), the number of lung cancers, the leading type of cancer for decades among males, has decreased due to the decreased use of tobacco products.

Furthermore, there have been favourable changes in self-reported health status, use of leisure time for physical activity, physical fitness and in the general quality of life. Self-rated working capacity has improved, especially in men (Helakorpi *et al.*, 2008). Two thirds of the Finnish working-age population, and one third of those aged 65 or over, evaluate their own health as 'good' or 'fairly good'. On the other hand, 44% of people aged 30–64 had at least one longstanding illness, and among persons aged 65 or over, 82% were found to have a similar condition. In comparison with data collected 20 years earlier in the Mini-Finland Survey 1989 (Aromaa *et al.*, 1989), the self-rated health of the population has clearly improved (Peltonen *et al.*, 2007).

Life expectancy has increased by 10 years in the last 30 years and over 30 years since the time of Finnish independence in 1917. At the moment, the average life expectancy for children born in 2000 is 83 years for females and 76 years for males (Statistics Finland, 2007). Thus, this positive trend sets up additional challenges for the Finnish health services due to the increasing number of aged citizens with an increasing number of health problems such as dementia and depression, accompanied by socio-economic problems (Aromaa and Koskinen, 2004).

Despite the favourable development in general health status in Finland, the risk of diabetes and metabolic disorders has increased (National Public Health Institute, 2008; Aromaa and Koskinen, 2004). The average body weight and body mass index has increased during past decades, especially among men. However, during the 5-year period 2002–07, the change in body mass index was no longer statistically significant. Still, the prevalence of obesity is high in the Finnish adult population (Helakorpi, 2009). Overweight and lack of exercise are among the most important risk factors of poor general health, which has reached alarming proportions among school children (Peltonen *et al.*, 2007).

Health services

In Finland, one of the explicit duties of the public sector is to take care of the health and well-being of the population, which is mainly provided through the organisation of social and health services. Thus, the majority of health services for the population are provided by the public sector, with the private sector providing about a quarter of services. Health services are also provided by occupational health care systems (Ministry of Social Affairs and Health, 2004).

The Ministry of Social Affairs and Health administers the overall functioning of social and health services. However, the responsibility for organising local health services, as well other basic services, lies with local government, which comprises the municipalities. In Finland, there are 336 municipalities, which are autonomous and have a considerable degree of freedom to plan and develop services based on their own considerations. However, central government generally steers the health care system by means of directing specific investments and the creation of new posts (Koskinen *et al.*, 2006.)

Health services are organised into primary health care and specialised health care. Primary health care is provided by health centres, established by a single municipality, or, in some cases, by neighbouring municipalities collaborating to provide combined services. Municipalities may also buy services from other municipalities or from the private sector. Municipalities are responsible for organising specialised medical care for local residents. To this end, Finland is divided into 20 hospital districts, each providing specialist consultations and care for its population. Each hospital district has a central hospital with departments for most main specialities. In addition, five university hospitals provide the most advanced medical care, as well as the training of medical and other health care personnel. It is the responsibility of municipalities to arrange and provide mental health services. In Finland, community care is the preferred mode of mental health care delivery and as a result, during recent decades institutional care has been reduced significantly (Ministry of Social Affairs and Health, 2004.)

Health promotion and illness prevention is a key feature of Finnish social and health policy, with the aim of supporting individual, family and community well-being. The ongoing development of health services generally is being driven by a number of state-level reforms, chief amongst which is the delegation of responsibility for some aspects of health care to municipal health services. Today, the most important development is the Development Programme for Social and Health Care, known as KASTE, which has been devised and will be implemented between 2008 and 2012 (Ministry of Social Affairs and Health, 2011).

The Ministry of Social Affairs and Health determines the course of the development of health services, drafts legislation and steers reform processes. It monitors the implementation and quality of services via the National Supervisory Authority for Welfare and Health (Valvira) and the Regional State Administrative Agencies. Valvira is responsible for ensuring the adequacy of services provided by health care professionals and health care operating units through guidance, supervision and standard setting. The Regional State Administrative Agencies are in charge of the basic services, for instance, the fields of social welfare and health care, environmental health care, education, consumer administration, rescue services and the delivery of emergency services.

Funding

Public financing of health services is done by means of levying local taxes, which are paid to the municipalities, and a National Health Insurance financing scheme based on compulsory insurance fees. Public funding is provided to municipal health care services. Municipalities fund most municipal health care services, except outpatient medicines and transport costs. National Health Insurance funds also pay for services bought from the private health care sector, occupational health care, outpatient medicines, transport costs, sickness allowances and maternity leave allowances (Vuorenkoski *et al.*, 2008, National Institute for Health and Welfare, 2010).

Critiques of the system

In general, the Finnish health care system offers good-quality health services for reasonable cost, with quite high public satisfaction. The biggest challenges for health care are presented by an ageing population, the rapid development of medical technology, budgetary constraints in general by the government, the growing expectations placed on the health care system and globalisation (Koskinen *et al.*, 2006). However, more strident criticisms are targeted at public health treatments, especially treatments for those with mental health problems. Finland has more cardiovascular diseases, diabetes and asthma than other OECD countries proportionately. These conditions are treated relatively often in inpatient care, and asthma mortality among children and adolescents is almost non-existent. However, mental health services appear to function less well in Finland than in the other similar OECD countries. In Finland, for instance, patients with mental health disorders return to psychiatric inpatient care, due to relapse, within 30 days, more often than in any other OECD country. Although relapse rates are high in other Nordic countries, those in Finland do give cause for concern. As has been pointed out by the OECD (2009), the data on which these comparisons are made may be questionable, as different methods of data collection exist and different inferences may be drawn.

Health outcomes between sections of the population vary significantly; therefore, it is essential to seek ways to improve this health disparity, especially in the most underprivileged groups (Koskinen *et al.*, 2006). There are also significant differences between the quality and delivery methods within health services in different organisations; for example, these include scope of services, user fees, waiting times and types of treatments provided. Moreover, the dual public financing system of municipal and National Health Insurance financing is considered as a challenge to the overall efficiency of service provision and may affect the quality of services (Vuorenkoski *et al.*, 2008).

Mental health need

Mental health problems are as prevalent in Finland as they are in other Western countries. The most common mental health problems amongst the Finnish population are various forms of depression, anxiety disorders and alcohol dependency. Depression is seen as a highly important public mental health problem on account of its high prevalence and the harm and damage it causes to individuals, families and the economy. A rise in the number of people with depression in recent years, especially among the young, is giving cause for concern. Psychological symptoms, major depression and burnout are also common, although there are no indications that mental health problems, in general, are becoming more prevalent than they were 20 years ago (Koponen and Aromaa, 2005).

According to Statistics Finland (2006), alcohol consumption has increased, giving rise to alcoholism, increasing numbers of people with cirrhosis and other medical problems linked to alcohol abuse, which are associated with early deaths among the middle-aged population. Generally speaking, increasing alcohol consumption and alcohol abuse are regarded as the biggest general health problem in Finland (Helakorpi, 2009).

The lifetime prevalence of all psychoses is estimated to be approximately 3% higher than other comparable countries; however, this may be due to data collection bias. Table 3.1 summarises the numbers of men and women presenting with the major conditions as a percentage of the total population.

TABLE 3.1 Prevalence (%) of mental disorders in Finland

Disorder/symptom	Women	Men
Major depressive disorder	6.3%	3.4%
Any anxiety disorder	4.8%	3.7%
Alcohol dependence	1.4%	6.5%

Source: Pirkola *et al.*, 2005

The number of accidental and suicidal deaths among males is one of the highest in Europe (Kumpula *et al.*, 2004), although suicide rates have decreased significantly recently, due to better recognition and treatment, particularly with better use of antidepressive medication. However, large numbers of common mental health problems remain unrecognised by health and social care services, which is a major challenge to the effectiveness of treatments and in the development of services (Lönnqvist, 2006; Suvisaari, 2010).

Historical development

In 1686, Karl XI, King of Sweden (Finland was an eastern part of Sweden) ordered that the care of lunatics was the duty of the church. At that time, most 'lunatics' were transferred from house to house and from farmer to farmer. To prevent them from escaping, they were bound to the walls of houses (Kaila, 1966). There is still a Finnish slang expression – *seinä hullu* (lit. 'wall greasy'), meaning totally insane.

The first institutional treatment for the mentally ill saw them housed with patients with leprosy, and later with poor, mentally handicapped and other socially abnormal individuals in institutions for paupers (Sarvilinna, 1938). When Seili hospital was founded in 1619, it was meant for both leprosy and mental patients. The location of Seili was on a small island, located in the archipelago of Turku, far away from other people and thus allowing the isolation of the patients from the rest of society. Kronoby hospital was founded in 1631, originally only for leprosy patients, but later beds were reassigned for mentally ill patients, and finally the entire hospital was, from 1785. Other hospitals were founded in the middle of the nineteenth century and later in the century, when municipalities received subsidies from the state to found psychiatric hospitals (Sarvilinna, 1938). The first law concerning the care of the mentally ill in Finland was introduced in 1840 by the Russian empire (Mäkelä, 2008).

Traditionally, psychiatric treatment in Finland centred around hospitals which were isolated, and the treatment was largely custodial and characterised by all means of coercion until the early 1900s. Conditions remained poor even after that time, and during the Second World War many inpatients died from malnutrition (Hyvönen, 2008). After the war, in the 1950s, an increasing number of long-term, chronic patients were placed into what was known as 'home care' on local farms. Also at this time, the ideas of psychotherapy became more popular amongst psychiatrists, leading to the first therapeutic communities (Kaila, 1966). In 1952, the new Act on Mentally Ill Patients was passed, which made municipalities responsible for the care of mentally ill patients. The country was divided into 20 districts, each of which was to have a psychiatric hospital and, additionally, a facility for psychiatric outpatients (Salokangas et al., 2000). The number of beds increased after this law came into effect; in 1955, there were 2.5 beds per 1000 inhabitants and this increased to a high point in 1970, with 4.3 per 1000 inhabitants being the highest in all of Europe, together with Ireland (Mäkelä, 2008).

Institutional care versus deinstitutionalisation

Finnish psychiatric care underwent an extensive transformation from the beginning of the 1990s. Major changes occurred in a relatively short period of time: at the end of the 1980s, there were 20 000 inpatient beds in Finland, but only 5600 by the year 2000. The process of change consisted of a deinstitutionalisation programme, the integration of mental health services with other health services and the transfer of the responsibility for organising services from central government to the municipalities. Alongside these administrative and structural changes, Finland underwent the deepest economic depression ever seen in industrialised countries, resulting in drastic cuts in the mental health budgets and hampering the development of services (Lehtinen and Taipale, 2001; Kärkkäinen, 2004; Ministry of Social Affairs and Health, 2005; Harjajärvi et al., 2006). Evaluations of the process of deinstitutionalisation conclude that the process was satisfactory and patients were quite satisfied with both the accessibility and quality of services (Korkeila, 1998; Korkeila et al., 1998(a,c); Lehtinen and Taipale, 2001); however, regional inequalities were found in the quality and availability of services (Ministry of Social Affairs and Health, 2005; Harjajärvi et al., 2006). Findings concluded that the Finnish mental health care system remains too hospital-based, and there is a lack of diverse and flexible community care services (NOMESCO, 2007).

Whilst the number of rehabilitation clients with mental health problems has increased rapidly over the last several years, the number of rehabilitation clients in all categories has only increased by 4.7% overall (Ministry of Social Affairs and Health, 2011). An example is that psychotherapeutic services were funded for a total of 14 100 clients in 2008, an increase of 8.3% over the previous year. Their number has doubled in the 2000s. The number of rehabilitation participants relative to the general population was highest in the Kainuu, Northern Ostrobothnia, Central Ostrobothnia and Lapland regions, and lowest in the Åland Islands, East Uusimaa and Päijänne-Tavastia. Medical rehabilitation services for the severely disabled play an important role in regions with a high relative population share of rehabilitation clients (Ministry of Social Affairs and Health, 2011).

Historically, mental health services have been directed by national programmes and projects. During the last two decades, many developments and research programmes in the area of mental health care have been carried out (e.g. the National Schizophrenia Project, 1981–87; National Suicide Prevention Project, 1986–96; National Depression Project, 1994–98; Meaningful Life Programme, 1998–2003). Programmes have also supported municipalities and mental health professionals in the setting up and improving of services so that they can better meet the needs of populations (Lehtinen and Taipale, 2001; Ministry of Social Affairs and Health, 2005). The National Plan for Mental Health and Substance Abuse Work (2009) defines the core principles and priorities for the future of mental health and substance abuse work until 2015. The plan emphasises the centrality of the service user, mental health and abstinence from alcohol and drugs are promoted, alcohol and drug-related harm are to be prevented and treated, and mental health and substance abuse services are to be organised, mainly in the community. Totally new suggestions include the 'low-threshold principle' of a single entry point for patients into services and the establishment of outpatient units that combine mental health and substance abuse services (Ministry of Social Affairs and Health, 2009).

The position of patients

In Finland, health care legislation does not distinguish between those who are mentally ill and those who are not. All patients, including those with mental health problems, are equal before the law. The Act on the Status and Rights of Patients (785/1992) lists the basic rights of patients and how their views and opinions are to be taken into account. All patients have to be cared for with respect and understanding (Chapter 2, Section 4a), and the act describes how patients' complaints are to be dealt with (Chapter 3, Section 10). Based on the Mental Health Act (1116/1990) and the Amendment of the Mental Health Act (1423/2001), a patient's opinion needs to be taken into account when deciding on involuntary treatments and interventions.

So far, there is no specific legislation on how patients or users should be involved in their own treatment. To date, user involvement has mostly been passive, and limited to participation in working groups to tackle specific issues (Tritter and McCallum, 2006; Kuosmanen, 2009). The Proposal for a National Framework for Mental Health Services in 2001 did not make any recommendations related to user involvement in mental health care (Ministry of Social Affairs and Health, 2001). However, the most recent effort by the Ministry of Social Affairs and Health to steer Finnish mental health and substance abuse treatment, the Mieli Working Group (2009), emphasises that the service user perspective needs to be taken into account when developing services (Ministry of Social Affairs and Health, 2009).

Attitudes to mental health problems

Typically, attitudes in Finland to mental problems are less favourable compared to other health problems. Historically, patients have been isolated from society in big psychiatric hospitals. Changes in mental health law and the systematic development of mental health services have only slowly changed attitudes towards mental problems.

TNS Gallup Oy (2009) conducted a national survey of Finnish citizens (the so-called Mielenterveysbarometri) for the Finnish Central Association for Mental Health (2009). Citizens' attitudes towards mental problems were measured by asking what kind of neighbours respondents would not like to live next to. Although attitudes among Finnish citizens have become more positive, still 28% did not want to live near nor have a neighbour with mental health problems living close to them. Those under 25 years had the most negative attitudes, of whom 41% held negative attitudes towards persons with mental health problems generally. Conversely, the attitudes of managers, higher officials and entrepreneurs were more positive. In 2007, 21% of managers, 27% of higher officials and 18% of entrepreneurs stated that they would not live next to a person with mental health problems (Finnish Central Association for Mental Health, 2010).

Furthermore, the Mielenterveysbarometri showed that a large majority of those with mental health problems feared that they ran the risk of losing their positions and status if they revealed their condition to friends or colleagues. Seventy per cent of those under 25 stated that they would not mention their own mental health problem to their fellow workers, and 45% would not tell their superior. Even mental health professionals confessed that they would prefer to remain silent if they faced the problem in their own personal life. Altogether, 300 patients and relatives and 330 psychiatrists and psychologists participated in the study (Finnish Central Association for Mental Health, 2010).

Expenditure on mental health

Total health spending in Finland amounted to €14.7 billion in 2007, amounting to slightly less than the average total health spend (8.2%) for OECD countries which was 8.9% that year. Total health expenditure increased by 3.2% from the previous year. At the same time, total expenditure on mental health care was €658 million, comprising primary mental health care (€85 million), psychiatric outpatient care/day-ward care (€169 million) and psychiatric inpatient care (€404 million). Expenditure on primary mental health care increased by 8.1%, while expenditure decreased on psychiatric inpatient care (4.6%), as well as on outpatient care and day-ward care (1.5%), from the previous year. Regarding the use of services, the number of outpatient mental health visits in primary health care increased by 4.3%, while the number of patients in psychiatric institutional care fell by 1% (National Institute for Health and Welfare, 2009).

Indirect costs of mental illness are difficult to estimate. However, sickness allowances due to mental health problems increased by 93% between 1990 and 2003 in Finland (Järvisalo *et al.*, 2005). Mental health problems are currently the most common reason for receiving a disability pension, and direct and indirect costs related to depression have increased. Costs of mental problems also include other indirect costs, such as child welfare costs to families with children and costs of special education due to mental health problems. These costs have also increased, and it is estimated that they will continue increasing into the future. Costs related to simultaneous mental and drug abuse problems amongst the young population, burnout in working life and exclusion from society are also all estimated to increase (National Institute for Health and Welfare, 2010). At the same time, costs related to severe mental problems, such as psychosis, have not changed. The annual cost of schizophrenia in Finland is approximately €1 billion (Duodecim, 2008) and the cost of antipsychotic medication was €92 million in 2007 (Social Insurance Institute of Finland, 2008).

Mental health law

General human rights and the autonomy of every individual are the main principles behind the Finnish Mental Health Act (1990). The subsequent 2001 Amendment to the act highlights patients' rights, liberty and the autonomy of all patients. All mental health legislation is concerned with minimising any restrictions to the person as much as possible. In addition, there are several other acts influencing mental health care in Finland, such as the Act on the Status and Rights of Patients (785/1992), the Act on Social Work with Intoxicant Abusers (41/1986) and Act on Primary Health (66/1972).

'Mental health work' is described in a very comprehensive way in the Mental Health Act (1116/1990). First, mental health work means the promotion of mental well-being, the ability to cope and the personal growth of the individual, and the prevention and alleviation of problems associated with mental illnesses and other disorders. Secondly, it includes social and health care services (mental health services) provided for persons suffering from a medically diagnosed mental illness or other mental disorder. Thirdly, it relates to improving the living conditions of the population, in order to help to prevent mental disorders, promoting mental health work and supporting the organisation of mental health services. To summarise, mental health work is defined as work which is done at all levels of society, not only by health and social care professionals.

According to the Mental Health Act (1116/1990), it is the responsibility of municipalities to organise mental health services, and community-based care, near to people's homes. However, forensic services are mainly organised by the state. Overall, the general planning, direction and supervision of mental health work is the responsibility of the Ministry of Social Affairs and Health. In addition, as described in the Mental Health Act, the provision of mental health services requires an effective system for supervision of all the professionals working those services. According to the Act on Status and Rights of Patients 785/1992, the patient has to be cared for based on mutual understanding between patient and professional.

Involuntary treatment

Involuntary treatment (treatment against the will of the patient) is carried out in situations where it is regarded as necessary in order to treat inpatients against their will in an inpatient psychiatric ward. All involuntary treated patients have a formal legal status. Thus, according to the Mental Health Act (1116/1990), a person can be ordered to have treatment in a psychiatric hospital against his/her will only if:
- the person has been found to be suffering from a severe mental illness, or
- if they are in need of psychiatric care, without which the mental illness will get worse, or
- it could seriously threaten their own or other people's health or safety, and
- if no other form of mental health service is available or is seen to be sufficient. It is also possible to admit a voluntary inpatient to involuntary treatment if no other form of mental health service is available or is seen to be sufficient.

The decision regarding compulsory admission is normally made by a general medical practitioner or another physician and the patient is transferred to hospital by paramedics. It is possible for the physician to request help in transferring the patient from the police, if this is considered necessary in terms of safety.

In hospital, the physician in charge of the assessment must produce a written statement concerning the patient no later than 4 days after the admission takes place. The assessment must include a well-founded opinion on whether or not the conditions for ordering the patient to treatment against his or her will are met. If it appears, during the observation period, that the conditions for ordering the patient to treatment are not met, the assessment must be discontinued immediately and the patient can be discharged. Patients also have the right to appeal to an administrative court (Välimäki *et al.*, 2003.)

A minor can also be ordered to treatment in a psychiatric hospital against his or her will if he or she needs treatment for a serious mental disorder which, if not treated, would become considerably worse or severely endanger the minor's health or safety or the health or safety of others, and if all other mental health services are inapplicable. The treatment of a minor must be provided in a unit which has the facilities required for that treatment. A minor must be treated separately from adults, unless it is considered that it is in the interests of the minor to act otherwise. The involuntary admission of a minor is legally more complicated than the admission of an adult, because a person under 18 is legally under the control of parents or parental substitutes. They should always be informed about involuntary admission and they also have the right to appeal to an administrative court (Mental Health Act 1116/1991).

In summary, the legal position is that patients should be treated by mutual understanding between the patient and the professionals involved; coercive measures may be applied only if they are necessary for the treatment of the illness, or for safeguarding patients' safety or the safety of others. Involuntary psychiatric hospitalisation is closely regulated by the Mental Health Act. However, the rules concerning the deprivation of liberty during inpatient treatment (by seclusion, restraint and restricted leave) are formulated in very general terms (Kuosmanen, 2009).

The structure of mental health care

To summarise, the majority of mental health care is provided by the public sector, and municipalities are responsible for arranging the provision of mental health services. Mental health care includes a variety of services, such as identification of mental problems and disorders, treatment at the primary care level, psychiatric outpatient and inpatient care at the specialised level. Psychiatric rehabilitation is provided by the public and private sectors and by non-profit and non-governmental third-sector organisations (Ministry of Social Affairs and Health, 2009).

Treatment of common mental problems and disorders is carried out by primary health care, especially in health centres. When primary health care is not satisfactorily effective, and where there are particularly serious mental health disorders, treatment is provided in specialised outpatient and inpatient care (Mental Health Act, 1116/1990). There is also service-provided accommodation available for mental health rehabilitees. Among the working-age population, occupational health care also supports the maintenance of mental health, as well as the prevention and early identification of problems. In Finland, there are two state-owned psychiatric hospitals providing mental assessments and treatment for patients whose care is considered dangerous or particularly complex.

Evidence of effectiveness

The psychiatric health care system has faced many changes in recent decades. Internationally, many countries have changed their approach to mental health services, moving away from inpatient hospital care and developing outpatient services (OECD, 2008). Since the early 1990s, in Finland, there has been a major shift away from institutional inpatient care for psychiatric patients towards outpatient community care (Lehtinen and Taipale, 2001; Ministry of Social Affairs and Health, 2005). Evaluations have shown that the process of deinstitutionalisation has been successful (Pirkola *et al.*, 2007, 2009). The effectiveness of the health care system can be monitored closely through registers that include very detailed data, down to single patient level.

The Current Care Board has produced evidence-based clinical practice guidelines for different areas of mental health care. Today, there are, altogether, 13 different guidelines on psychiatry, child psychiatry, adolescent psychiatry and geriatric psychiatry (Current Care, 2011). There is a special programme, administered by the Ministry of Social Affairs and Health, promoting the development of evidence-based nursing, and the Nursing Research Foundation has launched a programme to develop nursing guidelines. However, so far, none of the guidelines is on mental health issues (Nursing Research Foundation, 2011).

Critiques of the current system

Despite the recent development of mental health services, discrepancies have been revealed, especially related to psychiatric inpatient care. The Finnish mental health system is still hospital-based, and there is a lack of diverse and flexible community care services (NOMESCO, 2007). Involuntary placements and other forms of the deprivation of liberty are used at rates above the average of other countries (Salize and Dressing, 2004). Patients report psychiatric hospital care as being unstructured (Koivisto *et al.*, 2004) and providing a lack of activities that they can undertake during periods of hospitalisation (Kuosmanen *et al.*, 2006).

Patients have also reported inadequate information provision, poor interprofessional communication and a lack of opportunities for collaborative care, and they have perceived nurses in psychiatric hospitals as particularly inaccessible (Kuosmanen, 2009; Hätönen, 2010).

The contribution of nursing

In 2002, in total, 56 458 registered nurses lived in Finland (Stakes, 2003). The number of qualified nurses, i.e. registered nurses and mental health nurses working in psychiatric hospitals, decreased from 5399 in 1990 to 3984 in 2005 (Ailasmaa, 2007). The decreasing numbers are a clear outcome of the decreased number of psychiatric hospital beds leading to increasing numbers of nurses working in outpatient centres providing community-based care, although the vast majority of nurses are still working in inpatient settings (Ministry of Social Affairs and Health, 2009). The total number of nurses in Finnish mental health services is not exactly known, but it is probably about 7000–8000, which is the largest number in mental health services per head of population in the whole of Europe (WHO, 2007).

In reality, there are no comprehensive, fully reliable statistics about the total number, although it is known that 80% of the staff working in psychiatric inpatient services for children and adolescents are nurses (Ellilä, 2007) and it is obvious that the proportion would be approximately at the same level in all institutions providing psychiatric and mental health services.

Nurses working in mental health services can be divided into two main groups: registered nurses (RNs) with a degree in nursing (BA) training from universities of applied sciences, and practical mental health nurses trained in vocational schools. Psychiatric/mental health nurses have traditionally had a crucial role in mental health delivery, and they were officially registered as psychiatric mental health nurses. From late 1990, the curriculum of nursing education changed to a more generic model, with no specialist training. Today, RNs have at least 3½ years' general education with short theoretical and practical experience in mental health nursing. The length of mental health nursing experience varies between universities, but the degree programme in nursing does not include special training in mental health nursing. Hence, there is specialist training available in postgraduate studies in many universities on various areas of nursing, including mental health nursing, although doctoral studies are not available in universities of applied sciences (Ministry of Education, 2007). There are four master's programmes with specific studies focusing on mental health/psychiatric nursing available in four Finnish universities of applied sciences, starting from autumn 2011.

Nursing is, arguably, the fundamental profession in mental health care.

Nurses play an active role in contributing to the development of Finnish mental health services and implementing nursing care. Mental health nurses work in close relation with physicians, psychologists, social workers and other professionals in the public, private and third sectors (Ministry of Social Affairs and Health, 2004). Overall, the nurse's role is to promote health, prevent disease, to provide care and rehabilitate. A nurse, for example, plans and carries out nursing care, monitors the patient, administers medication and informs, guides and supports patients and relatives. Nurses work both independently and in multidisciplinary teams (Finnish Nurses Association, 2007; Ministry of Social Affairs and Health, 2001). Their professional expertise is based on knowing how to work ethically, making decisions in nursing, cooperating with the multidisciplinary team, developing leadership, nursing multiculturally, working socially and nursing clinically (Ministry of Education, 2007).

The nurses' role in Finland is independent and nurses are responsible for the decisions they make in daily nursing care. They have the most sustained and direct interactions with patients and their relatives. In the field of psychiatric nursing, the nurse's basic role is to take care of the health and well-being of individuals and groups and to support them to manage daily health problems which are encountered as a result of their illness (Finnish Nursing Association, 2007).

The most common role of the nurse in hospitals is as a primary nurse, key worker or 'own nurse', as it is commonly called in Finland (Salenius, 2005; Hjerppe, 2008). The role of 'own nurse' could be that of a therapist, as it was in therapeutic community-type wards from 1970–80. At that time, nurses had their own patients and they had regular therapy sessions with them almost daily (Alanen *et al.*, 1986). However, it was long inpatient treatment periods that made this possible. Nowadays, the role of the nurse has changed, although nurses working in outpatient settings may still see their work as therapists, as they see their patients weekly in outpatient clinics. They also work as community psychiatric nurses, following the case manager model (Ministry of Social Affairs and Health Care, 2004). Senior nurses with special education in administration, mostly at master's level, work in leading positions as managers in many areas of mental health services (Ministry of Social Affairs and Health, 2004).

In the doctoral thesis by Latvala (1998), it was reported that nurses follow three main work orientations in the basic process of psychiatric nursing in a hospital environment when helping the patient to manage in daily life, an enabling process that enhances personal control and encompasses awareness and commitment to change. The orientations were related to the definition of the goals of nursing, the definition of the patient's needs or problems and the helping methods used. The three different types of psychiatric nursing orientations were collaborative, educative and confirmatory nursing orientations. The confirmatory type represents traditional helping methods and establishes an authoritative relationship with the patient, as in the case of custodial care. A multidisciplinary influence is seen in educative orientation, as teaching is to be provided for the patient and the nurse is seen more as a teacher or guide. Confirmatory psychiatric nursing emphasises patient empowerment. Cooperative helping methods are used in collaborative psychiatric nursing.

Many nurses, working in the field of mental health nursing, educate themselves in the field of psychotherapy, creating one of the biggest professional groups of health care professionals with official psychotherapy training in individual, group or family psychotherapy (Valvira, 2009). Psychotherapy has traditionally been provided by self-employed persons in the private sector, whose customers or patients have been reimbursed for their treatment by the Social Insurance Institution, or in some cases by private insurance institutions where specifically allowed (Pirkola and Sohlman, 2005).

Nurses enjoy great popularity and respect among the general public in Finland. According to a large national survey published by Suomen Kuvalehti (2010), the nursing profession was ranked as the ninth-most-respected profession in the country. All the professions with higher ranking were also connected with health care or, alternatively, rescue work. Syrjäpalo (2006) also found that that psychiatric inpatients highly respected the work of their nurses. They felt that the care received from nurses was humane and patients were respected by them as individuals (although other studies suggest that they may be seen, at times, as inaccessible, as above). The patients participating in this particular study had similar opinions as nursing staff about the most important values of nursing care. The expectations of patients about what was important related to truth, humanity, and respect for human beings, their privacy and freedom.

Plans for the future

The national plan, published by the Finnish Ministry of Social and Health Care (Mieli, 2009), focuses on the development of mental health and substance abuse work and defines the core principles and priorities for the future until 2015. The fact that the plan is referred to as the 'national plan' gives it added emphasis and seeks to show that mental health and substance abuse problems are essentially related to public health, and should be taken into consideration in decision-making at all levels of Finnish society. Thus, mental health is a basic element of health and important in the general structure of the whole of society, human interactions and well-being.

The following 12 points summarise the main recommendations of the plan (Mieli, 2009). This is the first time that a comprehensive plan has outlined common national objectives for mental health and substance abuse work in Finland.

- The importance of the client's status is emphasised and the planning process for mental health services should involve members of the services' user movement, experts by experience, peers and family members.
- Decreasing stigmatisation of clients with mental health problems shall be supported by giving more public information about mental illnesses and by people with mental illnesses talking to the public, especially in schools.
- The poor economic situation of most clients with long-lasting mental health problems should be improved and involvement in employment could be improved by creating more part-time working possibilities and social enterprises.
- More emphasis shall be put on prevention of drug and alcohol abuse, and primary prevention is preferred to secondary and tertiary interventions.
- There shall be more importance put on the early recognition of, and interventions with, mental health problems in childhood and adolescence. School nurses and teachers will play the key role in this.
- Municipalities shall coordinate and use the mental health services of public, private and voluntary sectors flexibly, focusing on the cost-effectiveness of services and the needs of every service user.
- Mental health and substance abuse services will be organised for all age groups in a way that ensures the availability of basic and outpatient services.
- New key definitions for developing the service include the low-threshold principle of a single entry point for all clients using social and health centres.
- New types of outpatient units that combine treatment for both mental health and substance abuse problems shall be established and there shall be more attention given to the treatment of clients with dual diagnosis.
- In the case of involuntary admission and treatment, a system of external experts (possibly to provide second opinions) will be established and the use of involuntary admissions and coercive treatment methods shall be decreased by 40% by 2015.
- Special education for nurses and other health care professionals should be provided and the proportion of subjects, such as mental health nursing and psychiatry, should be increased in the curricula of nursing degree programmes.
- Master's-level education in mental health nursing should be established, leading to the position of advanced nurse practitioner or clinical nurse specialist.

Case scenario

A 23-year-old unemployed man is reported by his landlord as acting increasingly strangely. He has barricaded his room, talking about being spied upon by the CIA.

He can be heard shouting within his room in an angry and incoherent way. He has not been seen by a psychiatrist in the past, although his mother has told the landlord that he has been isolating himself and acting increasingly oddly over the last couple of years.

This case describes a very challenging situation for the health and mental health care system because of the nature of the situation: a man barricading his own home and not wanting anyone to visit that home. Thus, it seems apparent in this case that the person is in need of psychiatric treatment, because of a paranoid type of psychotic behaviour.

Voluntary admission to open care or inpatient care should be prioritised; however, it is evident in this case that the use of outpatient services would be very problematic if the person himself does not want help. Where his mother or other relative calls the local health centre or private health services for help, in Finland it is the duty of the physician in charge to assess the person and, if needed, to write a recommendation for admission to psychiatric care and, if need be, on an involuntary basis.

Generally, it is the health centre physician, after hearing from the client himself, his relatives and/or neighbours or other significant others, who would call paramedics for transport, and the man would be transferred to a health centre for observation. If the physician in charge considers that it is obvious that the transport to a health centre would fail because of the potentially violent nature of the person, then the physician can require the police to provide assistance. In the health centre, the physician examines the man and, if psychiatric treatment is considered necessary, then the physician draws up a written statement (referral for observation). This is only done if other possibilities for treatment are not suitable. In addition to the medical assessment, the physician can interview the patient's mother or other significant others. It is also possible that the physician would make a home visit, instead of transferring the man to a health centre.

According to the Finnish Mental Health Act, a person can be ordered to undergo treatment in a psychiatric hospital against his or her will only:
- if the person is diagnosed as mentally ill
- if the person needs treatment for a mental illness which, if not treated, would become considerably worse or severely endanger the person's health or safety or the health or safety of others, and
- if all other mental health services are inapplicable or inadequate.

The patient can be sent to hospital for observation on the basis of a referral for observation, based on an examination undertaken no more than 3 days earlier, if the conditions for ordering the patient to undergo treatment are likely to be met. In the psychiatric hospital, another physician will examine the patient. The physician can use other sources of information, e.g. the patient's mother, but this needs the patient's agreement. Prior to admission, nursing staff inform the patient of ward rules and patients' rights.

Pharmacotherapy begins early in the period of assessment. Nursing staff need to take relatives into account, who are encouraged to contribute to the care of their family member. The family is seen as a partner in care. If it appears, during the assessment period, that the conditions for ordering the patient to undergo treatment are not met, the assessment will be discontinued immediately and the patient shall be discharged if he or she so wishes. In the assessment period, nursing staff discuss and observe the patient's mental state every day. The physician in charge shall produce a written statement on the patient's assessment no later than 4 days after admission. As part of treatment, the patient may engage with different therapy groups, for example, occupational therapy, art therapy, physical therapy or psychological treatments. Discussions will also take place with a 'primary nurse'.s Nursing staff would also be responsible for providing a safe environment and good basic nursing care, and for arranging follow-up community care with a community psychiatric nurse. This might include home visits, psycho-educational work with relatives, supportive housing visits to a clubhouse, supported work in a day centre and in some cases psychotherapy.

Other forms of help that the patient would be able to access include:
- weekend breaks during treatment
- care meetings with family and patient
- peer support
- morning gatherings (milieu therapy)
- patient information (ward brochure, medication procedure, etc.)
- occupational therapy

Acknowledgement

The authors would like to thank Pekka Makkonen RN, MN.Sc for his help with this case study.

References

Act of Special Health Care in Finland (1062/1989). Available at www.finlex.fi/fi/laki/kaannokset/1989/en19891062.pdf (accessed 17 July 2011).

Act on Primary Health (66/1972). Available at: www.finlex.fi/en/laki/kaannokset/1972/en19720066 (accessed 17 July 2011).

Act on Social Work with Intoxicant Abusers (41/1986). Available at: www.finlex.fi/en/laki/kaannokset/1993/en19931289.pdf (accessed 17 July 2011).

Act on Status and Rights of the Patients (785/1992). Available at: www.finlex.fi/fi/laki/kaannokset/1992/en19920785.pdf (accessed 17 July 2011).

Ailasmaa R. Towards improved quality – improving nurses continuing vocational training in psychiatric hospitals and inpatient units. In: Välimäki M, Scott A, Lahti M, *et al.*, editors. *The*

Changing Face of Psychiatric Nursing – Care or Control? Turku: ePsychNurse.Net/Department of Nursing Science, University of Turku; 2007.

Alanen YO, Räkköläinen V, Laakso J, *et al.* Towards need-specific treatment of schizophrenic psychoses. *Monographien aus dem Gesamtgebiete der Psychiatrie, Psychiatry Series.* 1986; **41**: 1–295.

Amendment of the Mental Health Act (1423/2001). Available at: www.finlex.fi (accessed 5 March 2006).

Aromaa A, Heliovaara M, Impivaara O, *et al.* Mini-Suomi-terveystutkimuksen perustulokset. *Kansaneläkelaitoksen julkaisuja.* AL:32, Helsinki; 1989.

Aromaa A, Koskinen S, editors. Health and functional capacity in Finland. *Baseline Results of the Health 2000 Health Examination Survey.* Helsinki: Publications of the National Public Health Institute, B12/2004; 2004.

Ellilä H. *Child and Adolescent Psychiatric Inpatient Care in Finland.* Doctoral thesis. University of Turku, Department of Child Psychiatry; 2007.

Finnish Cancer Registry – Institute for Statistical and Epidemiological Cancer Research. *Cancer in Finland 2006 and 2007.* Cancer Statistics of the National Institute for Health and Welfare (THL); Cancer Society of Finland Publication no. 76, Helsinki; 2009.

Finnish Central Association for Mental Health (2010) Mielenterveysbarometri. Available at: www.mtkl.fi/?x752385=1230924 (accessed 13 June 2010).

Finnish Nurses Association. *Ethical Guidelines of Nursing.* 1996. Available at: www.sairaanhoitajaliitto.fi/sairaanhoitajan_tyo/ohjeita_ja_suosituksia/sairaanhoitajan_eettiset_ohjeet/ethical_guidelines_of_nursing (accessed 10 May 2010).

Finnish Nurses Association. *Nurses' Work.* 2007. Available at: www.sairaanhoitajaliitto.fi/sairaan hoitajan_tyo (accessed 9 May 2010).

Harjajärvi M, Pirkola S, Wahlbeck K. *Aikuisten mielenterveyspalvelut muutoksessa.* STAKES, Suomen Kuntaliitto, ACTA Nro 187; 2006.

Helakorpi S. *Suomalaisen aikuisväestön terveyskäyttäytyminen ja terveys, kevät 2008.* Kansanterveyslaitoksen julkaisuja; 2/2009.

Hjerppe M. *The Realisation of Primary Nursing as Assessed by Named Nurses.* Master's thesis. University of Tampere, Faculty of Medicine, Department of Nursing; 2008.

Hyvönen J. *The Finnish Psychiatric Health Services in the 1990s from the Point of View of Historical Continuity.* Kuopio University Publications D. Medical Sciences 440; 2008.

Hätönen H. Patient education to support the self-mangement of patients with mental illness. *Annales Universitatis Turkuensis.* 2010; D-891.

Järvisalo J, Andersson B, Boedeker W, *et al. Mental Disorders as a Major Challenge in Prevention of Work Disability: experiences in Finland, Germany, the Netherlands and Sweden.* Helsinki: Kela; 2005.

Kaila M. *Psykiatrian historia.* Porvoo: WSOY; 2004.

Koivisto K, Janhone S, Väisänen L. Patients' experiences of helping in a psychiatric inpatient setting. *J Psychiatr Ment Health Nurs.* 2004; **11**: 268–75.

Koponen P, Aromaa A. *Suomalaisten terveys kansainvälisessä vertailussa.* 2005. Available at: www.terveyskirjasto.fi/terveyskirjasto (accessed 19 May 2010).

Korkeila JA, Lehtinen V, Tuori T, *et al.* Frequently hospitalised psychiatric patients: a study of predictive factors. *Soc Psychiatry Psychiatr Epidemiol.* 1998a; **33**: 528–34.

Korkeila JA, Lehtinen V, Tuori T, *et al.* Regional differences in the use of psychiatric hospital beds in Finland: a national case-register study. *Acta Psychiatr Scand.* 1998b; **98**: 193–9.

Korkeila JA, Lehtinen V, Tuori T, *et al.* Patterns of psychiatric hospital service use in Finland: a national register study of hospital discharges in the early 1990s. *Soc Psychiatry Psychiatr Epidemiol.* 1998c; **33**: 218–23.

Korkeila J. *Perspectives on the Public Psychiatric Services in Finland. Evaluating the Deinstitutionalisation Process.* STAKES, Research Report 93; 1998.

Mental health services in Europe

Koskinen S, Aroma A, Huttunen J, *et al.*, editors. *Health in Finland*. National Public Health Institute KTL, National Research and Development Centre for Welfare and Health, STAKES, Ministry of Social Affairs and Health, Helsinki, Finland; 2006.

Kumpula H, Lounamaa A, Paavola M, *et al.*, editors. *Injuries Among Young Men*. Reports of the Ministry of Social Affairs and Health, Helsinki, Finland; 2006.

Kuosmanen L, Hätönen H, Jyrkinen A, *et al.* Patient satisfaction with psychiatric inpatient care. *J Adv Nurs*. 2006; **55**(6): 655–63.

Kuosmanen L. Personal liberty in psychiatric care – towards service user involvement. *Annales Universitatis Turkuensis*. 2009; D-841.

Kärkkäinen J. *Onnistuiko psykiatrian yhdentyminen somaattiseen hoitojärjestelmään? Psykiatrisen hoitojärjestelmän kehitys Suomessa ja sairaanhoitopiiriuudistuksen arviointi psykiatrian näkökulmasta*. Helsinki: National Research and Development Centre for Welfare and Health (STAKES), Research Report 138; 2004.

Latvala E. Potilaslähtöinen psykiatrinen hoitotyö laitosympäristössä. 1998. Available at: http://herkules.oulu.fi/isbn9514250680/html/x1047.html (accessed 13 July 2010).

Lehtinen V, Taipale V. Integrating mental health services: the Finnish experience. *Int J Integr Care*. 2001; **1**: e26.

Lönnqvist J. (2006) Mental health problems. In: Koskinen S, Aromaa A, Huttunen J, *et al.*, editors. *Health in Finland*. 67–69. National Public Health Institute KTL, National Research and Development Centre for Welfare and Health, STAKES, Ministry of Social Affairs and Health, Helsinki, Finland; 2006.

Mental Health Act (1116/1990). Mielenterveyslaki. Available at: www.finlex.fi (accessed 6 January 2008).

Mieli. *Plan for Mental Health and Substance Abuse Work: proposals of the Mieli 2009 working group to develop mental health and substance abuse work until 2015*. Helsinki: Reports of the Ministry of Social Affairs and Health, Finland; 2009: 3.

Ministry for Foreign Affairs of Finland. Virtual Finland. 2007. Available at: http://virtual.finland.fi/netcomm/news/showarticle.asp?intNWSAID=25876 (accessed 9 May 2007).

Ministry of Education. *Education and Science in Finland. Publication 15*. Helsinki: Ministry of Education; 2007.

Ministry of Social Affairs and Health. Nurses', public health nurses' and midwifes' competence requirements in health care: essential elements in practising health care. Helsinki: Brochures of the Ministry of Social Affairs and Health; 2000: 15.

Ministry of Social Affairs and Health. *Quality Recommendation for Mental Health Services*. Helsinki: Ministry of Social Affairs and Health, Association of Finnish Local and Regional Authorities; Handbooks 2001: 13.

Ministry of Social Affairs and Health. *Health Care in Finland*. Brochures of the Ministry of Social Affairs and Health; 2004: 11.

Ministry of Social Affairs and Health. *Mental Health in Finland*. Brochures of the Ministry of Social Affairs and Health; 2005: 1.

Ministry of Social Affairs and Health. *Plan for Mental Health and Substance Abuse Work: proposals of the Mieli 2009 working group to develop mental health and substance abuse work until 2015*. Reports of the Ministry of Social Affairs and Health; 2009: 3.

Ministry of Social Affairs and Health. National development programme for social welfare and health care (Kaste). 2011. Available at: www.stm.fi/en/strategies_and_programmes/kaste (accessed 21 October 2011).

Mäkelä J. *Houruinhoitoasetuksesta mielenterveyslakiin. Mielisairaanhoidon ja erityisesti tahdosta riippumattoman hoidon lainsäädännön muutokset vuosina 1840–1991*. Master's thesis. University of Joensuu, Finland; 2008.

National Institute for Health and Welfare. *Health Expenditure and Financing 2008*. Tilastoraportti

12/2010. Official Statistics of Finland. Health 2010. THL. Available at: www.stakes.fi/tilastot/tilastotiedotteet/2010/Tr12_10.pdf (accessed 21 October 2011).

National Institute for Health and Welfare. THL:n asiantuntijoiden arvioita peruspalvelujen tilasta. *Peruspalvelujen tila 2010 -raportin tausta-aineisto.* Raportti 9/2010. Terveyden ja hyvinvoinnin laitos. Helsinki.

National Institute for Health and Welfare. *Health Expenditure and Financing 2007.* Statistical Report 1/2009, Official Statistics of Finland, Health 2009. Available at: www.stakes.fi/EN/tilastot/statisticsbytopic/healthservices/expenditure/healthexpenditure.htm (accessed 21 October 2011).

National Public Health Institute. *The Report of the Expert Group on Cardiovascular Diseases and Diabetes.* Publications of the National Public Health Institute, B2/2008. Available at: www.ktl.fi/portal/2920 (accessed 21 October 2011).

NOMESCO. *Health Statistics in the Nordic countries 2005. Theme section: mental health.* Nordic Medico Statisticat committee 80; 2007.

Palosuo H, Koskinen S, Lahelma E, *et al.*, editors. *Health Inequalities in Finland: trends in socio-economic health differences 1980–2005.* Helsinki: Publications of the Ministry of Social Affairs and Health; 2007.

Peltonen M, Harald K, Männistö S, *et al. The National FINRISK 2007.* Study Publications of the National Public Health Institute, B34/2008.

Pirkola SP, Isometsä E, Suvisaar J, *et al.* DSM-IV mood-, anxiety- and alcohol use disorders and their comorbidity in the Finnish general population – results from the Health 2000 Study. *Soc Psychiatr Epidemiol.* 2005; **40**: 1–10.

Pirkola S, Sohlman B. *Atlas of Mental Health.* Statistics from Finland, National Research and Development Centre for Welfare and Health. STAKES, Helsinki; 2005.

Pirkola S, Sohlman B, Heilä H, *et al.* Reductions in postdischarge suicide after deinstitutionalization and decentralization: a nationwide register study in Finland. *Psychiatr Serv.* 2005; **58**(2), 221–6.

Pirkola S, Sund R, Sailas E, *et al.* Community mental-health services and suicide rate in Finland: a nationwide small-area analysis. *Lancet.* 2009; **373**(9658): 99–100.

Organization for Economic Co-operation and Development. *Mental Health in OECD Countries. The OECD Policy Brief.* 2008. Available at: www.oecd.org/dataoecd/6/48/41686440.pdf (accessed 21 October 2011).

OECD. OECD *Programme for International Student Assessment (PISA).* 2010. Available at: www.pisa.occd.org/pages/0,3417,en_32252351_32235731_1_1_1_1_1,00.htm (accessed 5 July 2010).

Salenius, P. *Omahoitajan toiminta lastenpsykiatrisella osastotutkimusjaksolla.* Master's thesis, University of Turku, Department of Nursing Science; 2005.

Salize J, Dressing H. Epidemiology of involuntary placement of mentally ill people across the European Union. *Br J Psychiatry.* 2004; **184**: 163–8.

Salokangas RKR, Stengård E, Honkonen T, *et al. Sairaalasta yhteiskuntaan.* Seurantatutkimus sairaalasta kotiuttamisen vaikutuksista skitsofreniapotilaan elämään ja hoitotilanteeseen, Stakes, Sosiaali- ja terveysalan tutkimus- ja kehittämiskeskus. Raportteja 248, Saarijärvi; 2000.

Sarvilinna A. *Mielisairaanhoidon kehityksestä Suomessa vuoteen 1919.* Yliopistollinen väitöskirja. Vakka-Suomen Kirjapaino, Uusikaupunki; 1938.

Syrjäpalo, K. Values and Appreciations in Psychiatric Care. Staff's and Patients' Views of Current Status of Care [thesis, in Finnish]. Oulu: University of Oulu; 2006. Available at: http://jultika.oulu.fi/Record/isbn951-42-8015-6 (accessed February 2012).

STAKES. *Health Care Professionals 31.12.2002.* Stakes Statistics 8/2003. Helsinki; 2003.

Statistics Finland. *Life Expectancy of Newborn Babies in Finland 1751–2006.* [Information brochure] 10 October 2007.

Statistics Finland. Causes of death in 2009. Available at: www.stat.fi/til/ksyyt/2009/01/ksyyt_2009_01_2011-02-22_kat_002_en.html (accessed 17 January 2012).

Statistics Finland. Population. 2010a. Available at: www.stat.fi/tup/suoluk/suoluk_vaesto_en.html/byage (accessed 5 July 2010).

Statistics Finland. Adult education survey. 2010b. Available at: www.stat.fi/til/aku/index_en.html (accessed 24 May 2010).

Statistics Finland. Educational structure of population. 2010c. Available at: www.stat.fi/til/vkour/2008/vkour_2008_2009-12-04_tie_001_en.html (accessed 3 July 2010).

Statistics Finland. Adoption, population and cause-of-death statistics. 2010d. Available at: www.stat.fi/til/adopt/2009/adopt_2009_2010-05-20_tie_001_en.html (accessed 24 May 2010).

Statistics Finland. Income and consumption. 2010e. Available at: www.tilastokeskus.fi/tup/suoluk/suoluk_tulot_en.html (accessed 5 July 2010).

Statistics Finland. Employment and unemployment in May close to one year ago. 2010f. Available at: www.stat.fi/til/tyti/2010/05/tyti_2010_05_2010-06-22_tie_001_en.html (accessed 3 July 2010).

Suomen Kuvalehti. *Arvostetuimmat ammatit.* 21 May 2010. Available at: http://suomenkuvalehti.fi/jutut/kotimaa/ammattien-arvostus-on-taas-tutkittu-kirurgi-yha-ykkonen (accessed 21 May 2010).

Suvisaari J. Epidemiology of mental health problems in Finland. In: Partanen A, Moring J, Nordling E, *et al.*, editors. *The National Plan for Mental Health and Substance Abuse Work 2009–2015. From Plan to Action in 2009.* National Institute for Health and Welfare (THL), Helsinki: Discussion Papers 16/2010.

The Finnish Medical Society Duodecim and the Finnish Psychiatric Association. *Schizophrenia. Current Care Summary.* 2008. Available at: www.duodecim.fi/käypähoito (accessed 18 May 2010).

The Social Insurance Institute of Finland. *Statistical Yearbook 2007.* 2008. Available at: www.kela.fi/it/kelasto/kelasto.nsf/NET/121208122509TL/$File/Vk_07.pdf?OpenElement (accessed 20 April 2010).

Tritter JQ, McCallum A. The snakes and ladders of user involvement: moving beyond Arnstein. *Health Policy.* 2006; **76**: 156–68.

Valvira. Statistics on psychotherapists in Finland. 2009. Available at: http://suomenkuvalehti.fi/jutut/kotimaa/ammattien-arvostus-on-taas-tutkittu-kirurgi-yha-ykkonen (accessed 9 December 2010).

Vuorenkoski L, Mladovsky P, Mossialos E. Finland: health system review. *Health Syst Transit.* 2008; **10**(4): 1–168.

Välimäki M, Kaltiala-Heino R, Kjervik D. The rights of patients with mental problems in Finland. *J Nurs Law.* 2003; **9**(2), 17–28.

Wahlbeck K, Huber M. *Access to Health Care for People with Mental Disorders in Europe.* European Centre for Social Welfare Policy and Research; 2009. Available at: www.ehma.org/files/PB_Access1-Mental%20health-apr_09.pdf (accessed 21 January 2012).

World Health Organization. *Highlights on Health in Finland 2004.* 2006. Available at: www.euro.who.int/document/e88101.pdf (accessed 10 May 2007).

World Health Organization. *Atlas: nurses in mental health. Report presenting the results of a global survey on the availability, education, training and role of nurses.* 2007. Available at: www.who.int/mental_health/evidence/nursing_atlas_2007.pdf (accessed 21 January 2012).

www.evl.fi/english (Evangelical Lutheran Church of Finland).

www.hotus.fi (Nursing Research Foundation).

www.kaypahoito.fi (Current Care).

Mental health services in Germany

Michael Schulz

Introduction

Germany is unquestionably one of the strongest countries economically in the EU, and in order to continue to be so it requires an educated, skilled and healthy workforce. Following the Second World War, military expansionism was replaced by economic development, and until 1990 the country was divided between the communist East and the democratic West Germany. Following reunification, considerable efforts were made to integrate various political, cultural and economic systems. In this chapter, what has taken place in recent years to improve mental health services is reviewed and critiqued. The author describes key features of the mental health care system and identifies some of its most progressive aspects. It concludes by considering some likely future directions.

National profile

In order to understand the nature and structure of Germany's mental health services, it is important to understand the political, economic and demographic context in which they exist. The Federal Republic of Germany is a country in Central Europe, bordered to the north by the North Sea, Denmark and the Baltic Sea; to the east by Poland and the Czech Republic; to the south by Austria and Switzerland; and to the west by France, Luxembourg, Belgium and the Netherlands. The territory of Germany covers 357 021 km² and is influenced by a temperate seasonal climate. With 81.8 million inhabitants in January 2010,

Germany is the most populous of the member states of the European Union, and it is also home to the third-largest number of international migrants worldwide. It is the 14th most populous country in the world, with a stable population size, but an ageing population and a smaller cohort of young people (Population Reference Bureau, 2004).

Germany is a federal republic with Berlin as capital. The lawmakers at the national level are the Bundestag, whose members are elected every 4 years by popular vote and the Bundesrat, which consists of 69 representatives of the 16 states (Bundesländer). After the Second World War, Germany was divided into the democratic West and the communist East (German Democratic Republic). The Berlin Wall became the symbol of this division. It fell in 1989 and Germany was reunited a year later.

German is the most widely spoken first language in the European Union. Germany is the world's fourth largest economy, producing automobiles, precision engineering products, electronic and communications equipment, chemicals and pharmaceuticals, and much more besides. Its companies have invested heavily in the Central and Eastern European countries which joined the EU in 2004.

With 236.46 people per square kilometre, Germany is one of the most densely populated countries in the world (Nationmaster, 2010). More than 16 million people are of non-German descent (first and second generation, including mixed heritage), about 7 million of whom are foreign residents. In 2007, 62% of immigrants living in Germany came from Europe (*see* Table 4.1). The largest ethnic group of non-German origin are the Turkish. Since the 1960s, West Germany and later the reunified Germany has been attracting migrants, primarily from Southern and Eastern Europe as well as Turkey, many of whom (or their children) acquired German citizenship over time. While most of these migrations were for economic reasons, Germany has also been a prime destination for refugees from many developing countries, in part because its constitution has long had a clause giving a 'right' to political asylum, but new restrictions over the years have since made it less attractive.

TABLE 4.1 European immigrants to Germany

Immigrants from European countries	% of all immigrants
All Europe	62%
Turkey	14.9%
Russia	9.4%
Poland	6.9%
Italy	4.2%

Source: Statistische Ämter des Bundes und der Länder, 2009

Germany has one of the world's highest levels of education, technological development and economic productivity. Since the end of the Second World War, the number of students entering universities has more than tripled, and the trade and technical schools are among the world's best. The International Monetary Fund (2010) estimates the gross domestic product (GDP) per capita in Germany is currently at US$40 875, with a per capita income of about $27 460 ($528 per week). Germany is a broadly middle-class society. Germans are also very socially mobile; millions travel abroad each year. The social welfare system provides for universal health care, unemployment compensation and other social programmes. Due to Germany's ageing population and struggling economy, the welfare system came under a lot of strain in the 1990s. This led the government to push through a wide-ranging programme of belt-tightening reforms, Agenda 2010, including the labour market reforms known as Hartz I–IV. Since 2000, income inequality and poverty have grown faster in Germany than in any other OECD countries. They increased by more in 5 years (2000–05) than in the previous 15 combined (1985–2000) (OECD, 2008).

More German adults and children are living in poverty – that is, living in a household with less than half the median income – today than in 1985. For the total population, the income poverty rate increased from 6% to 11%, while for children it increased from 7% to 16%. There was no increase among older people: their poverty rate remained stable at around 7% (for those aged 66–74) and 11% (those aged 75 and over) (OECD, 2008).

Changing health needs

In common with most other countries, Germany has an increasing older population. In 2009, 20.3% of the population was estimated to be older than 65 years (CIA, 2009). Patterns of morbidity and health care needs are changing as the proportion of the population reaching old age increases. Germany's ageing problem is extreme, because for the past 30 years its women have produced children at an average rate of less than 1.4 babies per lifetime. Why its fertility rate is so low is another issue – some blame the tradition that German schools run only from 8 a.m. until lunchtime, making it very hard for women to combine career and motherhood – but the effect is clear. While Australia's age pyramid bulges slightly in the age group from 30 to 44, Germany has a massive bulge in the ages from 35 to 54, with a far narrower base beneath. Now, more and more schools run until the afternoon, but the system is changing slowly.

A particular challenge to the health care system results from coexisting health problems (multimorbidity) among the elderly. Regarding prevention and treatment goals, the focus needs to shift from disease-specific outcomes to function in daily life and subjective outcome dimensions, such as self-determination (autonomy), social participation, and quality of life. Health research faces the task of developing prevention and health care models adapted to the needs of specific subgroups of older people. Strengthening personal, social and organisational resources is crucial. There are some major issues which will play an important role in the attempt to meet future health care needs.

- There will be a growing need for illness prevention/health promotion activities.
- There will be a rising need for inpatient and community-based health care.
- There will be a growing number of people who are in need of care. At the same time, there is an erosion of traditional family systems and family-based help. Daughters and wives frequently used to do that caring work in the past.
- There will be shortages in the health care workforce, especially in nursing.

The epidemiological profile of an ageing society will lead to a higher rate of age-related diseases, e.g. Alzheimer's disease. As suicidal ideation is a common phenomenon in the elderly, new strategies have to be developed to face that problem. Knowing that those people are very often not ill but lonely, it is not only a problem of medical treatment but also a problem of society and inclusion.

The National Health Service

The German health care system has the reputation of being one of the best in the world. There is an extensive network of hospitals and doctors covering even the remotest areas of Germany. Germany has a mandatory statutory health insurance (SHI) for employees (Bismarck model). Public health is mainly within the jurisdiction of the federal states. The federal states are also responsible for planning inpatient facilities and financing investments in hospitals. In 2006, total health care expenditures were €245 billion (Richter *et al.*, 2008).

There are 4.3 million people working in the health sector, amounting to 10.6% of the total workforce (Richter *et al.*, 2008). Of those working in health care, 50% are salaried employees employed in inpatient care. There are 3.5 practising physicians per 1000 residents (Netherlands 3.8, Norway 3.7, Sweden 3.5, UK 2.5, US 2.4) and 9.8 nurses per 1000 (Netherlands 8.6, Norway 31.6, Sweden 10.7, UK 11.9, US 10.5). In general, there is universal coverage for health services, although some restrictions may apply for certain services (Gaebel *et al.*, 2009).

Mental health services

Following a reform of psychiatry ('Psychiatry Enquete', 1975), community and outpatient services took precedence over inpatient services. The medical specialities of 'Psychiatry and Psychotherapy' and 'Psychosomatic Medicine and

Psychotherapy' are for adult mental health care. 'Child and Adolescent Psychiatry' is a separate medical speciality in Germany.

In addition to the acute inpatient mental health care sector, there is a rehabilitation sector in the fields of psychiatry, psychosomatic medicine and psychotherapy, which covers the majority of inpatient 'psychosomatic medicine and psychotherapy' beds (Bergmann, 2002). Bergmann points out that the latter is not the same as the Anglo-American 'psychosomatic medicine' subspeciality, as it concentrates on psychotherapy as its main form of therapy. Outpatient psychotherapy is mainly provided by medical staff and psychotherapists.

A recent survey by the German Federal Health Monitoring System (Gesundheitsberichtserstattung) assessed this complex system (Schulz *et al.*, 2008). It was found that there is a considerable degree of complexity in the remuneration system for mental health care. Given such a highly diversified system, cooperation between inpatient and outpatient services, between medical specialities and psychotherapists, and between the curative and the rehabilitation sectors becomes a critical issue for mental health care in Germany. A recent review reported on the history and impact of innovative mental health care structures in Germany, such as the Integrated Care programme for the care of people with schizophrenia, focusing on programmes that try to ameliorate this situation (Weinmann, 2009).

Quality monitoring

The adoption of quality-monitoring systems is a growing issue in German psychiatry. Psychiatric facilities are hospitals, and the certification of hospitals and clinical departments has recently become a legislative requirement, as a core measure of quality assurance. There are several systems in place, e.g. Kooperation für Transparenz und Qualität im Krankenhaus (KTQ). Many psychiatric hospitals are implementing such systems, but until recently there was a lack of clear data as to the performance of such organisations. The insurance companies are applying pressure for change in the system; for example, they want clinics to use quality assurance systems such as ISO 9000 or similar systems. However, there is ongoing discussion as to whether the use of such systems actually leads to better patient outcomes.

The different federal states have their own rules for government-led quality-assurance processes in psychiatry. For example, in the federal state of Nordrhein Westfalen, a medical civil servant chairs a visitation commission. Members are professionals from other clinics and service users. By law, they have to visit each clinic once a year. They arrive unannounced. They check that everything is correct regarding adherence to the rules concerning compulsory treatment, they talk to patients and they look at clinical records.

Mental health needs and health service provision

This section will focus on demographics, evidence of unmet need and the changing profile of need. Mental disorders are considered to be costly in terms of elevated rates of health care utilisation and increased disability days. For the general German population, there has been a lack of data on health care utilisation and disability rates. It is estimated that 10% of the German population are suffering from mental stress (Population Reference Bureau, 2010). Eight per cent of women and 4% of men were diagnosed with depression within the last 12 months. A good working mental health system is one where people who need services receive them promptly. Compared to other countries in the world, data suggests that the situation in Germany is not that bad. An analysis of a 17-country mental health survey conducted by the World Health Organization found that 67% of people in Germany with severe mental health disorders received mental health services that they deemed to be of a minimum standard and which they found satisfactory (Wang, 2007).

In order to establish the epidemiology of mental disorders and mental health care utilisation in Germany, a representative nationwide survey of mental health care was undertaken in 1998 (Jacobi *et al.*, 2004), followed by a representative questionnaire study (Alonso *et al.*, 2004). The survey in 1998 assessed the population aged 18–65 and showed a 12-month prevalence of any mental disorder of 31%, which is higher than the European average of 27.4% (Wittchen *et al.*, 2005). A similar survey to that carried out in 1998, for the adult German population, is currently being conducted and funded by the German Federal Health Ministry. It will also include a follow-up investigation of the 1998 respondents and an analysis of the age group over 65 years. There is a considerable increase in service utilisation of both inpatient and outpatient psychiatric services in Germany. The numbers of days and cases of sick leave due to mental disorders have increased by about 80%, according to health insurers' statistics. Mental disorders have become the single most frequent cause of early pensions, and the numbers of inpatient cases due to mental disorders has been rising, in contrast to a general trend towards a constant number of somatic hospital cases. It is currently being debated whether there is an increased incidence of mental disorders in Germany or whether altered diagnostic practices or an increased acceptance of being labelled with a psychiatric diagnosis play a role (Richter *et al.*, 2008). This issue remains unresolved and continues to be reviewed.

The number of outpatients in the fields of psychiatry and neurology nearly doubled in the decade 1994–2004 (Albrecht *et al.*, 2009). For inpatient mental health care, there are currently 217 special psychiatric hospitals and 217 departments of psychiatry at general hospitals, with a total of 59 382 treatment places (including beds and part-time inpatient treatment places) (Arbeitsgruppe Psychiatrie der Obersten Landesbehörden, 2007). There are 418 *Psychiatrische*

Institutsambulanzen (PIAs), which provide outpatient services in hospitals. Nearly all psychiatric hospitals or psychiatric departments run PIAs. The average length of inpatient stay for patients with mental disorders has decreased from 38.4 days in 1994 to 20.8 days in 2007. The number of cases has increased from 770 514 in 1994 to 1 093 641 in 2007 (Federal Health Reporting, 2010), mainly due to increased case numbers of patients with affective disorders. In inpatient psychiatric services, rural areas are still neglected compared with urban areas and the coordination between different specialities and different service providers needs to be improved, according to a recent analysis by the psychiatric experts of the state mental health authorities (Arbeitsgruppe Psychiatrie der Obersten Landesbehörden, 2007).

Attitudes to mental health problems

Negative attitudes and rejection by the public of the mentally ill, and people with schizophrenia in particular, are some of the main obstacles to improving services and promoting access to treatments. The most common consequences of discrimination for people with schizophrenia are social distance and exclusion, as well as being disadvantaged with regard to housing and employment opportunities (Crisp *et al.*, 2000; Link, 2000; World Psychiatric Association, 1998). The stigma of severe mental illness exacerbates the patient's burden due to his illness (Link *et al.*, 1997; Sartorius, 1998; Wiersma and van Busschbach, 2001). Additionally, negative public attitudes against people who are mentally ill undermine the establishment of mental health services in the community (Rössler and Salize, 1995). Stigmatisation of mentally ill people is also reflected in disadvantages in social legislation and health insurance practice (Haefner, 2000).

Public attitudes in Germany regarding mental illness have been the focus of a number of studies. Gaebel *et al.* (2002) conducted a public survey with a particular focus on schizophrenia. His group interviewed a total of 7246 German-speaking persons aged 16 and over in private households in six German cities by telephone using a standardised questionnaire. The respondents were asked about their knowledge about schizophrenia, their social distance towards people with schizophrenia and estimations of the social stigmatisation of mental patients in general. They found that 33.1% of the interviewees were able to name causes of schizophrenia, 76.5% believed that people with schizophrenia often or very often need prescription drugs to control their symptoms and 81.1% believe that most people would pass over the job application of a former mental patient in favour of another applicant. The authors concluded that the German public is not sufficiently informed about the causes of schizophrenia. From their point of view, improvements in the education of the public about mental illnesses and provision of the opportunity for personal contact with mentally ill people are important measures for promoting the acceptance of the mentally ill by the public.

An example of extending the awareness of the community regarding mental health problems was a project to enhance awareness of symptoms of depression and potential suicide, called Nuremberg Alliance Against Depression European Network (EAAD) (Hegerl *et al.*, 2008). The aim of this project was to improve the care of depressed patients and to reduce suicidality. The Nuremberg Alliance Against Depression was initiated in 2001 within the framework of the German Research Network on Depression and Suicidality (funded by the Federal Ministry of Education and Research). The alliance's concept is based on an intervention on four levels:

- co-operation with GPs
- an information and awareness campaign for the general public
- educational training for people such as teachers, priests, nurses and other caregivers for older people
- support for all self-help activities.

After 2 years of intervention, the number of suicidal acts, the study's main outcome criteria, was significantly reduced by 24%, compared to the baseline and to a representative control region. Since 2002, the successful four-level intervention, its concepts and materials have been adopted by other regions within Germany. Nearly 40 community-based local campaigns are forming the German Alliance Against Depression (GAD) and many more regions are interested.

Expenditure on mental health

National expenditure on mental health care is rising. Indirect costs are much higher than direct costs. In 2008, direct costs for mental health in Germany were €8.7 billion, which was approximately 11% of the overall expenditure on health. Spending on dementia amounted to €9.4 billion, while €5.2 billion was spent on depression. Over the last 6 years, the insurance system has faced a cost increase in mental health of €5.3 billion – 32% of the total expenditure on mental health services.

Schizophrenia is known as the most cost-intensive diagnosis in mental health. It is estimated that about 50% of all spending on mental health care is spent on this group, but only 30% are direct costs. Kissling *et al.* (1999) calculated the direct and indirect costs of schizophrenia. Using the 'bottom up' prevalence-based method with a random sample of 180 schizophrenic patients, direct and indirect costs were retrospectively documented for a 12-month period. The annual costs depended on the service and the extent of care provided. For patients treated predominantly on an outpatient basis, the cost was approximately €16 500, it amounted to €63 000 for a patient requiring hospital care and about €77 000 for a patient in job rehabilitation. The direct yearly treatment costs were, as expected, lowest for patients recruited in the private practice of a psychiatrist and predominantly treated on an outpatient basis (€2890), and were the highest in the psychiatric hospital (€32 300) and in job rehabilitation (€40 000). For patients recruited in the outpatient domain, doctors' fees and medication together were responsible for only 4.5% of the total costs, whereas the indirect costs (e.g. unemployment benefits and housing allowances) were responsible for 87% of the total yearly costs. Graf von der Schulenberg *et al.* (1998) calculated individual direct costs for schizophrenia to be €14 204 per annum.

For methodological reasons, the total costs caused by schizophrenic psychoses in Germany per annum can only be roughly estimated; however, a conservative estimate suggests that it is between €4.25 and €9 billion. The study shows that schizophrenia is a very expensive illness, the direct and indirect costs of which are on the whole comparable to those of the common somatic illnesses. The authors concluded that for economic reasons, sufficient financial resources should be invested in the research and treatment of this severe illness.

Services in the newer states and in rural areas are not equitably developed. Resources and services are unequally distributed between psychiatric inpatient services and outpatient psychiatric services: although psychiatrists and *Nervenaerzte* (general physicians with an expertise in psychiatry and neurology) together provide services to 65% of all outpatient cases, they attract only 23% of all financial resources. Curiously, psychotherapists, on the other hand, provide care to 17% of cases, but attract 44% of all expenditure for mentally ill people (direct costs) (Melchinger, 2008).

The indirect costs of mental health disorders are much higher than the direct costs and are usually underestimated. A low level of education can be a result of depression, as well as low productivity, which can be described as 'presenteeism'. Presenteeism is the opposite of absenteeism, in that it refers to the problems faced when employees come to work in spite of illness, which can have similar negative repercussions on business performance. It is estimated in Germany that 1 in 7 days of absence through sickness is due to a mental health problem. Since 1998, the hours of sick leave because of a mental health problem have risen by 80%. The economic loss is estimated at €8 billion (Salize *et al.*, 2002).

History of the development of mental health services
······················

At the beginning of the nineteenth century the first asylums were founded in Germany, one of the first being the Carl Wigand Maximilian Jacobi, an asylum in Siegburg, in 1825. It was run by the state of Prussia and it was a very well-designed and staffed building for 200 patients. This asylum was seen as a positive example of reform, and was well known in Europe as a good example of such. At this time, the asylum had 50 warders to take care of the patients. Different therapeutic approaches were provided, such as occupational therapy, gardening and working with textiles. Patients received good food, light and water and there were many possibilities for leisure activities, such as merry-go-rounds, playing musical instruments or using the bowling alley. However, there was a strong policy of selecting patients: if their condition did not improve within a few months, they were discharged. If they were very ill, they were not admitted at all. In the following decades, more and more patients were admitted and conditions became worse. In 1868, the regional government decided to build five new asylums. The last one was built in 1906 in Süchteln, a city near Cologne. It had facilities for 800 patients.

In 1842, there was also a new asylum built in Illenau bei Achern. A new kind of large asylum was created, known as *Landeskrankenhäuser*. This was an attempt to bridge the gap between caring and curing. These institutions had different wings for women and men and focused on all kinds of mentally ill people, no matter if they were very agitated or not. This type of institution was a prototype for other clinics all over Europe. Besides these asylums, there were also ecclesiastical and privately run asylums, mostly used for incurable patients.

During this period, there was no education system to train physicians as psychiatric specialists. Physicians lived on the site of the asylums and were also responsible for training the warders/nurses. In reality, it was not until 1920 that there was any systematic training for nurses provided, although Ernst Horn claimed to have a School for Warders back in 1819.

There were specific requirements for warders/nurses in the nineteenth century. They had to be in good health, strong, had to be able to read and write and were not allowed to be married. Until the end of the nineteenth century, they lived with their patients in the same rooms and had to work 18 hours a day. In 1897, the first journal for psychiatric nursing was published, called *Die Irrenpflege*.

Germany was home to some of the most important researchers in the nineteenth and twentieth centuries, who had a great impact worldwide on the understanding and treatment of mental illness. Wilhelm Griesinger (1817–68), a neurologist and psychiatrist, worked as professor of psychiatry in Tübingen,

Zürich and Berlin. Griesinger is remembered for his reforms concerning the mentally ill and the asylum system. He believed in the integration of the mentally ill into society, and proposed that short-term hospitalisation be combined with the natural support of social systems. He also provided valuable insights concerning the nature of psychopathic behaviour and was influential in anchoring the study and treatment of mental illness into medicine.

Of equal importance was Emil Kraepelin (1856–1926). As a psychiatrist, he is known as the founder of modern scientific psychiatry, psychopharmacology and psychiatric genetics. His theories dominated psychiatry at the start of the twentieth century. Kraepelin's work on classifying schizophrenia and manic depression is probably one of his most notable contributions. His theories on the aetiology and diagnosis of psychiatric disorders remain the basis for all major diagnostic systems in use today (e.g. DSM-IV and ICD-XI).

Between 1939 and 1945, it has been estimated that 200 000 people with mental illnesses and learning difficulties were murdered in what was then the region of the former 'German Reich'. Psychiatrists and psychiatric nurses played a significant role in planning and justifying these executions within National Socialist 'Euthanasia Programs'. Nurses commonly had special training in how to execute patients with wet towels, either by means of strangulation or suffocation, without leaving marks of any kind that would indicate the cause of death. Undoubtedly, it appears that at least a portion of German nurses accepted the National Socialist reinterpretation of professional nursing ethics and humanitarian principles, in that by obeying orders they were doing good.

However, German nursing also changed in less sinister ways due to external factors during the Nazi period, for example, in terms of the improved social status of nurses, the unification of professional nursing organisations, the passing of new laws affecting nursing and the politicisation of the profession (Steppe, 1992).

Steppe (1992) concluded that historical research undertaken in Germany points to clear lessons for contemporary nurses. Nurses in Nazi Germany were under the illusion, and were led to believe that, they were remaining true to their professional ethics, and were unaffected by the social changes that were taking place around them. Believing that they were apolitical and acting in the best interests of patients and the country, nurses' professional consciousness was so manipulated that they were soon subsumed as part of the larger political system. Steppe believes that we must be clear that nursing never takes place in a value-free, neutral context; nursing, she concluded, is a highly political activity and is always a socially significant force in any country. This means that nurses must be always alert to the political climate in which they work and the types of work they are asked to do. They cannot simply be participants in actions without questioning what is taking place around them. They are not simply observers, but must be actively involved in helping to shape the sociopolitical environments in which they work and those of service developments. Steppe pointed out that German nurses have a burden to carry as a result of what happened in their profession during its darkest hours. The lesson for all nurses in all countries, she stated, is that they must be ever vigilant to any signs of inhumanity or neglect of vulnerable people.

Soon after the end of the Second World War in 1945, social psychiatric issues were of only minor concern in Germany. There were several reasons for this. As a result of the murder of so many within the asylums after the war, there was only a need to provide long-term care to relatively few people and this was still carried out in large, old-fashioned institutions in remote areas (Rössler *et al.*, 1996). Moreover, just as in pre-war times, the surviving mentally ill had a very low social standing. As a result of the enormous economic depression that affected Germany after the war, and the fact that it was virtually bankrupt, many asylum inmates who had survived the war subsequently died of starvation. Because so many inmates died, overcrowding in psychiatric hospitals did not pose as great a problem as it did in the UK or US, hence there was no significant pressure to implement new services for the mentally ill (Salize *et al.*, 2007). Furthermore, the widespread suppression of any public discourse about the mass murder, and feelings of shame regarding what had happened to people with mental illness, contributed to the neglect and indifference towards the basic medical and social needs of patients with mental illness during the 1950s and 1960s. As a result, mental health care reform in Germany started much later than in other countries.

Move from asylum care

In Germany, it took until the middle of the 1970s for the psychiatric landscape to change. In a general climate of social and political reform, Germany turned towards community-based mental health care. In 1975, a federal expert commission's report on the quality of West German mental health care concluded that:

- Psychiatric inpatient care was provided almost exclusively by large and inadequately staffed state mental health hospitals or asylums.
- There was an almost complete absence of both psychiatric wards in general hospitals and of other community mental health services.
- There was a significant separation between mental health care and the general care system (Deutscher Bundestag, 1975).

Consequently, the commission recommended the urgent improvement of the old mental asylum system and defined four basic principles as a means of attaining structural reform:
1. the principle of community-based mental health care delivery
2. the principle of needs-based and comprehensive care for all people suffering from mental disorders

3. the principle of needs-based coordination of mental health care in defined catchment areas
4. the principle of quality standards and access to somatic care.

The continuing deinstitutionalisation process and the implementation of community mental health services was considerably affected by the reunification of East and West Germany in 1990, which required dramatic changes in the structure and quality of the mental health care system of the former German Democratic Republic (GDR). The 1990s saw a gradual but significant decrease in the number of psychiatric beds, although nurses continued to work mostly in inpatient settings. In 1991, legislation was passed which established staffing levels for inpatient psychiatric treatment. In 2003, the total number of psychiatric beds was a mere two thirds of the overall bed capacity in 1991, the first year as a reunified Germany, when psychiatric beds in East and West Germany totalled 80 275.

From 1970, psychiatry in the community has become the 'new program' (Dörner, 2009). Community psychiatry strives to establish for people suffering from mental health disorders, health care and treatment near to their places of residence. Consequently, the number of psychiatric units in general hospitals has enormously increased; large-scale dehospitalisation programmes have been established for reintegrating people with lasting mental disorders into local communities and more day clinics and day centres have been founded (Kohl, 2001).

The Psychiatric Help system for patients in Germany assumes that a person is able to participate in social life and is involved, or capable of being involved, in community activities. For those who lack this ability, there exists a dual system:
- First, health insurance covers primary medical care, hospital treatment and ambulant treatment.
- After that, different resources of social insurance and welfare guarantee the access to sheltered housing, work under protected conditions and leisure contacts, such as cafés, theatre projects, etc.
- As a non-professional alternative, there are self-help groups of 'psychiatry experienced persons' and discussion platforms called 'Trialog', where family members, patients and professional psychiatric staff can meet.
- Recently, the strict separation between hospital and ambulant services has ceased. Instead patients who attend facilities can return to their wards at night time, thus allowing them to stay in touch with the nursing staff they know and trust.
- Psychiatric hospitals have a pivotal role to play in managing care and advising patients about the various care and treatment options available to them, particularly after-care services.

A useful means of avoiding fragmented activities across and between the services of different service providers in a region (welfare, churches and health services) is what has become known as the Belegungskonferenz. This is a formalised presentation for patients, carers and guardians by various professionals and providers of services. Its main function is to inform patients about what is available and it addresses the following:

- the types of services available and how they are paid for
- the types of treatments available and how much each of them costs
- the role and responsibilities of each mental health professional
- how services relate to and engage with each other
- the types of social and church-based services and how to access them
- how to access help and advice when deciding on a range of services
- the role and purpose of one's key worker.

An important part of this presentation is the part that deals with how much these services cost. It can be enlightening for patients and carers to learn how much care and treatment actually cost. Apart from finding out about the costs, patients are also helped to choose a programme of care that is both reasonably priced and proven to be therapeutically effective. Once informed about what is available to them and how much it costs, it becomes apparent that patients have a large part to play in deciding their treatment whilst containing costs. Furthermore, many see it as their responsibility to select programmes of care that they believe will be most helpful for them, rather than having them prescribed. If this presentation continues to develop and manages to improve, it will have many advantages. It will help reduce the gap between hospital and ambulant care, it will also show patients what other services are available to them and it will offer patients more choice in deciding what is in their best interests. This openness will go some way towards informing the public of what mental health consists of and hopefully will encourage greater public participation in decision-making about mental health care. Lastly, it will recognise that patients are able to make decisions and take responsibility for their own future development.

Psychiatric nursing

These structural changes influenced the development of the role and function of the German psychiatric nurse (Schoppmann, 2005). Throughout this recent period, psychiatric nursing in Germany was mainly focused in inpatient settings, in contrast to psychiatrists, whose work consisted of predominantly community-based services. Not only was the role of the nurse beginning to be more clearly defined, so too were nursing skills. As the role of the nurse changed, so did the education and training of nurses. In Germany, all nurses undergo a 3-year training and are registered with the Public Health Department in the towns or counties, not with the government or a professional body.

All qualified psychiatric nurses must undertake general nurse training and, after some years, can then specialise in psychiatric nursing by undertaking a specialist part-time psychiatric training lasting 2 years, while continuing to work in practice. These courses are not state funded, and the individual nurses or their employers pay for this training. There are several institutions that provide such training, and most of them are closely allied to professional or religious organisations and are close to or attached to hospitals. All the courses must be state approved.

Once qualified, psychiatric nurses receive better payment than their general nurse colleagues, despite the fact that they may be working together in the same ward or clinical setting. It is not uncommon to have a psychiatric ward where there are two qualified psychiatric nurses and 10 general nurses. More recently, the development of post-basic psychiatric nurse education has catered for nurses wishing to work in different services. Although there are slight variations in the regulation of this education in different federal states (Bundesländer), courses take 2 years and contain theoretical as well as practical components. Nurses are expected, by law, to carry out the prescribed care of medical staff, even when working in community settings.

Involvement of user organisations

Until the 1980s, user and family organisations were rarely involved in the mental health care field in Germany. The psychiatric reforms that started at that time raised public awareness and strengthened the position of users and relatives, so that by the year 2000, user associations were active in all federal states. However, financial support for attending meetings is not generally available across the country, and so delegates and representatives of user associations are frequently unable to attend meetings at state-level mental health care advisory boards where important decisions are made (Hölling, 2001).

Current mental health care

Germany's National Health Service is not financed and/or managed by a federal authority administration. Instead, mental health care is organised as a subsidiary system, with federal authorities being entitled to organise service provision only in the event that private, voluntary or other organisations are unable to provide the service. Planning and regulating mental health care is the responsibility of the 16 federal states, which do so by passing state-level health legislation. The national government provides a basic legal framework by passing general health care or welfare legislation. As a result, German health care provision – particularly the provision of mental health care – is spread among many sectors and characterised by considerable regional differences.

Due to the low priority that was given to the evaluation of the shift from hospitals to community, little research was undertaken with respect to its success or otherwise. Without the guidance of research, the building up of new community services during the 1970s and 1980s was left entirely to providers. There was little evidence as to how much this innovation cost, who should be involved and what model of community care provision was most effective. During the 1990s, the majority of psychiatric research grants were directed not at mental health service research but at biological research programmes, which continue to dominate psychiatric research funding bodies in Germany, chief of which is the German Ministry of Education and Research (BMBF) (Salize *et al.*, 2007).

Mental health law

There exist two subsidiary systems, delivered by public resources: police laws to maintain public safety and order and the law on tutelage or guardianship.

Police laws to maintain public safety and order

In every Bundesland (federal state), there are police laws designed to maintain public safety and order. If someone threatens his or her neighbourhood by loud or menacing behaviour, the police might be involved in order to find out if the danger caused by the abnormal state can only be controlled by bringing the patient – even against his or her will – into a closed psychiatric ward. The decision of the police has to be based on a medical judgement (attestation) and has to be confirmed by a hearing with a judge who will visit the patient within 24 hours. If there is no such confirmation, the patient has to declare he or she will stay voluntarily in the ward or has to be released. For treatment behind locked doors, there are two more safeguards, i.e. the judge has to check the necessity of treatment after 6 weeks and again after 1 year at least.

In most cases, patients who start their psychiatric involvement will accept support as provided by the system, e.g. open wards, day clinics, dwelling supported by psychiatric services and regular contacts with therapists. With psychotic patients, it might occur that they skip medical treatment, develop symptoms again and run through the cycle several times. There is no legal provision for compulsory treatment in the community.

More frequently than the case of an individual presenting actual 'danger to the public', it is more common to find persons in need of treatment, but not in a situation requiring them to be hospitalised right away. Since 1992, the

Betreuungsgesetz (law on tutelage or guardianship) has been developed into quite a flexible tool, easily adaptable to personal needs and changing situations.

To commence processes according to this law, somebody (no matter who) can inform a court that the person needing help cannot arrange or look after his or her own belongings and activities (be they financial, medical or administrative issues) and care properly for him/herself. The court then asks for a judgement made by a court-appointed appraiser (social worker and psychiatrist) and consequently decides if a guardian should be placed in charge of the client and whatever are the necessary range of responsibilities. The latter can include the right to bring someone into hospital for treatment. This path is used frequently with patients who have had two or more illnesses that resulted in hospitalisation.

Legal safeguards in the law are: a review after 6 weeks of closed in-patient care, if this still is necessary; a second review after 1 year; and a general review after 7 years, at the latest, if tutelage or guardianship is still necessary. During these periods, patients are offered different support systems, such as primary medical care, hospital associated ambulant services, counselling, leisure and working facilities.

An advantage of the law is that it is valid for the whole of the Federal Republic of Germany, not fragmented according to different federal states. A disadvantage is the risk of a judicialisation of society, because it is much easier for courts to set up tutelage, with the consequent effects on the self-determination of an individual.

The role of nursing in mental health care

As nurses in Germany are not centrally registered, precise figures as to their numbers are not available. However, it has been estimated that approximately 40 000 psychiatric nurses are employed in various capacities and in different services. Although nurses are increasingly being employed in community settings, their work is still largely based on what takes place in hospitals. Even for nurses who have been undertaking nursing duties for some time, their role is poorly defined and varies from individual to individual. The biggest problem for and with community-based nurses is that their roles vary and also suffer from being ill-defined. The first postgraduate diploma programme in psychiatric nursing in Germany commenced in Bielefeld in 2011.

German psychiatric nurses typically have a preference for inpatient work, as what they are required to do is more clearly prescribed and they tend to collaborate with other mental health professionals. Treatment programmes are more specific and complex, and a lot of nurses specialise in certain types of work, e.g. dialectic behavioural therapy, which is used for those with borderline personality disorders. Many inpatient nurses opt to undertake counselling and psycho-education in hospital settings.

In common with many other countries worldwide, Germany is facing an exodus of nurses in the next 10–15 years due to their reaching retirement age. Until now, there has been no data available concerning the average age of psychiatric nurses in Germany. Schoppmann and Mayer (2010) undertook a small-scale survey of German psychiatric nurses working in managerial positions in psychiatric institutions, with the aim of ascertaining some demographic data. Sixty-two institutions took part, located in 14 federal states and employing 7838 psychiatric nurses. They found that the average age was 42.2 years. They also found that in institutions of adult psychiatry today, one in every four psychiatric nurses is over 50 years.

An evidence-informed practice approach in psychiatric nursing in Germany is developing slowly. In the 1990s, nursing in Germany developed into a graduate profession, but there remain only a few researchers in the field of psychiatric nursing and only a few papers published in international journals. A major leader in the field of psychiatric nursing research is Susanne Schoppmann, who has made some important scientific contributions to the German body of nursing knowledge following the publication of her doctoral thesis about self-injurious behaviour (Schoppmann et al., 2007). In another study, she sought to define and describe the role and function of nurses in a psychiatric clinic and made a considerable contribution to clarifying the role (Schoppmann and Lüthi, 2009). Schulz (the author of this chapter) started his research work in 2001 in a research department of a psychiatric clinic. He is currently involved in research dealing with aspects of coercion and stress in nursing (Schulz et al., 2009). He is also collaborating with Professor Richard Gray (UK) on a study to explore how adherence therapy to medication can be implemented in Germany (Gray et al., 2010).

An important recent educational development has been the establishment of the 'Dreiländerkongress' for psychiatric nursing. This is an annual conference focusing specifically on the profession of psychiatric nursing and over the past six years has become an important venue for debate and discussion in German-speaking countries.

Future services planning

A view can be taken that German mental health care services have, more or less, successfully accomplished a shift from hospital-based to community mental health care since the start of reforms in the 1970s. However, this development is in need of further improvement.

Community psychiatric nursing in Germany is still underdeveloped and there is much still to be done to define what nurses can actually do. As the community-based system provides services that are mainly run by psychiatrists or psychotherapists in clinics and for outpatients, services providing care in people's homes, such as home treatment teams, remain underdeveloped. Nurses should be seeking to go beyond existing clinical settings and develop roles which allow them to work in the environments where patients live and work.

In the past, German mental health care has proven its ability to deal with unexpected developments and to adapt to new situations. Unified forces are needed to uphold this standard in the future and to guarantee a continued high level of care for mentally ill people. Therefore the role of the psychiatric nurse, in particular, has to be developed with an evidence-based approach and with access to the full range of settings in which the care of mentally ill people is needed. For them to work effectively and efficiently, other mental health professionals will also have to develop their roles accordingly so as to avoid overlap and confusion.

In an ongoing struggle to adapt to changing administrative arrangements, legal frameworks and financial constraints, psychiatry in Germany is currently facing specific problems and is being seriously challenged to build on its considerable past achievements (Salize *et al.*, 2007). A major obstacle to achieving the aims outlined in EU policy documents lies in the fragmented system of mental health care provision and mental health care funding. This serious split in responsibilities has been labelled the 'German disease' due to its potential to hamper mental health care planning and cause under- and oversupply. As has already been pointed out, progress in German mental health services is slow and deliberate, and attempting to speed up the process might result in confusion and failure. Perhaps one of the major cultural differences between countries is their ability to cope with change in mental health services, and although they may share a common view of the desired direction of travel, how and when this is done is highly variable.

Case scenario

A 23-year-old unemployed man is reported by his landlord as acting increasingly strangely. He has barricaded his room, talking about being spied upon by the CIA. He can be heard shouting within his room in an angry and incoherent way. He has not been seen by a psychiatrist in the past, although his mother has told the landlord that he has been isolating himself and acting increasingly oddly over the last couple of years.

Much will depend, in this case, as to whether the young man is ready to see a general practitioner or a psychiatrist. Usually, neurologists and psychiatrists in Germany have an office in towns where ambulant patients can attend. This service is available for those who voluntarily attend, hence it does not provide for the needs of people who lack insight or who refuse to acknowledge that they require help. Hence, the German primary care system serves those people with common mental health problems who are self-motivated. Generally, private doctors, running an office of their own, will not come to visit patients at home, especially if they do not know them and a treatment contract has not been established. In most regions, there are no mental health nurses or assertive community outreach teams who could visit the patient in his own home.

As described above, under mental health law, there are two subsidiary systems available, provided by public resources, that may be applied to this young man in his situation:

- police laws that maintain public safety and order
- in the case of actual 'danger to the public', persons in need of treatment can be hospitalised right away.

As the reader will note, this case study appears to deal with the possibility of bringing a psychotic person with acute symptoms into hospital. As yet, there exist few facilities for stabilising him at home by means of community-based services. This is typical of the situation in Germany: there is a lack of low-threshold and fast-reacting professional care, such as day-and-night crisis intervention teams or short-time crisis beds, sometimes found in other countries, such as in Soteria in Switzerland. This situation illustrates the point that without progressive attitudes on the parts of governments and professionals, service development is often left incomplete.

Hospitalisation, on the other hand, is not always as negative an experience as is sometimes made out. Closed wards can be a shelter or a place of safety, and the presence of nurses can provide a sense of protection and calmness, especially for those who resist pharmacological treatment. Medication against one's will can only be prescribed if there is immediate danger of aggression or violence. For such a patient, their greatest need is for practical care, e.g. food, drink, hygiene and the presence of a caring person, especially at night. The first nurse to deal with the patient is ideally the one who should stay with them throughout their stay in hospital. Primary nursing, as this approach is referred to, has been found to be particularly helpful, especially in a situation where the patient is highly distressed, lacking insight and confused. In developing a special relationship, nurses have an enormous amount to contribute in circumstances like this.

The primary nurse will guide the patient through the nursing process, using a care plan with assessment, nursing diagnosis (in some hospitals) and intervention. He or she will work closely together with other members of the interdisciplinary team, such as the psychiatrist, the social worker, the occupational therapist, the psychologist and the physiotherapist. The patient may also become involved in group programmes, e.g. psycho-education. Some clinics offer adherence therapy delivered by nurses.

The patient will stay on average for 18 days in the clinic. In the case of aggression or violence due to his disturbed mental state, mechanical restraint could be used, but has to be monitored in a careful way. Whether doors are closed or not depend not on the individual's symptoms, but on the hospital where he will be treated: there are some hospitals which have wards that are locked only rarely. If the person needs financial support from the community, the social worker can help provide such support.

Medication is still the most prominent therapeutic intervention. Psychiatric hospitals often provide atypical antipsychotic medications, which are very expensive. After discharge, the community-based psychiatrist very often prescribes typical, rather than atypical, antipsychotics, because this is cheaper. If the patient needs psychotherapy, it is difficult to get treatment. In some regions he would have to wait for longer than 6 months.

In some psychiatric hospitals, patients and professionals have the possibility of working out joint crisis plans. The process is like a contract and patients and hospital workers plan what to do if a new crisis arises in the future and hospital treatment will be necessary.

In some places in Germany, it would be possible for the patient to be visited by community psychiatric nurses after discharge, but where such resources are available in a region, they have to be prescribed by a psychiatrist and, also, allowed by the insurance.

After discharge, the Psychiatric Help programme for patients is available to support them to participate in social life and to be involved in community activities (see above for details).

The Belegungskonferenz is a formalised presentation for patients, carers and guardians by various professionals and providers of services. Its aim is to inform patients about what services are available in the community (see above for details). Apart from finding out about the costs, patients are also helped to choose a programme of care that is both reasonably priced and proven to be therapeutically effective. The strength of this approach is that decisions are made with patients in the presence of their relatives or carers, medical and nursing personnel and any agency that may be involved in their care. Their combined efforts can only assist patients in what they elect to do and the level of support available in helping them to do it.

References
Albrecht M, Fürstenberg T, Gottberg A. *Strukturen und Finanzierung der neurologischen und psychiatrischen Versorgung*. Berlin: IGES Institut; 2007. Available at: www.bvdn.de/main/projekt_fset.php?SID&bild_id=3682 (accessed 25 May 2009).

Alonso J, Angermeyer MC, Bernert S, *et al.* Prevalence of mental disorders in Europe: results from the European Study of the Epidemiology of Mental Disorders (ESEMed) project. *Acta Psychiatr Scand.* 2004; **109**(Suppl 420): 21–7.

Arbeitsgruppe Psychiatrie der Obersten Landesgesundheitsbehörden (AOLG). *Psychiatry in Germany: structures, services, perspectives.* 2007. pp. 1–112. Available at: www.lpk-w.de/archiv/news2007/pdf/070803_gmk_psychiatrie_bericht_2007.pdf (accessed 22 July 2010).

Bergmann G. On the development of psychosomatic and psychotherapeutic medicine in Germany. *Wien Med Wschr.* 2002; **152**: 507–15.

Central Intelligence Agency. *The World Factbook.* 2009. Available at: https://www.cia.gov/library/publications/the-world-factbook (accessed 20 July 2010).

Crisp AH, Gelder MG, Rix S, *et al.* Stigmatisation of people with mental illnesses. *Brit J Psychiatry.* 2000; **177**: 4–7.

Deutscher Bundestag. *Bericht über die Lage der Psychiatrie in der Bundesrepublik Deutschland.* Bundestags-Drucksache 7/4200. Bonn: Bundestag; 1975.

Dörner Klaus. Irren ist menschlich. Lehrbuch der Psychiatrie und Psychotherapie. Neuausg. 2002, 4., korrigierte Aufl. Bonn: Psychiatrie-Verl; 2009.

Gaebel W, Baumann A, Witte AM, *et al.* Public attitudes towards people with mental illness in six German cities: results of a public survey under special consideration of schizophrenia. In: *Eur Arch Psychiatry Clin Neurosci.* 2002; **252**(6): S. 278–87.

Gaebel W, Janssen B, Zielasek J. Mental health quality, outcome measurement, and improvement in Germany. *Curr Opin Psychiatry.* 2009; **22**(6): 636–42.

Graf von der Schulenburg JM, Uber A, Höffler J, *et al.* Untersuchungen zu den direkten und indirekten Kosten der Schizophrenie. *Gesund Ökono Qual Manag.* 1998; **3**: 81–7.

Gray R, White J, Schulz M, *et al.* Enhancing medication adherence in people with schizophrenia: an international programme of research. *Int J Ment Health Nurs.* 2010; **19**(1): 36–44.

Haefner H. Stigma, Diskriminierung und die Folgen. In: *Das Rätsel Schizophrenie. Eine Krankheit wird entschlüsselt.* Munich: Beck; 2000. pp. 171–80.

Hegerl U, Wittmann M, Arensman E, *et al.* The 'European Alliance Against Depression (EAAD)': a multifaceted, community-based action programme against depression and suicidality. *World J Biol Psychiatry.* 2008; **9**(1): 51–8.

Hölling, I. About the impossibility of a single (ex-)user and survivor of psychiatry position. In: *Acta Psychiatr Scand Suppl.* 2001; **104**(Suppl. 410): S. 102–6.

International Monetary Fund. *World Economic Outlook Database.* April 2010 ed. Available at: www.imf.org/external/pubs/ft/weo/2009/01/ (accessed 28 February 2012).

Jacobi F, Wittchen HU, Holting C, *et al.* Prevalence, co-morbidity and correlates of mental disorders in the general population: results from the German Health Interview and Examination Survey (GHS). *Psychol Med.* 2004; **34**: 597–611.

Ketelsen R, Zechert C, Driessen M, *et al.* Characteristics of aggression in a German psychiatric hospital and predictors of patients at risk. *J Psychiatr Ment Health Nurs.* 2007; **14**(1): 92–9.

Kissling W, Höffler J, Seemann U, *et al.* Direct and indirect costs of schizophrenia. *Fortschr Neurol Psychiatr.* 1999; **67**: 29–36.

Kohl, F. Grundlinien der psychiatrischen Krankenhaus- und Institutionsgeschichte in Deutschland – Teil 2: Von der Begründung der Universitätskliniken zur Entwicklung der heutigen "Versorgungslandschaft", *Psych Pflege heute.* 2001; **7**(1): 16–21.

Link BG. Die Folgen des sozialen Stigmas für das Schicksal psychisch Kranker. *ZNS Journal.* 2000; **21**: 32–41.

Link BG, Struening EL, Rahav M, *et al.* On stigma and its consequences: evidence from a longitudinal study of men with dual diagnoses of mental illness and substance abuse. *J Health Soc Behav.* 1997; **38**: 177–90.

Melchinger H. Ambulante psychiatrische Versorgung. Umsteuerungen dringend geboten. *Dtsch Ärztebl.* 2008; **46**: A2457–60.

OECD. *Growing Unequal? Income Distribution and Poverty in OECD Countries.* 2008. Available at: www.nationmaster.com/graph/geo_pop_den_peo_per_sq_km-density-people-per-sq-km&date=2005 (accessed January 2011).

Population Reference Bureau. *Population Handbook.* 5th ed. 2004. Available at: www.prb.org/pdf/PopHandbook_Eng.pdf (accessed December 2010).

Richter D, Berger K, Reker T. Are mental disorders on the increase? A systematic review. *Psychiatr Prax.* 2008; **35**(7): 321–30.

Rössler W, Salize HJ, Riecher-Rössler A. Changing patterns of mental health care in Germany. *Int J Law Psychiatry.* 1996; **19**: 391–411.

Rössler W, Salize HJ, Voges B. Does community-based care have an effect on public attitudes toward the mentally ill? *Eur Psychiatry.* 1995; **10**: 282–9.

Salize HJ, Dressing H, Peitz M. *Compulsory Admission and Involuntary Treatment of Mentally Ill Patients – Legislation and Practice in EU-Member States.* Research project – grant agreement no. SI2.254882 (2000CVF3-407). Final report. 2002.

Salize HJ, Rössler W, Becker T. Mental health care in Germany. *Eur Arch Psychiatry Clin Neurosci.* 2007; **257**: 92–103.

Sartorius N. Stigma: what can psychiatrists do about it? *Lancet.* 1998; **352**: 1058–9.

Schoppmann S, Herbert MH. Altersstruktur psychiatrisch Pflegender in Deutschland. *Pflegewissenschaft.* 2010; **3**: 149–55.

Schoppmann S, Lüthi R. Insights from inside: the duties and activities of nurses at the psychiatric clinic Münsterlingen (CH). A qualitative study. *J Psychiatr Ment Health Nurs.* 2009; **16**(7): 606–20.

Schoppmann S, Mayer H. Altersstruktur psychiatrisch Pflegender in Deutschland. *Pflegewissenschaft,* 2010; **54**(2): 149–55.

Schoppmann S, Schröck R, Schnepp W, *et al.* 'Then I just showed her my arms . . .' Bodily sensations in moments of alienation related to self-injurious behaviour. A hermeneutic phenomenological study. *J Psychiatr Ment Health Nurs.* 2007; **14**(6): 587–97.

Schoppmann S. A German perspective on paradigmatic issues in psychiatric nursing. In: Tilly S, editor. *Psychiatric and Mental Health Nursing – the field of knowledge.* Oxford: Blackwell; 2005. pp. 203–12.

Schulz H, Barghaan D, Harfst T, *et al. Gesundheitsberichterstattung des Bundes – Psychotherapeutische Versorgung.* Heft: Robert Koch Institut; 2008. p. 41.

Schulz M, Damkröger A, Heins C, *et al.* Effort-reward imbalance and burnout among German nurses in medical compared with psychiatric hospital settings. *J Psychiatr Ment Health Nurs.* 2009; **16**(3): 225–33.

Statistische Ämter des Bundes und der Länder: Gebiet und Bevölkerung – Ausländische Bevölkerung, Stand. 2009. Available at: www.statistik-portal.de/Statistik-Portal/de_jb01_jahrtab2.asp (accessed 22 March 2011).

Steppe H. Nursing in Nazi Germany. *West J Nurs Res.* 1992; **14**(6): 744–53.

Wang PS. Use of mental health services for anxiety, mood, and substance disorders in 17 countries in the WHO world mental health surveys. *Lancet.* 2007; **370**(9590): 841–50.

Weinmann S, Puschner B, Becker T. Innovative structuring in German care for schizophrenics. *Nervenarzt.* 2009; **80**: 31–9.

Wiersma D, van Busschbach J. Are needs and satisfaction of care associated with quality of life? *Eur Arch Psychiatry Clin Neurosci.* 2001; **251**: 239–46.

Wittchen HU, Jacobi F. Size and burden of mental disorders in Europe: a critical review and appraisal of 27 studies. *Eur Neuropsychopharmacol.* 2005; **15**: 357–76.

World Psychiatric Association. *Fighting Stigma and Discrimination Because of Schizophrenia.* New York, NY: World Psychiatric Association; 1998.

www.gbe-bund.de (Federal Health Reporting).

Mental health services in Greece

Evmorfia Koukia

Introduction

Greece is currently in the grip of an unprecedented economic crisis, having had a long history of borrowing more than it can realistically pay back. Among its many problems is the fact that labour costs are too high and exports much less that many other EU countries. This has and will have untold consequences for the funding and maintenance of public health services. The shape of current mental health services has been strongly influenced by the scandal of institutional neglect on the island of Leros. This chapter illustrates how local context and culture can influence the detail of how mental health services operate. Although significant changes have been made, the author concludes that there is still much to be done to address the needs of all people, regardless of where they live. She argues that in order for mental health services to progress, enlightened service providers are required who can work as equals, share resources, challenge tradition and respect what people find helpful as opposed to what professionals think people need.

National profile and context

In order to understand the manner in which Greek mental health services are provided, it is important to first understand the political, economic and demographic context of Greece itself. Greece, also known as Hellas, and officially the Hellenic Republic, is situated on the southern end of the Balkan Peninsula. The country has the 10th-longest coastline in the world, many surrounding islands and a total area of 131 957 km². Greece's topography is highly diverse. One fourth of the land is lowland, one fifth forested and the rest mountainous. Islands in the Aegean and Ionian seas occupy one fifth of the territory. The capital is Athens. Greece has 54 prefectures (*nomoi*), which constitute the units of local government and are headed by a prefect (*nomarchis*), who is elected approximately every 4 years. In all, there are 13 regions, each one consisting of a number of prefectures. Greece is a parliamentary democracy with a unicameral parliament consisting of 300 delegates. The leader is the prime minister, and Greece has been a member of the European Union since 1981 and the Economic and Monetary Union since 2001. This chapter describes the existing mental health services in Greece, with a particular emphasis on the 20-year psychiatric reform programme.

Population and demographics

In 2001, Greece's total population was 10.9 million (National Statistical Service of Greece, 2001) and the population growth rate annually is approximately 0.146%. Almost two thirds of the Greek people live in urban areas, consisting of Athens, Thessaloniki, Patras, Larissa, Volos and Heraklion. Throughout the twentieth century, because of the economic situation, millions of Greeks migrated to the US, Australia, Canada, the UK and Germany. This trend was reversed after some fortunate changes in the Greek economy since the 1980s. However, the past 2 years have seen a reversal of fortune, and the Greek economy, due to a number of factors including the economic recession, is once again struggling to sustain the population and the services it requires.

Data on the extent of the immigrant population in Greece remains unreliable, and as yet, exact figures have not been calculated. However, approximations suggest that upwards of 8.5% to 10.3% of the total population are immigrants, constituting about 1.15 million immigrants. In 2001, a study undertaken by the Mediterranean Migration Observatory showed that 7% of the total population residing in Greece was without Greek citizenship. It further provided a break-down of the immigrant population as follows:

- People from the Balkan countries (Albania 56%, Bulgaria 5%, and Romania 3%) make up almost two thirds of the total foreign population.
- Migrants from the former Soviet Union (Georgia, Russia, Ukraine, Moldova, etc.) comprise 10% of the total.
- The greatest cluster of the non-EU immigrant population is to be found in the municipality of Athens, some 132 000 making up 17% of the local population.

Approximately 97% of the population belong to the Greek Orthodox faith, although there are minority groups that belong to other faith traditions. For instance, in Thrace there is a Muslim community ranging from 98 000 to 140 000 (between 0.9% and 1.2% of the population). Albanian immigrants (approximately 700 000) are predominantly Muslims and live largely in and around Thrace. Judaism has existed in Greece for more than 2000 years; today, the Greek Jewish community, comprised of those descendants who survived the Holocaust, is estimated to number around 5500 people. Greek members of the Roman Catholic faith are estimated at 50 000, Old Calendarists account for 500 000 followers. There are a wide variety of religions with smaller followings, indicating that Greece is a tolerant country, particularly with respect to practicing one's faith. These faith communities do play a part in supporting members who are old, infirm and lonely and without which the mental health of some people would be considerably worse than it is.

The first and only official language spoken is Greek, and immigrants are expected to learn the language, especially if they hope to get employment or are in need of services. Minority languages, e.g. Turkish, Bulgarian and Romani, continue to be spoken by regional immigrant groups in various parts of the country. Among the Greek-speaking population, speakers of the distinctive Pontic dialect came to Greece from Asia Minor after the Greek genocide and have constituted since then a sizeable group.

The economy of Greece, although currently going through a period of crisis, is estimated to be the 27th-largest economy in the world. The gross domestic product per capita is US$30 856 (IMF, 2009). The public sector accounts for about 40% of GDP, and the maintaining of services is now severely strained due to rising unemployment levels and public overspending.

By the end of 2009, as a result of a combination of international (financial crises) and local factors (uncontrolled spending prior to the October 2009 national elections), the Greek economy faced its most severe crisis since 1993, having the second-highest budget deficit (12.7%) as well as the second highest debt-to-GDP ratio in the EU. This rising debt caused an economic crisis for the country, which placed the largest strain to date on the Euro-nation. In early 2010, the Greek government admitted having difficulties servicing its large sovereign debt and petitioned the intervention of the IMF. This situation may have a future detrimental impact on the development of health services in general and mental health services in particular.

Changing health needs

In common with other countries worldwide, Greece has an ageing population. In 2001, 16.71% of the population was 65 years and older, 68.12% between the ages of 15 and 64 years, and 15.18% were 14 years and younger. The crude death rate (CDR) is at 10.33 deaths per 1000 population, and the life expectancy is one of the highest among OECD countries (78 years for males and 84 years for females). The consumption of health and social care services, as is the case elsewhere, increases as people get older. The family is the agency totally responsible for the care of dependent relatives of all ages. This fact results from two important factors: firstly, older people do not receive adequate care from any other source, and secondly, such are the requirements of the Greek culture that families are expected to care for their vulnerable members, particularly those who are ill. If a family is unable to care for a relative for whatever reason, the person is cared for by the social security system. Long-term care for the elderly is provided mainly by the private sector, a fact that imposes an extra financial burden on the family. Older mental health patients, especially, face major problems in terms of provision of care, quality of care and where it is provided. The reform of the existing psychiatric system has created new resources, like vocational rehabilitation for the mentally ill and apartments in proximity to psychiatric centres, in various regions of the country.

During the last 10 years, Greece has seen a dramatic increase in the number of illegal immigrants, thus creating extra demands on health and social care services. Immigrant families do suffer economic deprivation, due largely to unemployment or poorly paid work, and some do have poor physical and mental health, while others may choose not to have public health care insurance. According to Greek legislation, illegal immigrants may ask to be admitted to a public hospital only if an emergency arises. In Greece, a number of independent/non-governmental organisations provide a variety of services which include free medical and pharmaceutical care, social and psychological support, legal shelter and employment advice to refugees, economic immigrants, the poor, the homeless and the uninsured.

The National Health Service

The Greek National Health Service (NHS) was established in 1983, heralding major restructuring in terms of the provision of services and legislation. The government plan in doing so was twofold: to place all health care under the state in order to ensure equality of health care delivery, and to contain the rise of the private sector. Law N. 2889/2001 allowed for the creation of 17 administrative health regions throughout the country, while law N. 3329/2005 directed how these regions were to be managed, their aims and how they were to be funded.

The Ministry of Health and Social Solidarity is responsible for the financing of the National Health Service. According to OECD health data (2009), Greece in 2007 spent 9.6% of GDP on health. When one considers the levels of need, this allocation on health is inadequate. However, insurance- and tax-based revenues, as well as private ones, also contribute to the running of the Greek health care system, with additional mandatory contributions being paid by employers

and employees to supplement these funds. Public and private medicine operate alongside each other in a complementary pattern, rendering the Greek
health care system a mixed health care economy, constituted from the health
care branches of the various social insurances and the National Health System
(Ethnico Systima Ygeias) (ESY). ESY (1983) guaranteed free health care for all
residents of Greece, regardless of whether they were Greek nationals or not.
Article 21 of the Foundation Law of ESY provided for the inclusion of mental
health services within the overall national health system. Although residents are
entitled to health services, the viability of such services is somewhat limited by
their uneven distribution, particularly for those who live in rural areas, especially
the many Greek islands. When calculated on a per capita basis, health care costs
in Greece are among the lowest in the European Union member countries.

The combined social security system is designed to cover the total population. This system comprises a number of insurance organisations, the main ones
being the Institute of Social Insurance (IKA; 50% of the urban population),
Organization of Agriculture Insurance (OGA; 25% of the rural population), Funds
of Merchants, Manufacturers and Small Businessmen (TEVE-TAE; 13% of the
population), OTE, DEH, banks (2.5% of the population working in telecommu-
nications, electricity and banks) and civil servants (7% of the population). The
rest of the population (nearly 9%) is covered by the public sector. Additionally,
5%–8% of the population has made private arrangements through private insurance companies for their welfare needs.

Since 1985, Greece has seen a steady rise in the growth in the number of
establishments providing private facilities. Psychiatric care relies to a large extent
on psychiatrists providing private practice, either contracted with various social
insurances or paid directly by the patient. Unfortunately, direct payments to
medical doctors by their patients are a usual occurrence in the Greek health
care system as a means of securing better quality of care provision. These off-
the-record, out-of-pocket payments are quite a frequent phenomenon in public/
private hospitals and outpatient care facilities as well.

It is important to appreciate that the Greek health care delivery system consists of both primary health care and public health services. Primary health care
(PHC) services are provided through outpatient departments of hospitals, rural
health centres, provincial clinics and polyclinics of the social insurance institutions, as well as by physicians in private practice and private hospital outpatient
departments. Secondary health care services, on the other hand, are provided
through public hospitals (free of charge), private hospitals and clinics/hospitals
owned by major social insurance funds.

In 2006, the bed-to-population ratio was 3.9 per 1000, which is one of the
lowest of the Western European nations. By far the majority of these beds are
located in the capital, Athens. The number of doctors per capita increased rapidly

to reach 5.4 physicians per 1000 population in 2006, whereas the number of nurses, 3.2 nurses per 1000 population, is much lower than the average 9.6/1000 in OECD countries. The Greek health care system is characterised by a critical shortage of professional nurses.

Mental health need and demographics

Epidemiological data has shown that, at any one time, 14%–16% of the general population of Greece suffers from a psychiatric disorder, with 5% of the population suffering from chronic depression or anxiety. In 2008, suicide rates and self-inflicted injuries in all ages were estimated to be 2.85 per 100 000, one of the lowest in the European Union. In contrast, suicide rates amongst psychiatric patients are extremely high (bipolar disorders 20%, schizophrenia 10%–15%, neurological disorders 8.69 per 100 000) (WHO, 2008). The low suicide rate in Greece has been attributed to cultural and social factors. For instance, families stick together and support each other, especially during times of crisis. This kind of social and psychological support by family and friends plays a protective role in diminishing the effects of social isolation and feelings of loneliness that may eventually lead to suicidal behaviour.

Attitudes to mental health problems

Until the development of community mental health services, attitudes to mental health problems presented a number of cultural barriers that prevented many people and their families from seeking help. Among these barriers, the greatest were ignorance, stigma and wide-scale negativity on the part of the general population. Knowledge about mental illnesses in general, but especially schizophrenia, is poor, and even the term itself provokes a negative attitude in both relatives and friends, especially amongst those who live in rural areas and who have had little education. They believe patients with schizophrenia are dangerous, should be avoided and are incapable of working with normal people. The admission of a patient to a public or a private mental hospital is seen as a stigmatising experience for the whole family. Because of this, until 1985, hospitalisation in the nine public or private mental hospitals tended to occur only when the person had become so ill that there was no alternative. At that time, community-based services were not an option as they did not exist.

In 1978, the Department of Psychiatry at Athens National University, under the supervision of the professor in psychiatry, Michael Madianos, established the first community mental health centre in the country. Madianos *et al.* (1987) sought to discover the attitudes of 1574 adult members of the public towards people with mental health problems. The study revealed that there existed five main areas of concern: social discrimination, social restriction on what people could do, an absence of social care, an inability to integrate and a poor understanding of the causes of mental health problems. The existence of these in the general public gave rise to feelings of being rejected, fearfulness and suspicion on the part of mental health patients, thus creating a situation in which patients felt unable to recover or feeling forced to accept that there was very little for which to recover. After 10 years, Madianos et al. (1999) undertook a follow-up study in which they compared the attitudes towards mental illness of the general public and those personnel who worked in the same community mental health centre. The results showed statistically significant differences between the two samples; however, both groups expressed more positive attitudes towards the mentally ill than had been the case previously. Both groups were more favourably disposed towards social integration than had previously been the case, they held less authoritarian attitudes to social restriction and they possessed a good level of knowledge about the aetiology of mental illnesses. It was especially noteworthy that female respondents were more open-minded and expressed more positive attitudes than their male counterparts. Hence, it was apparent that in addition to making facilities more available in the community for patients and their families, this was instrumental in educating the public to change their attitudes towards people with mental health problems.

In 1989, Marina Economou, associate professor of psychiatry at the University Mental Health Institute, following an initiative started by the World Psychiatric Association, commenced a study that focused on reducing and ultimately eliminating stigma and discrimination in mental health care. She entitled her study 'Programme against Stigma'. The programme was the first of its kind in Greece and its aim was to fight the myths and misunderstandings that have traditionally been associated with mental illness. It also held that in order to develop community-based services, the attitudes and beliefs of the public were significant factors in whether or not people would benefit from such services. The criticism of this study was that it was carried out in urban areas where the majority of people live. Economou et al. (2009) conducted the first national survey to investigate the level of stigma against patients with schizophrenia. The results showed that Greek residents continued to display stigmatising attitudes towards patients with schizophrenia, especially those in rural and semi-urban regions. The deeply entrenched beliefs that Madianos et al. (1987) found were still present, and many respondents believed that schizophrenic patients were dangerous and were so fearful that they would not initiate conversations with them. Knowledge about schizophrenia was found to be poor, and attitudes were attributed to news programmes and documentaries they had seen on television, which was the main source of their information. With respect to the attitudes held by nursing students, Madianos et al. (2005) found that, following a placement during their training in mental health settings, their attitudes had changed considerably. It appeared that exposure to mentally ill people and seeking to assist them had the effect of engendering more positive views about such people as well as assisting them to acquire a better understanding of the psychological needs of people, especially those who are ill. Nurses generally, on the completion of this placement, felt more strongly that psychiatric patients should be helped to socially integrate; nurses also behaved in a less authoritarian way towards patients. More thought is required in order to assess how best general attitudes among the population at large could be altered, as it is now clear that a major part of a person's recovery from mental health problems depends on the attitudes of those around them.

Expenditure on mental health

According to the *Mental Health Atlas* (WHO, 2005), there is no reliable data on the precise budget allocation for mental health in Greece. It is possible that as better accounting is being implemented in health care, more reliable data will be forthcoming in the near future. One possible reason it is so difficult to assess the expenditure on mental health is that funding comes from a variety of sources, e.g. taxes, social insurances, private insurances and patients' direct payments. As a consequence of this, it is not possible to assess which services are both efficient and effective and provide 'value for money', as they are all seen as necessary. It is possible that the fragmentation of funding contributes to the fragmentation of services and the inequality of access by individuals and families.

History of the development of mental health services

Until the development of asylums in the nineteenth century, the mentally ill were cared for at home and were mostly contained indoors. The care of the patient was the responsibility of the family. In undertaking this work, which was often arduous and expensive, families were stigmatised and often shunned by neighbours and relatives for having 'mad' relatives. In some cases, where families were not sufficiently conscientious or were unable to care for their relatives, the mentally ill were left to wander aimlessly, become permanently homeless and were often mistreated by the people. Throughout most of the eighteenth century, monasteries played a central role in providing comfort and care to those in need of psychiatric treatment.

The growth of the asylum system

The foundations for mental health services were laid during the late Byzantine era, when a number of monasteries became shelters or sanctuaries, sometimes referred to as monastery asylums, for those suffering from various forms of mental illness. The Byzantine Empire (or Byzantium) was the predominantly Greek-speaking eastern part of the Roman Empire throughout late antiquity and the Middle Ages. It was a highly successful empire in terms of economic growth, military power and political influence; it also valued and provided for the health and well-being of all its citizens (Beckwith, 1986).

Around 1821 saw the beginnings of the War of Greek Independence, when the Turks occupied and sought to conquer Greece. At that time, the care of the mentally ill was wholly the responsibility of monasteries, and what was provided was termed 'moral treatment'. The shared belief in God, by both the patients and the staff, and religious practices were deemed to be therapeutic. In subsequent years, when monasteries and families were unable to provide care for their relatives, a number of mentally ill people were confined in jails, the main one being Kydatheineon in Plaka, Athens. Towards the end of the nineteenth century, scientific psychiatric care was embraced in Greece and 11 purpose-built asylums were developed. Despite attempts to see mental illness as a condition like any other health problem, the mentally ill continued to be stigmatised and were the cause of many families feeling ostracised within their communities. If mentally ill people took it upon themselves to walk in public places, they ran the risk of being ridiculed or subjected to cruelty.

The asylum period started in the late nineteenth century and lasted until the end of the first half of the twentieth century. The first mental health hospital was founded in 1834 in Corfu, then under British occupation, and had 425 beds. In 1862, the first mental health legislation was introduced, and in 1884 the building of the first private mental hospital in Athens for fee-paying patients, the Dromokaition, commenced and it accepted its first patients on 10 January 1887. The university mental hospital Aeginition was established in 1904, and at the beginning of the 1920s the first public asylum, the Psychiatric Hospital of Attica, was built in order to provide care for all mentally ill patients.

Within a very short period following the opening of psychiatric facilities, Greek asylums became overcrowded and the standards of care and treatment provided fell. The exception was Dromokaition, which due to its private character, refused to admit more patients than it was able to cater for. Other institutions were unable to be as assertive and so they felt obliged to accept all the patients referred to them. The onset of the Second World War saw large numbers of patients being admitted into overcrowded conditions and with a decline in what was acceptable as psychiatric care.

The introduction of psychotropic drugs in the 1950s saw an improvement in the care and treatment of the mentally ill and a radical change took place in how health care staff and patients related to each other. Unfortunately, the continued overcrowding of asylums impeded any progress that could be made and the lack of resources ultimately resulted in psychiatric care declining even further.

In the meantime, Leros Mental Health Hospital was founded in 1959 on the island of Leros and officially opened in 1965. This island was considered to be a strategic area historically, due to its geopolitical position and its large natural harbours. After the Second World War ended and Italian occupation ceased, immigration and unemployment on Leros became crucial problems. The founding of the mental health hospital was seen as a solution to these growing socio-economic problems, and unfortunately between 1958 and 1981, 4500 patients were transferred to the island and forced to live in the most inhumane and untherapeutic conditions. The building of a psychiatric institution did little to remedy the slow economic decline of the island.

In 1968, during the dictatorship years, the Ministry of Health presented a plan for health care reform, the aims of which included the improvement of the quality of psychiatric care. However, by the end of the plan in 1973, ironically the year the new Mental Health Law was introduced, almost none of these goals had been achieved. With the restoration of democracy in 1974 came more demands for the reform of health care. In the late 1970s, psychiatric provision was based in nine overcrowded public mental hospitals; there being a total absence of community-based services, there were some regions with a complete absence of access to any sort of psychiatric care.

The 1970s saw a rapid development in extramural mental health services with the first day hospital opening in Athens in 1977. The following year, the first psychiatric unit in a general hospital was established in Alexandroupolis, and in 1979 the first community mental health centres in Kessariani and Byron (boroughs of Athens with a combined population of 150000) were established by the Department of Psychiatry at the University of Athens. There was no psychiatric emergency service in Greece until 1978, when the Department of Psychiatry of Athens National University formed a relationship with Eginition Hospital and provided the first 24-hour emergency service. By 1980, psychiatric care was based in nine public mental health hospitals, 40 private mental health hospitals and the services mentioned above. In 1980, the Greek government undertook the task of reviewing the whole mental health system, with special attention being paid to Leros Mental Health Hospital.

Deinstitutionalisation (1984–2015)

It became apparent that a radical review of the mental health care system was needed and more focused planning required, as opposed to the piecemeal approach that had been adopted up till then. Two main priorities were identified:

first, the decentralisation of psychiatric services, and second, the development of a 5-year plan (1984–89) that would direct how reforms could be implemented. The Commission of the European Communities provided financial and technical support to assist in realising the 5-year plan, and as a result, in 1984 the Greek government received €120 million. The objectives of the 5-year plan consisted of the following:

- the decentralisation of mental health services and the development of community-based services
- the deinstitutionalisation of long-stay patients in the mental health hospitals
- the training of mental health professionals in the new role-care models.

Special attention was given to Leros hospital because of the concern expressed worldwide about the conditions that existed there, and 13 community hostels were established throughout Greece in order to provide residential care for the more than 100 former psychiatric patients who lived there. The 5-year plan was extended up to 1995 with the same objectives. Particular emphasis was given to Leros hospital, and in 1989 the Hellenic Psychiatric Association informed the Greek Ministry of Health that a further 1150 inpatients from there were to be removed from Leros and rehoused in various sheltered housing schemes throughout the country. As a result of the 10-year reform programme, 1984 to 1996, a gradual development of community-based mental health services (CMHC) was observed, including community mental health centres, outpatient departments and child guidance clinics. As shown in Table 5.1, between 1984 and 1996, significant developments took place across a number of services.

In the same study, it was reported that during the period 1984–96, there was an increase in the ratios of professional personnel/100 beds of all specialities: psychiatrists (+214.0%), psychologists (+107.5%), social workers (+148.3%), nurses (+21.7%) and occupational therapists (+300.0%). During the same period, admissions decreased from 10 560 in 1984 to 9798 in 1996 (−7.2%) and discharges increased from 7504 in 1984 to 9805 in 1996 (+30.6%).

From the results shown above, it can be seen that during this period several goals were achieved, however a number of others had still to be attained, such as equality in geographic distribution. In 1996, there were still 19 prefectures in several regions where no mental health system existed. Additionally, despite the development of rehabilitation services, these were inadequate to meet the needs of the discharged mental patients and the chronically mentally ill already living in the community. Legal and administrative difficulties, such as the sectorisation and coordination of the 54 prefectures and the ways that they interpreted community services, created a number of obstacles in the implementation of the reform programme. Because of the location of the university psychiatric department, additional community services were added, while rural areas continued

TABLE 5.1 Mental health resources

	1984	1987	1990	1993	1996	1999	2006	% change 1984–2006
No. of beds in general hospitals	36	99	281	306	327	407	646	+1694.5
No. per 1000 population[1]	0.004	0.01	0.03	0.03	0.03	0.03	0.06	
No. of community mental health centres[2]	7	15	19	23	33	41	45[3]	+542.8
No. of child guidance clinics	8	12	22	24	24	28	30	+275.0
No. of outpatient departments in general hospitals	20	38	43	51	56	56	70	+250.0
Total no. of extramural services	35	65	84	98	113	125	145	+314.3
No. per 100 000 population	0.34	0.63	0.81	0.95	1.10	1.20	1.32	
No. of places in day hospitals/care centres	55	295	258	381	369	390	941	+1610.9
No. per 1000 population	0.005	0.02	0.02	0.04	0.04	0.04	0.08	
No. of places in psychosocial rehabilitation services	195	315	779	1603	1643	1780	3080	+1479.5
No. per 1000 population	0.01	0.02	0.06	0.1	0.2	0.2	0.3	
No. of beds in alternative residential facilities	15	25	359	540	1052	1962	4026	+2674.0
No. per 1000 population	0.001	0.002	0.03	0.05	0.1	0.2	0.3	

[1] Psychiatric beds in general hospitals, extramural facilities, and psychosocial rehabilitation places and residential beds (per 1000 population).

[2] Fifteen community mental health centres also provide services for children and adolescents by multidisciplinary teams.

[3] Thirty-four operational.

Source: Madianos and Christodoulou, 2007

to be neglected. Between 1984 and 1996, an increase in the number of neuropsychiatrists was observed, especially in urban areas. The limited number of professionals working in rural mental health centres is still considered to be inadequate, and there appears to be no plan to remedy this situation in the near future.

There was a significant increase from 0.34 in 1984 to 1.32 in 2006 in the total number of extramural facilities per 100 000 inhabitants. The reduction in number of beds in public mental hospitals coincided with a reduction in number of beds in private psychiatric hospitals as well. The growth in community services during that period was unprecedented and the transformation of services dramatic; with the exception of day hospitals' capacity per 1000 inhabitants, which appears to be rather low (0.08 in 2006), places in other facilities like rehabilitation services, residential alternatives and community-based centres increased enormously.

The development of the psychiatric profession

The emergence of psychiatry in Greece took place during the second half of the nineteenth century and the development of a psychiatric medical speciality evolved between 1880 and 1930. It was characterised by Western models of care due to the significant number of Greek psychiatrists studying abroad. In 1905, the Department of Neurology and Psychiatry of the University of Athens was founded in Eginition Hospital. Until 1981, Greek psychiatry was mainly organic-focused and was officially referred to as 'neurology-psychiatry'. This was combined with the fact that psychiatric care was based in public asylum-like hospitals and private inpatient clinics. The education of psychiatrists was based on residency training and there was an absence of any psychotherapeutic treatment. Medication played a key role in psychiatric care and community care, as an alternative did not appear until the end of the 1970s. In 1963, the Department of Psychiatry of the University of Athens became independent from the Neurological Department, but since then both departments have been housed in Eginition Hospital.

The university's Department of Psychiatry is responsible for the formation of educational programs at undergraduate and postgraduate levels, which are provided in seven universities. However, a significant number of graduates pursue their studies abroad. After the completion of basic medical studies, doctors are required to enter their names on a waiting list for the psychiatric speciality of their choice. Curiously, as mental health services moved into community settings, mental health education did not keep pace. For instance, the training of primary care physicians is still undeveloped, and the psychosocial dimensions of community mental health care and rehabilitation are poorly addressed in psychiatrist training. There are no opportunities in any of the Greek medical schools to study psychosocial rehabilitation. The number of medical doctors in Greece is above the Western European average, but the fact that almost 88% of psychiatrists work in large cities shows the lack of services in rural areas, due to the reluctance of mental health personnel to work there. In common with other countries, mental health professionals are like many other workers, in that they tend to go to where they are likely to get higher-paid jobs, can choose what they want to do and generally plan a life that suits their requirements and those of their families. In doing so, this creates a serious lack of mental health specialists with knowledge and experience in rural areas, where there are often more long-term, complex and enduring needs.

Nurses in mental health care

The first nurse who took care of mentally ill patients was Agape Hatzidaki-Kouratora, who worked in the gaol of Kydatheineon in the early nineteenth century. Later on, she was appointed to the public Psychiatric Hospital of Athens. Nurses working in the asylums were untrained; very few had completed elementary education and they were unable to provide professional care due to a number of obstacles. Her work was further complicated by the fact that there were few effective medicines that were designed to assist people with major psychiatric illnesses, living conditions within the hospital were primitive and the limited number of staff coupled with the increasing number of patients made the work, though always challenging, far from satisfying.

It was not until the early 1890s that doctors made the first attempts to train nurses in order to provide a more caring approach. Up to 1946, there was no training whatsoever in psychiatric nursing in nursing schools. At this time, a lecturer, who had obtained her postgraduate degree in psychiatric nursing abroad, recommended the creation of a 7-week training programme for nursing students at the Psychiatric Hospital of Athens.

Early attempts at providing training for nurses were seen in 1950, when four qualified nurses from the Health Visiting School decided to work at the Psychiatric Hospital of Athens and to lay the foundations for what was to become psychiatric nursing services. In the mid-1950s, a small number of qualified nurses were appointed to the existing mental hospitals, Dromokaition situated in Athens and in the hospitals of the islands of Crete, Corfu and Leros. Qualified nurses were still scarce, and the care of the growing number of patients was still carried out by unqualified staff in unbearable conditions (Missouridou, 2009).

The term 'keeper', as used in other countries, most notably England, was widely used until 1965. From the beginning of the First World War, and for at least two decades afterwards, the working conditions were truly miserable, characterised by long shifts with little time off, low payment and dealing with dangerous patients. In 1955, it was decided to introduce an 8-hour day for all nurses in Greece.

The official history of mental health nursing education began in 1967, when

Aphrodite Ragia, one year after her postgraduate education in psychiatric nursing at the United Nations, initiated lectures in psychiatric nursing at the School of Nurses in Evangelismos Hospital. She compiled the first lecture notes in psychiatric nursing and gave lectures in various schools. During this time, she was invited by the Military School of Nurses to train the first head nurse of the psychiatric wards and began the 'psychiatric speciality' designed exclusively for nurses. In 1979, the first University School of Nursing was established in Athens. In the 1980s, Ragia, with a group of other university professors, introduced the postgraduate and, later, doctorate studies in mental health designed for nurses and other professionals with a university degree.

In the same decade, a real shift took place in focusing the work of the nurse from containment to therapy. The emphasis was now given to therapeutic relationships with the patients and the beneficial nature of nurse–patient interaction was being explored. In 1988, psychiatric speciality-designed 3-year courses were recognised as a legal requirement. Nowadays, the Greek educational system has many different levels of education for nurses. The following are the types of programmes available for the training of psychiatric nurses, a situation that many find confusing and serves to undermine the identity of mental health nurses:

- A great number of auxiliary nurses opt for a *2-year preparation* course, on completion of which they can have almost the same responsibilities as fully qualified nurses. Currently, 47 schools (Ministry of Health) and 168 schools (Ministry of Education) provide these courses.
- The largest number of nurses undertake a *3-year education* in the faculty of nursing of a technological college, currently provided at eight technological colleges.
- A small number of *3-year educated* nurses can undertake a psychiatric speciality offered in mental hospitals (1 year's duration).
- Fewer nurses still undertake a *4-year university degree* (one nursing school, University of Athens).
- There are a minimal number of nurses holding master's and doctoral degrees in mental health.

In addition, the modernisation of the Greek mental health system, with its emphases on community-based facilities and rehabilitation services, has greatly highlighted the need for primary care mental health nurses. Yet the training of nurses for primary care settings has not been given any priority. There is an apparent lack of expert nurses in this field, resulting in community facilities being staffed with untrained and unspecialised nurses. This situation is in urgent need of attention if recent mental health policies are to be effectively operationalised. In addition, the number of nurses in Greece is substantially lower than other European countries; especially the number of psychiatric nurses, which currently stands at three per 100 000 population (WHO, 2005). The majority of psychiatric nurses work in the public sector, and as has already been stated, there is a significant lack of specialist nurses in rural areas. As is the trend in Greece, the public mental health hospitals in large cities attract the majority of qualified nurses.

The changing position of service users

In ancient Greece, a mentally ill person was someone who was possessed by the supernatural spirits of Mania and Lyssa, and illness was seen as a punishment inflicted by the gods. Hippocrates was the first philosopher to introduce the notions of aetiology and treatment in medicine and to show the logical relationship between the two. He introduced a triad of mental disorders: melancholia, mania and phrenitis, being the first to reject the 'spirit theory' or 'spirit possession' of mental health illness. Plato spoke of two types of mental illness, one divinely inspired and the other a physical disease. Aristotle, too, proposed a physical explanation for mental illness. In the Middle Ages, the Greek Orthodox church returned to the notion of 'possession theory' and considered the mentally ill to have been possessed by the devil, with the treatment being exorcism, undertaken by the clergy. During the 400 years of the Ottoman occupation of Greece, madness was seen as a combination of theological, philosophical and scientific elements. This approach formed the basis of thought and practice for a significant period of time in Greece.

It was due primarily to this situation that stigma was heightened. Not only did whole communities turn against mentally ill people and wish them removed from their neighbourhoods, families were ostracised and isolated. It was not uncommon for 'the mad of the village' to become the centre of wild and offensive amusement, and audiences would gather solely to ridicule and torment them. Even at the beginning of the establishment of mental hospitals, some villages prevented the mentally ill from being removed there, preferring instead to hold on to them for entertainment. It was during the late nineteenth century that the term 'psychopath' was introduced, which meant a disorder of the soul. Actually, the term 'mental illness' was not widely used in the scientific nomenclature until the late twentieth century. Terms such as 'client' or 'service user', though sometimes used, have not met with approval by mental health personnel. Up until the mid-1990s, patients' views and comments had no part to play in the planning of care or treatment. However, in the course of the last decade there have been signs that things are beginning to change and that the experiences and knowledge of patients and families are being taken seriously, and various movements have come into existence to cater for their needs.

The Pan-Hellenic Association of Families for Mental Health (SOPSI), which was founded in 1993, is a non-profit organisation whose members come from families of people with mental illnesses. The association is trying to increase society's awareness of the mentally ill. The Hellenic Observatory for Rights in the Field of Mental Health is a network of people (users of psychosocial services, users' relatives, mental health professionals and citizens) founded in 2006 which strives to promote the participation of users of psychosocial services in decision-making, and to defend the rights of mentally ill people facing social exclusion.

At the beginning of 2010, the Hellenic Hearing Voices Network was set up as an alternative way of approaching the care of people who hear voices and experience paranoia. Involvement of all these groups, and the contribution that they make, is serving to change the existing ways that mental illness is seen and is expanding the part that service users can play in mental health services.

Current mental health care

Since 1983, Greece has had a number of 10-year national plans for mental health services, co-funded by the EU; the last one, originated in 1998, is called Psychargos and has served as both the legislative framework and the national policy since 1999. It is divided into three phases: Phase A, 1998–2001; Phase B, 2002–06; and Phase C, 2006–15. The main objective of this programme was the deinstitutionalisation of the remaining 3000 long-stay patients, the development of 616 mental health services, including community-based structures and rehabilitation units, and the closure of the remaining mental hospitals. Closure was planned for five out of nine psychiatric hospitals by the end of 2006 and the remaining by the end of 2015.

Secondary and tertiary care are provided in a number of psychiatric hospitals, psychiatric departments in general hospitals and university clinics. Some private hospitals also provide tertiary care. Currently, the total number of psychiatric beds nationally stands at 8.7 per 10 000 population. The breakdown is: psychiatric beds in mental hospitals, 4.3 per 10 000 population; psychiatric beds in general hospitals, 0.3 per 10 000; and psychiatric beds in other settings, 4.1 per 10 000 individuals (WHO, 2001).

Madianos and Christodoulou (2007) explored the effect of the psychiatric reform programme and found that between 1984 and 2006 the number of long-stay patients decreased by 80.8%, from 5677 long-stay patients in 1984 to 1091 in 2006. Table 5.2 shows the trends in the number of patients in eight of the remaining public mental hospitals, and the planning for mental hospital closure is presented (1984–2012). Eginition Hospital (not included below), a university hospital, was due for closure in 2006, but is still in the process of being wound down.

TABLE 5.2 Bed numbers: 1984–2012

Mental hospital	1984	2000	2004	2006	2012
Attica	1950	831	640	728	To be closed
Dromokaition	880	555	419	493	To be closed
Thessalonika	1000	581	526	254	To be closed
Petra Olympou	500	260	51	Closed	–
Chania (Crete)	416	250	167	Closed	–
Corfu	416	280	120	Closed	–
Leros	1905	538	495	469	130
Tripolis	420	220	124	78	–
Total	7487	3515	2542	2022	130

Source: Madianos and Christodoulou, 2007

As can be seen, the implementation of the European Union initiatives and the Psychargos programme contributed to the discharge of a great number of long-stay psychiatric patients. For this to happen, there was a great need for many community-based and rehabilitation services, and, indeed, there has been an enormous increase in the amount and variety of community services between 1984 and 2006, including community mental health centres, outpatient departments in general hospitals, rehabilitation services, residential alternatives and child guidance clinics.

Hospital-based services

Despite the reduction in beds in recent years, the Greek health care system continues to be focused on hospital-based services. The facilities providing psychiatric care include the following:

● Outpatient hospital departments/emergency departments in public general hospitals (NHS hospitals financed by state budget and social insurance funds). These services are offered during particular days on a rotating basis and all patients have access.
● Psychiatric departments in public general hospitals (NHS hospitals).
● Public psychiatric hospitals (NHS hospitals).
● University psychiatric hospitals and university outpatient hospital departments in general hospitals, financed by the Ministry of Education.
● Private psychiatric clinics.
● Military hospitals. Only military personnel and their families have access to these hospitals, which are financed by the Ministry of Defence.

The major problem is the uneven geographical distribution of these facilities. Most services are concentrated in urban areas like Athens and Thessaloniki.

The reform resulted in new specialised services in various regions like the island of Crete or Macedonia and Thessaly, but the problem of the increased patient flow towards major cities remains. The referral system still malfunctions and the implications from the closure of the psychiatric hospitals remain to be seen.

Community facilities

Primary care is offered by a small number of community mental health centres and the outpatient clinics of psychiatric departments in general hospitals. The implementation of the psychiatric reform programme (1984–2006) significantly changed the face of public health psychiatry and aggressively focused on dein-stitutionalisation and rehabilitation. By 2010, a significant number of extramural services had been developed, although most are located in urban areas.

Even though the reforms created a number of facilities under state respon-sibility, the private sector still remains strongly attached to a payment system called 'fee-for-service'. Public health continues to rely on users' salaries and social insurance funds. Social security includes different insurances, each of which has its own requirements. Health care delivery remains a problematic area. The lack of coordination and quality assessment and the poor quality of manage-ment has resulted in a number of inefficiencies having to be addressed by the government.

Over the past 20 years, the continuing reduction of long-stay patients in mental hospitals, the closure of several large psychiatric inpatient facilities and the increased development of community-based care have meant that people are now forced to use community services, as other options are not available. Of course, it is not just direct mental health care services that people require; many of them also require occupational rehabilitation and training. The demands of finding employment for patients recovering from mental health problems, at a time when levels of unemployment are high nationally, will prove problematic and possibly result in many of them being condemned to living lives blighted by economic deprivation.

Common treatments

Medication treatment is the main intervention for all mental health patients and all mental health problems; consequently, in the last decade, drug expenditure in Greece has increased dramatically. Medicines are subsidised by the social security system at a high rate (nearly 25%). This situation has caused some con-cern at ministerial level within the Greek Department of Health, with the result that directives have seen issued to limit and control pharmaceutical expenditure. To ensure this takes place, the Health Procurement Committee (HPC) was established in January 2009 with the sole remit of implementing measures for pharmaceutical constraint.

In the last 20 years, psychotherapeutic interventions (e.g. cognitive, behavioural, psychoanalytic, psychodynamic, art therapy, etc.) have become a common part of treatment. A growing number of psychiatrists, nurses, psychologists and social workers are now participating in psychotherapeutic training programmes and devising services where these interventions are central. Even though there is no legislation in Greece to integrate all these programmes and to give official license to 'therapists', these interventions play a critical role in patients' treatment. There is evidence that the once-reductionist medical model which predominated within the Greek mental health system is gradually being replaced by psycho-education coupled with psychosocial approaches.

Quality monitoring and effectiveness of mental health services

In the Greek health system, the evaluation of the quality of extramural services has not yet been formally undertaken, although there are plans to do so. The public character of the existing health care system, coupled with the absence of skilled administrative employees and the fact that there is often a significant delay in the incorporation of newly introduced technological systems, explains why there is obvious resistance to the application of an evaluation procedure. In 2005, in an effort to control the progress of Psychargos III, the Ministry of Health, in cooperation with the Ministry of Education, started conducting investigations to examine whether or not responses to policies were having a positive impact on improving the health of people (Public Law 1590/16-11-2005).

Studies evaluating the impact of the reform, the policies and funding programmes intended to promote the community care of mental health patients, are scarce. Since the beginning of the reform, very few studies have been conducted concerning the evaluation of the rehabilitation programmes (Stylianidis, 1992; Stylianidis and Ghionakis, 1997). These studies have shown the positive impact of the rehabilitation process in patients' life quality, functioning and staff–patient interaction. Studies that have focused specifically on the discharge of patients from Leros hospital and their placement in community apartments have also shown a significant improvement in patients' quality of life (Zissi and Barry, 1997; Paxinos, 2005). Stylianidis *et al.* (2008) conducted research concerning the evaluation of the impact of care transfer from psychiatric hospitals to community residential homes as part of a wider evaluation project of all services provided by the Scientific Association for Regional Development and Mental Health (EPAPSY). The results have shown that the rehabilitation process had a significant, positive impact on patients' level of functioning. In 1997, a novel legislation provided for a new governmental agency. This agency was to be responsible for the evaluation of quality control, economic elements and health technology assessment (Liaropoulos and Kaitelidou, 2000). Due to the continuing pressure for the minimisation of spending, combined with the emergent need for improvement in quality of health services, the evaluation of the existing services has become imperative. Greater emphasis must be given to the patient and to the satisfaction of his/her needs.

Service users' experience of services

There is virtually no research concerning service users' experiences of mental health services. In Greece, when discussions on what patients get from services take place, it is always assumed that what is reported is truly what they feel, despite never asking them. The unsatisfactory nature of this situation has been pointed out on several occasions and in numerous ways, but as yet with little results. There are a number of reasons this is so, including the following:

- Lack of financial resources gives rise to lack of incentives to carry out such evaluations.
- Lack of resources can lead to the belief that nothing can be done about problems that are discovered.
- In 1999, Law 2716/1999 was introduced by the Human Rights Committee, which made certain statements to the Ministry of Health concerning the violation of patients' rights. Unfortunately, this committee ceased to exist in 2010.
- ARGOS, a network of 36 non-profit NGOs, has since 1990 been responsible for the planning and organisation of Leros Mental Health Hospital. It has played an important part in the deinstitutionalisation of chronic mental patients and people with mental retardation, in promoting their psychosocial reintegration into smaller communities, and the reform of the mental health care system. However, the future of this organisation is not certain.

In 2007, ARGOS sent a letter to the European Commissioner pointing out the main problems which in their estimation were having a direct impact on the improvement of mental health services. Among the problems they raised were:

- long delays in the payment of mental health workers
- poor monitoring of care facilities
- a continuous lowering of standards
- a reluctance on the part of any agency to intervene
- most mental health centres suffer from inadequate staffing. The lack of managerial and financial autonomy of the centres impedes the implementation of different policies.

Despite the promises of improvement, organisations like the Pan-Hellenic Federation of Families for Mental Health (POSOPSY) continue to point out that the barriers faced by patients and their families, in some parts of the country, are as bad as they have always been.

Staffing

In the era of the reform of the mental health care system in Greece (1984–2006), there was a change in the geographical distribution of mental health personnel. Additionally, the gradual reduction in the number of beds was accompanied by an increase in the number of mental health staff in public mental hospitals. The greatest changes were observed in the ratio of psychiatrists and psychologists per 100 beds, as shown in Table 5.3.

TABLE 5.3 Hospital personnel and length of stay

	1984	1987	1990	1993	1996	2000	1984–2000 change, %
Personnel per 100 beds	7487	6889	5460	5460	5007	3315	−55.7
Psychiatrists	2.01	2.80	3.15	3.58	6.31	6.30	+213.4
Psychologists	0.53	0.68	0.68	0.70	1.10	9.32	+337.7
Social workers	0.58	0.67	0.83	0.90	1.44	1.93	+69.9
Nurses	30.9	33.0	36.2	38.0	37.6	60.0	+94.2
Occupational therapists	0.25	0.44	0.53	062	1.00	1.00	+75.0
Length of stay (days)	408.5	457.7	334.6	257.1	221.0	108.0	−73.5

Source: Madianos, 2002

Mental health law
•••••••••••••••••••••••

The main mental health law was enacted in 1979 with the specific aims of improving the arrangements for the care of the chronic mentally ill regarding compulsory hospital admission and ensuring that their rights were protected. In the following years, several new laws have been added with special reference to vocational rehabilitation, employment experience for people with special needs and social welfare benefit policy for the noninsured mentally disabled (Stefanis *et al.*, 1986).

Greek law also provides possible actions to detain a person in hospital against their will in certain circumstances. Where a patient does not have the capacity to consent, then either the legal guardians (blood relatives, relatives by marriage, spouses or persons who have custody of the person) or the juridical magistrate himself will request or promote a reception order to the court for psychiatric evaluation. The patient is brought to the mental health hospital or ward in the custody of the police; the officers are often required to be present at the psychiatric evaluation. If this evaluation indicates a need for involuntary hospitalisation, a court order must be obtained.

For involuntary admission, the following conditions must be met:
- There is strong suspicion of a psychiatric disorder.
- It is impossible to obtain the consent of the patient, while at the same time the severity of the illness may lead to a serious deterioration of their condition.
- The involuntary admission is considered essential for their mental health state, in order for the appropriate treatment to be administered.
- There is an obvious risk of harm to self or others.

In fact, only the court can order the patient's involuntary admission. The publication of any juridical decision must be issued within 10 days, taking into account the medical opinion of two psychiatrists. Until then, the patient is involuntarily detained in the mental health ward or hospital. This is a provisional incarceration in the form of obligatory hospitalisation.

After the issuing of the juridical decision, the length of the involuntary hospitalisation may not exceed 6 months. After the first 3 months, the psychiatrist in charge of the mental health ward, together with another psychiatrist, presents a written report to the juridical magistrate concerning the mental health condition of the patient. The juridical magistrate shares the report in court, requesting either the interruption or the continuation of the patient's hospitalisation. The renewal order may extend this period by a further 3-month period (to a maximum of 6 months).

Law 2716/17-5-1999 was the first mental health law that included regulations for a significant number of mental health issues:
- the organisation of mental health facilities
- the formation of a committee responsible for the protection of the rights of a person with mental health problems
- the sectorisation of mental health services
- special settlements for mental health extramural facilities, such as community mental health centres, inpatient psychiatric departments, day centres, mobile units, psychosocial rehabilitation units, mental health services for children
- adequate and appropriate staffing levels
- patients with special needs.

In 2004, 12 mental health sectors were introduced in order to resolve administrative and managerial issues (Public Law 937/23-6-2004). With Public Law 1537/15-10-200, any newly introduced mental health facility was officially incorporated in each mental health sector. In 2004, the Hellenic Regulatory Body of Nurses was established with the aim of uniting all nurses of differing educational backgrounds. This body works on behalf of mental health nurses, and in addition to clarifying their role in a changing world, it seeks to ensure that nurses have the opportunities for undertaking relevant training, accessing supervised clinical experience and having the opportunity to work independently.

The new Medical Ethical Code was initiated in 2005. In Article 28, there is a specific description of the exact acts that constitute the practice of the psychiatrist (Public Law 287/28-11-2005). Under these regulations, psychiatrists must follow concrete guidelines for the treatment of mentally ill patients. Since 2001, the Nurse Ethical Code has only one paragraph for psychiatric nurses' responsibilities concerning the provision of care with respect to patients' will, on the condition that the patient is totally capable to decide on his/her own situation (Public Law 167/25-7-2001). This fact constitutes a serious lack in legislation concerning psychiatric nurses' responsibilities (Hellenic Regulatory Body of Nurses).

Current role of nursing in mental health care

All of Greece has a shortage of professional mental health nurses, and what nurses there are face a number of professional problems. By moving the majority of services into community settings, it would seem logical that that is where the majority of nurses should be. However, as can be seen in Table 5.3 above, a high number of nurses remain in hospital settings, and furthermore there are no organised educational programmes devised to assist these individuals. Training in psychosocial rehabilitation in other nursing programmes is either poor or does not exist at all. All that can be said is that the work of practical nurses in mental health settings remains largely controlled and monitored by doctors, a situation that does little to advance the professional standing of nurses.

Koukia et al. (2009) reported that the principal constraint, as perceived by nurses to their independence and autonomy, is their accountability to the law and to other professionals. Beginning with basic nursing education that has to meet their expected role in an inpatient unit, Greek nurses revealed several areas with which they have concerns. Firstly, in many situations nurses have to rely on their instincts and previous experience to help them cope with patients' psychiatric problems, for which they have no preparation or education. There is an urgent need for mental health nurses to be trained in certain therapeutic skills in order to fulfil the role they occupy. The areas that seem to be a priority in Greek nursing education are the managing of crises, and training in specific therapeutic techniques, e.g. problem solving, counselling and communication skills. Without adequate training, progress in the improvement of Greek mental health services will continue to cause concern. It is imperative that continuing professional education is provided for nurses. If nurses could prescribe medication, they would be able to deliver much faster services, engage in early interventions and periodically monitor progress, thus adding considerably to what currently exists.

Of course, in the absence of education and training, being able to acquire these skills is impossible.

Service users' views of mental health nursing

The quality of the relationship between service users and mental health nurses is an unexplored field in Greek mental health services. On the occasions that service users have been invited to comment on services, their main complaint is that there is a chronic shortage of nurses. Not only have they requested an increase in nurses generally, but they have specifically identified primary care as being significantly short of psychiatric services and mental health nurses.

Effectiveness of mental health nursing

To date, few concentrated attempts have been made to identify the specific work of nurses in mental health care. The reason for this is that what they do is dependent on what doctors direct them to do, not what they consider important or necessary. Koukia et al. (2009) conducted a study concerning the work of nurses and types of interventions they deliver in inpatient psychiatric wards. The results indicated that nurses spent a great deal of their time controlling the behaviour of patients, usually in situations where there was a minimum number of nurses on duty, where medical staff only worked in the mornings and where there were long periods of time when there was no access to a doctor. The lack of protocols, procedures, guidelines and professional and legal autonomy leave nurses with a sense of inefficiency.

Relationship with other professions

The most frequently made criticism by Greek nurses is the lack of support for them from nursing management and medical staff. Doctors usually provide little information and do not give clear instructions on how to manage difficult patients; furthermore, they are usually not available when difficulties occur. In most cases, the instructions nurses receive is to administer injections of sedative medication in case of an extreme episode. This fact, in addition to the nurses' limited autonomy as a result of the existing legislation, results in nurses feeling confused about their roles and inadequate about initiating anything that has not been directed by a doctor. Curiously, nurses state that they have good relationships with doctors, even though they would prefer to have a more central role in the delivery of more effective care (Koukia et al., 2009). The newly introduced extramural services will have to be staffed by multidisciplinary teams in the future, thus requiring that more professionals than doctors and nurses collaborate to provide these services.

Future plans for mental health care

Greece, among other countries in the European region, has signed and endorsed the Mental Health Declaration for Europe and the Mental Health Action Plan for Europe. Additionally, the Greek Ministry of Health under a new contract, referred to as the Spidla Agreement, is involved to ensure that the psychiatric reform programme continues until the end of 2015. In undertaking this, Greece has committed itself to address these major priorities:

- The Government has to complete the deinstitutionalisation of mental health patients and continue the psychiatric reform.
- Staffing and financing of existing and newly introduced facilities must continue.
- Evaluation of performance and quality of mental health services must be undertaken, regardless of the financial cutbacks.
- Qualitative research should focus on the results and the obstacles of the implementation of the psychiatric reform programme. The urgency to evaluate the effectiveness of interventions in community mental health settings is obvious.
- More focused primary care and prevention programmes have to be implemented in various regions, especially in rural areas.
- The decentralisation of the existing system must be combined with equal financial and geographical access for all citizens.
- The level of poverty and the difficulties that many disabled people have in finding paid employment are priorities. More emphasis is required to improve the outcomes for vocational rehabilitation programmes.
- More availability and better-quality training in mental health for primary care personnel.
- A much more focused approach to health promotion and prevention.

The need for a reform of the Greek mental health care system became imperative in 1983. Law 1397/83, Article 21 provided the grounds for deinstitutionalisation and decentralisation of psychiatric services from 1984 to 2006. With respect to this reform, thousands of psychiatric patients were discharged; furthermore, admissions to mental health hospitals decreased and the number of beds in the public sector was reduced. Finally, community-based and rehabilitation services were founded in many areas of the country.

Despite these impressive changes, a number of constraints, inefficiencies and poor practices require immediate attention. The main problem of the Greek psychiatric reform is the inadequate attention that has been given to both financing and staffing the project. The significant reduction in funds from the Ministry of Health and Social Solidarity affects the efficient functioning of the extramural services. There is also a serious lack of mental health units in rural and semi-rural areas. Prevention of mental illness, evaluation of the quality of mental health services and staff training in community psychiatry are some of the key matters which require reorganisation and programming. Additionally, patients' and families' evaluation, as well as evaluation of the quality of care provided, indicate that the mere provision of services is insufficient; it is the quality and effectiveness of these services that matter to people in the long run. Without these changes, the reform of the mental health system can only be said to be partially achieved. The continuance of what, until recently, has been the state of mental health services in Greece cannot be allowed to continue; otherwise, the danger of the complete failure of the reform programme is likely.

Case scenario

A 23-year-old unemployed man is reported by his landlord as acting increasingly strangely. He has barricaded his room, talking about being spied upon by the CIA. He can be heard shouting within his room in an angry and incoherent way. He has not been seen by a psychiatrist in the past, although his mother has told the landlord that he has been isolating himself and acting increasingly oddly over the last couple of years.

Either the landlord or a relative, in this case the mother, will contact the community services in their neighbourhood. Firstly, the community mental health centre's staff would try to persuade the person through his mother to come to the CMHC. If there is no such community facility in the neighbourhood or if the person denies any specialist intervention, the mother should call the police. The police will pick up the person, but firstly a reception order from the juridical magistrate needs to be issued, and then he will be admitted to an institution. The routine approach is that two psychiatrists will examine him in the emergency department of a mental or general hospital in order to diagnose his condition. Then he will remain in the hospital for at least 1 month, in order to receive treatment; there he will be under the care of a supervising psychiatrist who will decide the details of the treatment.

Usually, prescribing medication would be the first intervention once in hospital. Psychotherapeutic intervention on a public or private basis will follow during the first period (normally 2–4 weeks) and vocational rehabilitation if needed, after which the patient will be discharged from the hospital. Usually, the final stage of intervention will be the placement of the patient in a residential facility. This procedure is followed when either the family is incapable of accommodating the patient or he is unable to live on his own and pay the rent in an apartment. At this point, the main intervention that a nurse provides, in a hospital or in a community centre, is counselling and support for the patient and his family. She can also follow up the medication prescribed by the doctor and assist in addressing the possible side effects. If the nurse works in home-care nursing, she follows up the patient in his residence for a long period of time.

Concerning the follow-up of the patient, the nurse will have to refer to the community centre in the region in which the patient resides. If there is no community centre, the patient is given two options: either the outpatient clinic of the hospital will follow him up, or a private medical doctor will take charge of him. Otherwise, the patient has the choice to continue treatment in the hospital or the community centre only if they contain a day-care facility or a vocational rehabilitation unit.

Acknowledgements

I would like to acknowledge my debt and appreciation to Michael G. Madianos, professor of psychiatry, University of Athens, for stimulating support in the process of writing the chapter.

I would also like to thank Panagiota Sourtzi, associate professor of nursing, University of Athens, and Nikolaos Gonis, biologist, for their valuable help.

References

Beckwith J. *Early Christian and Byzantine Art.* New York, NY: Yale University Press; 1986.

Economou M, Richardson C, Gramandani C, *et al.* Knowledge about schizophrenia and attitudes towards people with schizophrenia in Greece. *Int J Soc Psychiatry.* 2009; **55**(4): 361–3.

Koukia E, Madianos M, Katostaras T. On-the spot interventions by mental health nurses in inpatient psychiatric wards. *Issues Ment Health Nurs.* 2009; **30**(5): 327–36.

Liaropoulos L, Kaitelidou D. Health technology assessment in Greece. *Int J Technol Assess Health Care.* 2000; **16**(2): 429–48.

Madianos MG. Deinstitutionalization and the closure of public mental hospitals. *Int J Ment Health.* 2002; **31**(3): 66–75.

Madianos MG, Christodoulou GN. Reform of the mental healthcare system in Greece, 1984–2006. *Int Psychiatry.* 2007; **1**(4): 16–19.

Madianos MG, Economou M, Hatjiandreou M, *et al.* Changes in public attitudes towards mental illness in the Athens area (1979/1980–1994). *Acta Psychiatr Scand.* 1999; **99**(1): 73–8.

Madianos MG, Madianou D, Vlachonikolis J, *et al.* Attitudes towards mental illness in the Athens area: implications for community mental health intervention. *Acta Psychiatr Scand.* 1987; **75**(2): 158–65.

Madianos MG, Priami M, Alevisopoulos G, *et al.* Nursing students' attitudes change towards mental illness and psychiatric case recognition after a clerkship in psychiatry. *Issues Ment Health Nurs.* 2005; **26**(2): 169–83.

Madianos MG, Tsiantis J, Zacharakis C. Changing patterns of mental health care in Greece (1984–1996). *Eur Psychiatry.* 1999; **14**: 462–7.

Missouridou E. Exploring the past: mental health nursing in Greece. *J Psychiatr Ment Health Nurs.* 2009; **16**: 18–26.

Paxinos I. Perceptions of quality of life among residents of community residential units of Leros Hospital. *Tetradia Psychiatrikis*. 2005; **90**: 47–55.

Stefanis CN, Madianos MG, Gittelman M. Recent developments in the care, treatment, and rehabilitation of the chronic mentally ill in Greece. *Hosp Community Psychiatry*. 1986; **37**(10): 1041–4.

Stylianidis SF, Pantelidou SM, Chondros PC. Evaluation of the rehabilitation process in Greek Community Residential homes: resettlement from Greek Psychiatric Hospitals. *Int J Psychosoc Rehab*. 2008; **13**(1): 31–8.

Stylianidis S. The experiment of Evia: an attempt between understanding and action. *Tetradia Psychiatrikis*. 1992; **40**: 108–18.

Stylianidis S, Ghionakis N. *La situazione in Grecia ed il caso Leros. La cronicita ed I loro bisogni*. Bergamo: CIC Edizioni Internazionali; 1997. pp. 51–8.

World Health Organization. *Atlas: country profiles*. Geneva: World Health Organization; 2001.

World Health Organization. *Mental Health Atlas 2005*. Athens: WHO; 2005.

World Health Organization. *European Health for All Database (HFA-DB)*. 2008. Available at: www. euro.who.int/en/what-we-do/data-and-evidence/databases/european-health-for-all-database-hfa-db2 (accessed 13 December 2011).

Zissi A, Barry MM. From Leros asylum to community-based facilities: levels of functioning and quality of life among hostel residents in Greece. *Int J Soc Psychiatry*. 1997; **43**(2): 104–15.

Mental health services in Ireland

Ann J Sheridan

Introduction

This chapter describes the evolution of Irish mental health services. In ancient times, Ireland had one of the most progressive approaches to people who suffered from disorders of mind and spirit. The chapter provides a brief overview of the population, economic activity and changing pattern of health need. An historical overview of mental health care, along with a critical depiction of the key health professionals associated with it, is also presented. The current system of mental health care and service provision is then explored, along with future plans for provision of services in Ireland.

National profile and context

The Republic of Ireland, referred to throughout this chapter as Ireland, is an independent country making up the majority of the island of Ireland. Its only land border is with Northern Ireland (NI), a part of the United Kingdom located on the northeastern part of the island. Ireland, along with the United Kingdom and Denmark, became a member of the European Economic Community, now the European Union (EU), in 1973 and is now one of 27 countries in that economic union. Along with the majority of other EU countries, it adopted the euro currency in 2002.

Population and demographics

Over the last four decades, Ireland's population has almost doubled, growing from 2.9 million in 1966 to 4.2 million in 2006, with current estimates that it will increase to 5.1 million by 2041. However, Ireland remains one of the least densely populated countries in Europe, with an overall population density for the state of 60 people per square kilometre. Dublin has the highest population density, with 4304 per square kilometre, followed by Cork (3015) and Limerick (2582). Counties Leitrim and Mayo, both on the western seaboard, have the lowest density at 18 and 22 people per square kilometre, respectively (CSO 2007). While a significant proportion of this population growth is attributable to natural increases, over the past decade historically high net inward migration combined with natural increases has resulted in an unparalleled average annual population increase of over 80 000 or nearly 2% per annum (CSO, 2008a). The past two decades have also seen increasing urbanisation in Ireland, with 61% of the population currently dwelling in urban areas. Conversely, this increasing urbanisation is occurring at the same time as the population of the five major cities is decreasing.

Although the past four decades have seen a decline in the total fertility rate in Ireland, it continues to have one of the highest fertility rates in the EU. As a country, Ireland also has one of the youngest populations in the EU, with 20% of its population between 0 and 14 years and 46% between 15 and 44 years. Additionally, it has the second-lowest proportion of those over 65 years in the EU. Recent high levels of immigration have resulted in increased ethnic and cultural diversity, and this has impacted on the population age structure. The age distribution of ethnic minority groups in Ireland is markedly younger than the overall population, and this is due principally to recent immigration patterns (CSO, 2008b).

Along with changes in ethnic/cultural diversity are changes in the religious composition of the population. Muslims, although still a relatively small group, are now the third-largest religious group in the state behind Catholics and Church of Ireland. Over the past decade, the Islamic population in Ireland has continued to increase and now stands at 32 500, continuing the growth observed in 1991 and 2002.

Economically, Ireland was recently ranked 11th in the world, with a per capita GDP of US$45,100. The service sector was the main contributor to national income, accounting for 45% of GNP. The construction industry had been significant over the past decade, with a price boom in domestic housing unparalleled in any other OECD country from the late 1990s to 2009. Ireland is heavily dependent on the export market, and its main trade partners are the United States, the United Kingdom and Belgium (McDaid et al., 2009). It is also heavily reliant on inward foreign investment and is therefore very vulnerable to external events, as has been demonstrated during the recent financial downturn. Between 2008 and the time of writing, house prices have fallen by up to 50% in some parts of the country, construction of new housing has almost ceased and unemployment has risen sharply.

Health status and changing health need

The health status of the population has improved since the 1970s, with mortality rates decreasing markedly in most disease areas. Average life expectancy for males in 2006, at 77.47 years, was slightly above the average of the EU countries, while that for females, 82.2 years, was just slightly lower than the EU average of 82.7 years (McDaid *et al.*, 2009). Infant mortality rates are low, at 3.71 per 1000 births, as are maternal mortality rates at 3.8 per 100000 live births. The principal causes of mortality are circulatory diseases, followed by cancer, which accounted for 62% of all deaths in 2005. Lung cancer (21%) was most common, followed by colorectal cancer (12%) and breast cancer (8%).

Although health status is improving, these improvements are not reflected equally across all sections of society. The adverse impact of social deprivation on health continues to be evident among the socially disadvantaged and other groups, including prisoners, the travelling community and the homeless population. In 2008, Farrell *et al.* reported that 38% of those classed as being at risk of poverty were suffering from a chronic illness, compared to 23% of the general population. Harkin (2001) reported that all causes of mortality were two to three times as high in lower socio-economic groups. Likewise, the Chief Medical Officer (2002), reporting five years' (1991–96) data from the National Psychiatric In-Patient Reporting System, provided evidence of an increasing socio-economic gradient in incidence of all psychiatric conditions from professional to unskilled manual group. This report also identified that the prison population suffers from a disproportionately high rate of psychiatric and drug-related problems. All mental health indicators are much worse for prisoners than for the general population, and are particularly high for female prisoners (CMO, 2002). Members of the travelling community have significantly poorer health status than the general population. Within this community, travellers of all ages have much higher mortality rates than people in the general population. Suicide rates and rates for other psychiatric conditions are also increased disproportionally in this population (CMO, 2002).

The health status of the adult homeless population is also less than the population average. Homeless adults suffer from a substantially greater burden of ill health, including depression, hypertension, hepatitis, alcoholism and illicit drug use. Furthermore, they also experience significant difficulty in accessing the health services they require (CMO, 2002).

In Ireland, more people are now living longer than at any time in the past, and it is estimated that by 2041 25% of the population will be over the age of 65. While this increase in longevity represents one of the greatest achievements of the last century, it will also pose significant challenges. The WHO's Global Burden of Disease assessment predicts a very large increase in disability caused by increases in age-related chronic disease in all regions of the world. In a few decades, the loss of health and life worldwide will be greater from non-communicable or chronic diseases (e.g. cardiovascular disease, dementia and Alzheimer's disease, cancer, arthritis and diabetes) than from infectious diseases, childhood diseases and accidents (US Department of Health and Human Services, 2007).

Health system

In Ireland, the Department of Health and Children (DOH&C), under the direction of the minister for health and ministers for state, has overarching responsibility for health and personal social services (McDaid *et al.*, 2009). The Irish health system is predominantly funded through the tax system and while having features similar to the UK NHS, does not equate directly with it.

Structurally, the health services are organised, funded and managed by the Health Services Executive (HSE), established following a major reform programme in 2005 which reconfigured the health system into a single national entity accountable directly to the minister of health. Prior to this, the health system was governed by the Health Act (1970), which created eight health boards funded directly by the Department of Health. The HSE has three key divisions: population health; hospitals; and primary, community and continuing care. It is organised into four administrative areas: Dublin North East, Dublin Mid-Leinster, Southern and Western. It has a budget of more than €13 billion and is the largest employer in the state, employing more than 65 000 staff directly and a further 35 000 indirectly. However, the system continues to include elements of its past and can best be described as a tripartite system comprised of public health services, voluntary health services and private health services.

Public services are funded, organised and managed directly by the HSE; voluntary agencies are also funded primarily by the HSE, but are owned and managed by separate boards of management. Voluntary agencies existed prior to the establishing of the public health system and constituted the major health provision in Ireland. These voluntary services, including the majority of acute care hospitals, the three major maternity hospitals and three paediatric hospitals, were originally owned and run independently by religious orders or corporate bodies. They currently provide public services as well as private services on a contractual basis with private health insurance companies and medical consultants.

In addition to the acute care services, the majority of intellectual disability services are provided by voluntary agencies which are funded by the HSE. Private health services, which receive no state funding, include both acute care and psychiatric hospitals. These agencies are privately owned and managed and are funded entirely by private sources, generally private health insurance schemes. However, in the case of psychiatric services, the HSE purchases services and beds within these private hospitals as part of the public service provision. General practitioners, dentists and opticians are private providers. They provide public services under contract with the HSE through the General Medical Scheme (GMS) and private services based on a fee per consultation basis. The majority of GP practices in Ireland continue to be either single handed or small group practices.

While all members of the population can access the public health system, only about one third can do so free of charge. The remainder of the population has to make some form of payment at the point of access, including fees for general practitioner services, medications, attendance at accident and emergency, inpatient acute services, dental treatment and ophthalmic services. Almost half of the population contribute to voluntary private health insurance schemes.

Mental health need and services

According to the World Health Organization (2004), mental health problems account for approximately 20% of the total disability burden of ill health across Europe, and they estimate that approximately one in four people will experience mental health difficulties at some point in their lives. To date, Irish data relating to the incidence and prevalence of mental health issues is limited. Results from the first National Psychological Wellbeing and Distress Survey (NPWDS) were published by the Health Research Board in 2007 (Tedstone-Doherty et al., 2007) and identified that 12% of adults aged 18 years and over were at risk of psychological distress.

The 2006 Irish census and the National Disability Survey identified information relating to disability resulting from emotional, psychological or mental health disability. In the 2006 census, a total of 61 499 people aged 15 years and over identified themselves as having a disability associated with a psychological or emotional condition. Of these, 25 803 people (13 105 males and 12 698 females) stated that they were unable to work due to permanent sickness or disability, and the unemployment rate for people with a psychological or emotional condition was 28%, much higher than the national unemployment rate of 8.5% (O'Shea and Kennelly, 2008).

The National Disability Survey (2006) identified that people with an emotional, psychological or mental health disability accounted for 34% of the population reporting a disability, the vast majority of these, 67%, were between the ages of 18 and 64 years and just over 23% began being affected by their disability between the ages of 18 and 34 years. People with an emotional, psychological or mental health disability also reported the highest usage of aids for their disability (medical services – GP, community nurse = 77%; counselling = 25%; medication = 66%; support groups) with 90% using at least one aid (National Disability Survey, 2006). While health budgets in most European region countries have increased, the proportion of the health spend devoted to promoting and maintaining mental health, and treating mental illness, has in real terms decreased. In 2007, a total of €1.04 billion was allocated to the HSE for mental health service provision in Ireland and this accounted for approximately 6% of the total health spend.

Suicidal behaviour remains an important public health issue in Ireland. Over the last decade, there has been increasing concern with regard to the suicide rate, with deaths by suicide accounting for 26% of all deaths by external causes. In 2001, 458 deaths by suicide occurred, representing a rate of 10.6 deaths per 100 000 population. Central Statistics Office (CSO) figures for year of registration of death for 2009 (referred to as provisional) show an increase from 424 in 2008 to 527 in 2009. This is an increase of 24% on the previous year. The impact of the economic downturn in Ireland in 2008, and particularly in 2009, has led to substantial increases in both self-harm and suicide numbers. While suicide in Ireland is a predominantly male problem, and the highest rate occurs in young men aged 20–24 years (34.7 per 100 000), the overall suicide rate remains high (above 20 per 100 000 population) for those up to and including men aged 60–64 years.

Attitudes to mental health problems

Mental illness is associated with profound stigmatisation, which can and does result in cultural dispossession and alienation, with social exclusion occurring as an end point of stigmatisation (Johnstone, 2001; Reidpath *et al.*, 2005). The relationships between mental illness, social isolation, loneliness and stigma are complex, with many elements such as housing, low income, unemployment and restricted social networks being both a cause and a consequence of mental illness (Repper and Perkins, 2003; Prince and Gerber, 2005). While loneliness is frequently identified as a serious issue, as yet, little evidence exists of the degrees or nature of loneliness experienced by individuals with serious mental illness. However, initial results from a randomised controlled trial of supported socialisation for people with serious mental illness being undertaken in Ireland is producing evidence that this population have significantly higher rates of romantic, social and family loneliness when compared to the general population (Tait and Lester, 2005).

Social networks are essential in that they not only enable a person to become part of the social structure to which they belong but also affect their health.

Increasingly, social exclusion is being recognised as an important determinant of population health, with its negative impact arising out of restricted access to the social goods and services that act to support health.

A study by the National Disability Authority (2007) identified that the most negative attitudes towards disability related to people with mental health difficulties. In relation to education, only 36% of respondents agreed that children with mental health difficulties should be in the same school as other children, with 21% of respondents saying they would object if children with mental health difficulties were in the same class as their child. Just 7% of respondents thought employers would be willing to employ people with mental health difficulties, and respondents reported they would be least comfortable having people with mental health difficulties as work colleagues. In relation to parenting, 41% of respondents thought people with mental health difficulties should have children if they wish. These recent results make it evident that while concerted efforts have been made in recent years to raise public awareness of mental health and illness through media campaigns and education, much remains to be achieved in addressing public attitudes to mental health issues and in reducing the associated stigma.

Historical development of mental health services

Ireland has long been the subject of British interest and governance, and in effect it existed in some form from the fourteenth century up to the achieving of independence in 1921. The exercise of dominion by Britain over Ireland throughout the centuries has impacted on all aspects of life, including the care of the mentally ill.

Over the past two centuries in Ireland, the mentally ill have been identified as a group deserving of some special provision relating to their care and treatment. In earlier centuries, prior to the occupation of Ireland by Britain, laws existed which made specific provision for the insane. The Brehon Laws, which originated in pre-Christian Ireland, had effect up to the Elizabethan period, and according to Robins (1986) attempted to ensure the provision of care for the insane person by their family or the community. While the laws contained various penalties for failure to care for the insane person, it is difficult to establish if these laws afforded protection to the mentally ill. It is more likely, however, that those who were unable to care for themselves due to mental illness were incarcerated in pits, barns and outhouses, and beyond the provision of food were left there to die (Robbins, 1986).

With the re-establishing of direct British rule in Ireland in the early eighteenth century, no formal system of public provision for the sick, including the mentally ill, existed. The mentally ill were catered for in institutions including houses of correction, gaols, houses of industry and workhouses. These institutions, established to address the effects of poverty and criminal behaviour, had as their principal aim the reforming of the moral character of criminals and the poor. In the absence of other means of providing for the sick, these institutions provided accommodation and welfare to a substantial number of sick people, including the mentally ill. It soon became apparent that these institutions, aimed as they were at reforming the moral character of criminals and other offenders including the 'undeserving poor', were unable to cater for the mentally ill. Within a short period of time, 'violent lunatics' were confined to cells and frequently shackled in an attempt to prevent them harming themselves or others. Confinement and control were the only available options to the keepers of the houses of corrections and gaols, just as it had been in earlier times for families of the insane.

Throughout the eighteenth century in Ireland, the care of the mentally ill remained within the remit of these institutions. Apart from a few incidents of isolated provision by private philanthropic individuals and societies, no system of public provision of care existed.

By the end of the eighteenth century, however, the political situation in Ireland altered significantly. The introduction of the Act of Union in 1800 abolished the Irish Parliament, and on 1 January 1801 united the two kingdoms of England and Ireland 'forever'. The results of this union heralded a new era in institutional provision, including the establishment of the asylum system (Key 1982; Finnane, 1981). The establishment of the asylum system in Ireland pre-dated its British counterpart; however, it was by no means an indigenous development. This valorisation of the progressive institution, including the asylum, considered light, air and separate spaces for eating, sleeping and working not just as an end in themselves, but as a means to an end in creating a new person in Ireland who was, according to British measurement, rational, law-abiding and industrious (Saris, 1996). Thus, in the view of Saris (1996), the establishment of the nineteenth-century asylum system was deliberatively constructed to provide a productive environment that rectified deficits in unproductive individuals and therefore acted as a primary means of ordering Irish society.

The Richmond Lunatic Asylum, the first public asylum in Ireland, was opened in 1815 and was intended to provide for the reception of lunatics from all parts of the Kingdom of Ireland (Reynolds, 1992). By 1835, 10 asylums had been constructed in the first stage of development of the Irish asylum system. The second phase of asylum development was initiated in 1852 and was in response to the seemingly ever-increasing numbers of insane in Ireland requiring accommodation, a large proportion of whom were considered 'incurable'. In contrast to the earlier asylums, these new institutions were bigger, providing accommodation for up to 500 inmates in an attempt to relieve the by-now-chronic problem of overcrowding (Finnane, 1981).

The twentieth century

The final phase of development and consolidation of the asylum system occurred at the beginning of the twentieth century with the building of extensions to a number of district asylums and the building of auxiliary asylums. Again, these extensions and auxiliary asylums were primarily designed to deal with the problems of overcrowding within the district asylums and to provide accommodation for the large number of inmates deemed incurable.

By the first decade of the twentieth century, the asylum had become the primary means of providing for the insane (Finnane, 1981; Reynolds, 1992). Within a century, from the opening of the first public asylum in 1815, Ireland had come from a situation where there was virtually no public provision for the insane, to one where accommodation was being provided for approximately 17 000 patients in public asylums throughout the island of Ireland (Finnane, 1981). Furthermore, it was estimated that accommodation for up to a further 1000 patients was provided by private asylums. However, rather than providing a solution to insanity and the care of the mentally ill, it appears that the asylum system itself became self-sustaining. From its inception, there were significant annual increases in the numbers of insane requiring accommodation and treatment within them, and within a short period of time the system became overwhelmed.

By the early years of the twentieth century, the asylums were modelled increasingly on the existing hospital systems for the physically ill. This process served to legitimise the emerging specialities of psychiatry and psychiatric nursing. Attaining professional status for the treatment of madness and consequently for those who treated it brought with it a responsibility to seek new ways of understanding insanity and of dealing with it (Porter, 2002). Having the treatment of mental illness recognised as a legitimate medical pursuit required the doctors associated with it to attempt to discover causes and thereby be able to develop new treatments which would ultimately result in a cure. This somatising of mental illness was also influenced significantly by the emergence of laboratory science and the developments taking place in physiology and other biological sciences (Porter, 2002).

However, it would be erroneous to attribute the medicalisation of madness solely to the medical profession. While there is agreement that the status, dominance and power of the medical profession was a crucial factor in medicalisation, so too were the influence and activities of various social movements and groups who advocated for better treatment and care of the mentally ill and of 'third party players' (Conrad, 2005). Knowingly or unknowingly, these groups facilitated and indeed in some cases advocated for the assigning of medical definitions for problems which had previously been within the jurisdiction of other state apparatuses (Conrad, 2005). Third-party players such as insurance companies further contributed to the legitimising of certain conditions as medical through their decisions to recognise the condition as a legitimate medical one and to agree to pay for the treatments associated with it.

Psychiatric nursing

The care of the insane within early asylums was provided primarily by keepers or attendants. No special training or preparation was provided, and their role was more akin to domestic servants (Reynolds 1992; Malcolm, 1989). The Medico-Psychological Association (MPA), founded in 1841 as the Society of Medical Officers for the Insane, represented the views of asylum superintendents of Great Britain and Ireland. At its annual conference in 1875, a paper presented by Dr Stewart identified the absence of an adequately trained medical and nursing staff within the asylum system as one of the primary causes of the lack of advancement of psychological medicine in Ireland. In 1889, a special committee of the MPA was formed to examine the possibilities of establishing a formal system of training for asylum nurses, their recommendations were adopted by the MPA in 1891 and the first examinations leading to the award of the Certificate of Proficiency in Nursing and Attending on the Insane were held in 1892. Irish asylums were quick to engage with this new scheme.

The first records of attendants in Ireland being formally prepared for the examination of the MPA were in 1894 at the Richmond Asylum in Dublin (Sheridan, 1999). The number of nurses who undertook training in Ireland continued to increase, and by 1900, 334 nurses trained in Irish asylums had been awarded the certificate (Sheridan, 1999). Despite the continuing political and social unrest in Ireland, nurses from Irish asylums continued to undertake the examination of the MPA and by 1914, within 20 years of its introduction, a total of 945 nurses from Irish asylums had successfully completed the examination, with women continuing to outnumber men.

The Nurses' Registration Act in the UK received royal assent in 1919, and while Ireland was still under British rule, the act provided for the separate and distinct registration of nurses in Ireland by authorising the establishment of a General Nursing Council (GNC) for Ireland. While the GNC in Ireland had recognition by and reciprocal arrangements with the GNC for the remainder of the UK, the rules concerning entry to the Irish register were different in that those asylum nurses holding registration with the MPA could seek admission to the register of the Irish GNC without undertaking any further examination as 'existing nurses', and in this provision the GNC (Ireland) differed from its counterparts in the UK (Sheridan, 2006).

Courses in mental nursing continued to be offered by the now Royal

Medico-Psychological Association (RMPA) until 1951, and in reality two parallel systems existed for 28 years. The MPA became the RMPA in 1926. From 1935 onwards, the number of Irish registrants recorded in the RMPA register began to decline, while those registering with the GNC Ireland began to increase. Only in 1950 was a new Nurses Act introduced which dissolved existing statutory bodies, including the General Nursing Council and Central Midwives Board, and replaced them with a single body to be known as An Bord Altranais (Irish Nursing Board).

Gendering of psychiatric nursing roles

Within the institution of the asylums, segregation of male and female staff and patients had existed virtually since its inception, and elements of this segregation continue even in the present day. Within the institution, a substantial proportion of nurses' working time was occupied in activities relating to the smooth and efficient running of the institution. These activities were different for male and female nurses. Male nurses were largely involved in activities such as farming, grounds maintenance and tailoring, while females were primarily concerned with activities of a general domestic type such as laundry, kitchen duties and maintaining the ward environment. The close association of nurses with patients was also evident in leisure and social activities, and again these activities reflected the sexually segregated nature of both the psychiatric hospital and work activities for nurses as much as for patients (Sheridan, 2003).

During the 1960s, this segregation began to take on a new dimension. A significant recommendation for psychiatric nurses to emerge from the report of the Commission of Inquiry on Mental Illness (1966) was a recommendation to ensure males were provided with training to better position them for selection for higher posts. The report recommended that training in group leadership and clinical skills be initiated across services for male staff and that this training should be equated with the obtaining of a post-registration qualification in general nursing for the purposes of selection for higher posts. While recognising that relatively few men were facilitated to undertake general nurse training due to the prevailing systems in general hospitals, which did not provide training for male nurses, except those from religious orders, this recommendation can be viewed as constituting positive discrimination in favour of males as not all females undertook general nurse training. This view of positive discrimination in favour of males is further supported when the commission addressed the issue of patient and staff integration, and it stated that:

> many authorities accept that male nurses are often very suitable as group leaders, organisers of activities of various kinds, tutors and nurse-administrators and in these fields they can provide services to both male and female patients

and the Commission recommends that it should be made possible for them to do so. (Commission of Inquiry, 1966, p. 132)

While females continued to outnumber males by approximately 6 : 1, as promotional posts became available males became increasingly likely to be appointed to senior administrative and education roles. This situation was further consolidated by the existence of a 'marriage bar' for female staff and a system of promotion on seniority. Upon marriage, females were paid a marriage gratuity and could not continue to occupy a permanent or pensionable position. They could continue to work, but only as a 'temporary' member of staff. In effect, this bar on married women changed their status to that of non-permanent, preventing them from accruing service years and a work-related pension. This marriage bar was finally removed in 1979.

While employment equality legislation has done much to improve the working conditions of nurses in all health service sectors, it had particular relevance within psychiatric services. The Employment Equality Act (1977), like many other initiatives pertaining to employment, was primarily prompted by Ireland's membership of the EC and was designed to protect against discrimination on the basis of sex or marital status, in relation to terms and conditions of employment, access to employment, training schemes, benefits, facilities, services and promotion (Mental Health Commission, 2011).

The implications of the Equality Act required a number of fundamental changes to be implemented in Ireland, and significant among these was the use of the title 'nurse'. Traditionally in psychiatric nursing, nurses had been segregated based on their sex, with females caring for female patients and males for male patients. Under the provision of the act, the term 'nurse' was to be used without any restriction based on the sex of the holder of the title and resultantly deployment to clinical settings based on sex was required to cease. The removal of this sexual segregation of nursing staff also required changes in the system of promotion, which until then had been based on seniority (length of service). The system of promotion on merit initially recommended in 1972 was adopted.

Over the intervening decades, improvements in terms and conditions of employment have continued. The removal of the marriage bar in 1979 along with the crediting of years worked by females initiated an increase of promotion of women to management posts. Although the number of females obtaining ward sister/clinical nurse manager posts increased, no significant change in appointments to director of nursing posts occurred. Men, although only accounting for approximately 30% of the psychiatric nursing workforce, continued to occupy the most senior psychiatric nursing roles in management and education.

Changes following independence

For Ireland, achieving political independence from the UK resulted in more than just political separation. The desire of the newly established Irish government was to further Ireland as a separate nation that was 'Gaelic and Catholic'. In the immediate post-independence period, the then head of government considered giving the Vatican the power of veto over legislation contrary to faith and morals in return for papal recognition of the new state (Cooney, 1999). As Catholicisation of the Irish Free State proceeded, the Roman Catholic hierarchy became influential in prompting the government to introduce legislation aimed at preserving the moral character of the citizens of Ireland. The influence of the Catholic hierarchy and its antipathy to communism and socialism extended to areas such as behaviourism and psychoanalysis. This antipathy was important in influencing both the nature and pace of change within psychiatry in Ireland. The Roman Catholic church worldwide was hostile to dynamic psychologies, with the proscription on hypnosis remaining in place until 1955 (Healy, 1996), although this was not unique to Ireland (Oosterhuis, 2005). The rejection of dynamic psychologies by the Roman Catholic church was associated with the focus of therapy on self-directedness, autonomy and self-regulation vis-à-vis sexuality in particular; a position at variance with the church's teaching on obedience and adherence to rules. Ireland's position as a devoutly Catholic country, with the dominance of the Roman Catholic church in all state matters, continued to militate against the introduction of a range of therapies which were becoming accepted practice elsewhere in Europe. Furthermore, in the absence of a strong academic tradition within Irish psychiatry, academic psychiatry in Ireland did not emerge until 1971, and this also undermined progression within Irish mental health services.

Throughout the early years of the twentieth century, there is evidence of continuing concern with regard to provision for the mentally ill. As in previous decades, overcrowding and understaffing within the asylums continued. However, more concerning was the reported absence of treatment within asylums. In an article by Barrett (cited in Kelly, 2008), he considered 'the most lamentable feature of the present asylum system as the absence of treatment'. He further highlighted issues associated with 'poor diet, repulsive and prison like surroundings and hideous clothing'.

While recognising that the turbulence associated with the founding of a new state creates the need to establish new systems and identify core values, and of necessity to focus on issues of relevance to the whole population, when coupled with competition for scarce resources, this inevitably results in the overall development of many public services being haphazard. However, the continued lack of priority afforded to mental health services in Ireland at either policy or legislative levels contributed in this case to the continuation of an outdated system, and has to date resulted in the continuing haphazard and compromised nature of development within mental health services in Ireland.

Mental health legislation

While Ireland was under British rule, it was included in the legislative initiatives associated with the management of the mentally ill. However, following the establishing of the Irish Free State, Ireland diverged increasingly from the remainder of the United Kingdom in that the various revisions of mental health legislation did not apply to Ireland and provisions of the 1867 act remained in force until 1945, when the Mental Treatment Act (1945) was passed (Healy, 1996). This act repealed all previous legislation other than that related to the care of criminal lunatics and wards of court. The 1945 act, as well as having the aim of addressing legislative deficiencies in Irish mental health law, sought to strengthen delivery of appropriate care to individuals as well as reduce numbers within the institutions, reduce stigma associated with mental illness and introduce new provisions for the reception and detention of patients, including the introduction of a new 'voluntary admission' status (Kelly, 2008).

The first comprehensive report dealing specifically with the needs of the mentally ill commissioned since the founding of the Irish Free State, was the Commission of Inquiry on Mental Illness, set up by the minister of health in 1961 and producing its final report in 1966. This report provided an overview of the current state of psychiatric services in Ireland during the 1950s and 1960s and indicated a legacy of inertia. At that time, Ireland had the highest rate of bed provision in the world for the mentally ill, at 7.3 per 1000 of population, and it was estimated that there were approximately 18000 beds provided in district mental hospitals (excluding private institutions, which provided approximately another 1000) throughout the country, most of which had been built in the previous century. It was also acknowledged that these hospitals had inadequate facilities and services, and they lacked the purposeful activity and therapeutic atmosphere considered necessary in a modern mental hospital (Commission of Inquiry, 1966). In reality, very little had changed within the mental hospitals compared to the asylums at the turn of the twentieth century. The mainstay of provision continued to be institutionally based, and while some community-based services, principally outpatient services, did exist, these continued to be located within mental hospitals.

The development of community psychiatric nursing services began to emerge in the 1960s, with initial schemes established in Carlow and St. Brendan's Hospital in Dublin (formally the Richmond Asylum) in 1960. By 1966, five community psychiatric nurses were in post nationally, and by 1983 this number had increased to 166 (Report of Review Group on Community Psychiatric Nursing, 1983).

For Ireland, accession to the EEC was instrumental in initiating change.

Accession brought with it the commitment of the Irish government to bring its national policies in line with those already established within the community of Europe; this necessitated far-reaching changes in existing social, health and employment legislation. However, as in previous eras, these changes were destined to take time.

Current provision of mental health services

Over the past four decades, the number of patients residing in psychiatric hospitals in Ireland has decreased from 19801 in 1963 to 3389 in 2006 (Health Information Quality Authority, 2005). However, the most significant changes in the profile of mental health service provision in Ireland have occurred during the last 25 years. The publication of the report *The Psychiatric Services – Planning for the Future* in 1984 initiated a reorientation of psychiatric services away from the existing institutionally based system towards a community-based service. The main tenets of this report were the recommendation of comprehensive, community-orientated and sectorised services, with the community-based team as the focal point. The term 'sectorisation' describes the process of providing a comprehensive psychiatric service for each sector of a designated geographical or catchment area serving a predetermined population. *Planning for the Future* recommended that each sector have a multidisciplinary team, with each team having a psychiatrist, psychiatric nurses, psychologist, social worker, occupational therapist and a health administrator. Furthermore, it was considered that the components of a comprehensive service should be coordinated effectively so that as patient needs change, movement is encouraged from one type of facility to another without delay (Department of Health, 1984).

It was envisioned that this configuration would allow every person requiring access to psychiatric services to have it with minimum disruption to their normal way of life. These recommendations made explicit that in most instances patients should not be admitted to a psychiatric hospital; furthermore, when admission was required, it should be to a unit in a general hospital and take place only when treatment in the community was not an option.

While the components of a comprehensive service outlined in *Planning for the Future* included prevention and early detection of mental illness, assessment, diagnostic and treatment services, inpatient care, day care and outpatient care, community-based residences, rehabilitation and training, a considerable focus of the report was placed on establishing a range of community-based residences. These residences included hostels, domestic-scale residences and flats, lodgings, supervised hostels, high-support hostels and accommodation attached to day facilities. The emphasis placed on providing alternative accommodation for psychiatric patients highlighted that a primary driver of the 1984 policy was the relocation and rehabilitation of large numbers of psychiatric inpatients to community-based residence. It was considered that community residences would fulfil a therapeutic and rehabilitative function, and it was initially envisaged that patients, particularly those with persistent/enduring mental illness, would progress through the spectrum of 'support', graduating from higher to lower levels of support, with the ultimate aim for the majority of deinstitutionalised individuals being complete independence.

In line with this policy priority, the number and composition of community residences have grown considerably over the past 25 years. In 1984, there were 121 community residences, with 900 places; 20 years later in 2004, the number of people living in community residences exceeded 3000 (Mental Health Commission, 2007). As planned, this development had the intended effect of reducing the number of long-stay patients resident in psychiatric hospitals over a relatively short time period, as advocated in *Planning for the Future*. As a result of this policy, community residences now constitute a very important element of mental health services provision in Ireland, shaping the lives of over 3000 people and utilising considerable personnel and financial resources.

Given the position of community residence or hostels as a core feature of community psychiatric services, the Mental Health Commission commissioned a study in 2007 to examine the nature and quality of community residential accommodation and the extent to which it met the needs of residents. The results of this study identified that in general, residents were satisfied with their treatment and care and their current accommodation. Perceptions of residents about their life in hostels were generally positive, and they reported that they had control over their lives and were happy with their level of independence. However, this study also reported that the climate and culture of the residences reflected more those of a 'mini-institution' than of a home-like environment, especially in the high-support residences. The medium- and low-support residences, while somewhat more relaxed, frequently employed restrictive rules and regulations, and there appeared to be little in the way of individualised treatment and care. It was further reported that there was evidence of an excess of care in some cases, for example, the restrictive nature of residential facilities and the lack of autonomy of the residents given their current level of functioning (MHC, 2007).

In moving away from psychiatric hospital-based accommodation, inpatient acute admission units based in general hospitals were developed, and to a large extent these have now replaced old psychiatric hospital accommodation. In 2008, there were 20752 admissions to psychiatric units and hospitals, representing a rate of 489.5 per 100 000 total population. The number of first admissions increased from 5853 in 2007 to 6194 in 2008, an increase from 138.0 per 100 000 total population in 2007 to 146.1 in 2008. Readmissions accounted for 70% of all admissions, a slight decrease from 2007 (72%). Females had a slightly higher admission rate, at 492.7 per 100 000, than males, at 486.2 per 100 000. With regard to age group and marital and occupational status, the 45- to 54-year age group had the highest rate of all admissions, at 768.5 per 100 000 total population, while the 20- to 24-year age group had the highest rate of first admissions, at 212.9 per 100 000. Single people accounted for over half (54.5%) of all admissions, and the unskilled occupational group had the highest rate of all (975.6) and first (209.5) admissions. Depressive disorders (30%), schizophrenia (19%) and alcohol-related disorders (12%) accounted for 61% of all admissions (Health Information Quality Authority, 2005).

The highest level of activity in community-based mental health services occur within outpatient clinics. In 2004, the last year for which data is available, over 81 000 patients attended 14 000 outpatients' clinics which were held in over 240 locations throughout the country (MHC, 2006). The nature of activity within these clinics generally consists of consultation with doctors and psychiatric nurses; administration of Depo medication and monitoring of blood levels to ensure optimum effectiveness and/or indicators of adverse effects for specific medication. In addition to the above, some outpatient clinics will also provide access to and interventions with social work, psychology and occupational therapy professionals. However, while elements of all services exist in all areas of the country, there is a high degree of variability, in that not all services are available in all areas.

Day hospitals were established following the 1984 report with the intention that they should provide a comprehensive range of treatment on a short-term basis of the same intensity to acutely ill patients as that provided by inpatient services. It was intended that the day hospital be located within the community, be the base of the multidisciplinary team and admit patients as close to referral as possible, thus assisting in the prevention of hospitalisation. In addition, supportive psychotherapeutic treatment was to be provided in day hospital premises on a sessional and time-limited basis (Byrne and Onyett, 2010). In 2004, there were a total of 58 day hospitals, providing a total of 1022 places. Total attendances at day hospitals in 2004 were 162 233.

In addition to the role of the day hospital in providing acute care, emphasis has also been placed on community-based crisis interventions, including home-care approaches for acutely ill patients and assertive outreach for those with more enduring illness with complex presentations. The focus of assertive outreach is qualitatively different from conventional community treatment in that it concentrates its efforts on the delivery of community support through a team approach, high staff-to-patient ratios and the use of a range of naturally occurring community resources (i.e. family, neighbours, friends, employers, voluntary services and educational establishments). Its primary aim is to maintain and support the person within their own community. While the day hospital and assertive outreach/home-care teams focus primarily on acute illness and episodes, day centres place more emphasis on the social and rehabilitative aspects of care. Within day centres, rehabilitation and activation services may be provided and frequently include occupational therapy, social skills training and various therapies, including art and drama therapy. The majority of those who attend a day centre live in supported accommodation, and for a significant proportion, attendance is long term.

Current mental health law

While significant changes occurred throughout mental health services over the four decades from the 1960s to 2000, the 1945 Mental Treatment Act continued to be the mainstay of legal provision. Following a number of false starts, eventually in 2001 the Mental Health Act was formally enacted by the Irish Houses of the Oireachtas (Irish Government) on 8 July and achieved full implementation on 1 November 2006. The Mental Health Act of 2001 is primarily concerned with two aspects of psychiatric provision in Ireland: involuntary detention of persons with mental disorders in approved psychiatric centres and the mechanisms of ensuring standards of mental health care (Kelly, 2007). The act uses the term 'mental disorder', and included in the definition of this broad term are mental illness, severe dementia and significant intellectual disability. Mental illness is defined as:

> a state of mind of a person which affects the person's thinking, perceiving, emotion or judgment and which seriously impairs the mental function of the person to the extent that he or she requires care or medical treatment in his or her own interest or the interest of other persons. (Mental Treatment Act, 2001)

Mental health services are defined as 'services which provide care and treatment to persons suffering from mental illness or a mental disorder under the clinical direction of a consultant psychiatrist'.

The Mental Treatment Act (2001) iterates core principles which underpin the implementation of the act, apply to all patients whether voluntary or compulsory and must be considered when decisions are being made about admission, care and treatment. These principles are as follows:

- The best interest of the person must be the principal consideration in any decision about his/her care and treatment including decisions about admission, as well as having regard to the interest of others at risk of harm if the decision is not made.
- In any proposal about admission, renewal order or treatments, as far as is

practical, the person is entitled to notification and to make representation in relation to the issue and consideration must be given to these representations before the decision to admit is made.

● In all decisions under the 2001 Act, regard must be had for the need to respect the right of the person to dignity, bodily integrity, privacy and autonomy.

Under the terms of the Mental Health Act (2001), a person can be admitted to an approved centre voluntarily, or an order for an involuntary admission to an approved centre can be made on the grounds that the person is suffering from a mental disorder. Under the terms of the act, involuntary or compulsory admission must be limited to those who need it, and all persons being compulsorily detained must be offered the option to be admitted voluntarily. It is important to note that the act excludes from involuntary admission a sole diagnosis of personality disorder, social deviance and drug or alcohol addiction unless the person also has a mental disorder (Keys, 2008).

Application can be made for involuntary admission by a spouse, relative or an authorised office which includes a member of the Garda Siochana (Irish Police Force). The person making the application must be over 18 years of age. In circumstances where no one in any of these categories can be found, an application can be made by anyone else who fulfils the requirements set out in Section 9, Subsection 2 of the act. However, the applicant must have observed the person within 48 hours of making the application. Exclusion to who can make application for compulsory detention also applies, for example, separated spouses.

The act also provides for removal of the person to hospital and provides power to the Gardai (police) to assist with removal where necessary. The person being detained must receive a copy of the detention order, a general description of the proposed treatment, explanation of their rights to contact the inspector of mental health services, have their detention reviewed by a circuit court judge, by a mental health tribunal or appeal decision in the circuit court, entitlement to legal representation and the right to choose to be a voluntary patient. In addition, a copy of the detention order must be sent to the Mental Health Commission within 24 hours. All compulsory admissions are reviewed by a mental health tribunal, whereby the admission is reviewed by an independent psychiatrist and a legal representative is assigned to the patient.

Where a person has been admitted to mental health services in a voluntary capacity but their condition deteriorates requiring compulsory detention, Section 14(2) of the Mental Health Act (2001) provides for a 24-hour holding power. In this respect, the act states that:

> A consultant psychiatrist, a medical practitioner or a registered nurse on the staff of the Approved Centre shall be entitled to take charge of the person

concerned and detain him or her for a period not exceeding 24 hours (or such shorter period as may be prescribed after consultation with the Commission) for the purpose of carrying out an examination under subsection (1) or, if an admission order is made or refused in relation to the person during that period, until it is granted or refused.

However, the act does not provide for any authority to treat during this period, and in the absence of consent, treatment is justified only under the common law doctrine of necessity and the best interest of the individual (Keys, 2008).

Mental Health Commission

Under the provisions of the 2001 Mental Health Act, the Mental Health Commission, an independent statutory body, was established in April 2002. The principal functions of the commission, as specified in the act, are to promote, encourage and foster the establishment and maintenance of high standards and good practices in the delivery of mental health services and to take all reasonable steps to protect the interests of persons detained in approved centres (Section 33). The remit of the commission incorporates the broad spectrum of mental health services, including general adult mental health services, mental health services for children and adolescents, older people, people with learning disabilities and forensic mental health services (MHC, 2008).

The Mental Health Act (2001) also makes provision for the establishment of an inspector of mental health services, who is to visit and inspect every approved centre (hospitals or other inpatient facilities) at least once each year and any other premises where mental health services are being provided. The 2001 act also addresses the issues of bodily restraint and seclusion, participation in clinical trials, appointment of clinical directors and instigation of civil proceedings (Kelly, 2007).

Where a person believes that they are unlawfully detained, they or another person on their behalf may have recourse to the common law writ of habeas corpus, which is embodied in Article 40.4 of the Irish Constitution.

Roles of health professionals

In Ireland, psychiatric nurses represent the largest professional group in the mental health workforce. The majority of nurses and other mental health professionals are employed directly by the Health Services Executive (HSE). In 2010, the register of nurses maintained by An Bord Altranais (Irish Nursing Board) reported an overall total 13 084 nurses with a psychiatric nursing qualification – 9256 female and 3828 male. As a significant proportion of nurses on the Irish nursing register will have more than one registration recorded, registration data does not provide a reliable source of the actual numbers of psychiatric nurses engaged in practice.

Data pertaining to the actual numbers of psychiatric/mental health nurses employed and engaged in practice, as well as those for other professional groups within mental health services, is collected and collated by the Health Services Executive (HSE). Most recent figures available from the HSE in December 2010 indicate that a total of 5184 psychiatric nurses were employed by the HSE and engaged in mental health service provision; this represents a small decrease in numbers since 2005, which was then 5295.6.

While data does exist about other health professionals working within mental health services, it is extremely limited. Presently, data exists on the numbers of consultant psychiatrists employed but does not appear to exist for non-consultant medical staff, including registrars and senior registrars. Data relating to the number of social workers employed within mental health services is available; however, data relating specifically to the numbers of psychologists, occupational therapists, counsellors, psychotherapists, social care workers, music therapists, art therapists, rehabilitation workers or health care assistants is not currently available. Table 6.1 provides the number of consultant psychiatrists and social workers employed within mental health services for 2005 and 2010.

TABLE 6.1 Consultant psychiatrists and social workers employed in mental health services in 2005 and 2010

Mental health professionals	Actual WTE* December 2005	Actual WTE* December 2010
Consultant psychiatrists	283.5	356.8
Social workers – psychiatric	31.9	33.4

Source: HR Management Information Health Service Executive

* WTE = whole-time equivalents

The data available relating to the composition of the health care and other associated professionals in mental health services, while not comprehensive, indicates a service that relies heavily on roles which traditionally originated in and were consolidated by the asylum systems, and are associated with the dominant ideology of illness. When viewed in conjunction with other factors, including how mental health services are defined in the Mental Health Act (2001) as 'services which provide care and treatment to persons suffering from mental illness or a mental disorder under the clinical direction of a consultant psychiatrist', the slow pace of progress in developing mental health services nationally, as well as implementing the recent mental health policy, *A Vision for Change* (2006), this continued reliance on traditional health professional roles suggests a service that continues to operate predominantly from a disease rather than a recovery orientation.

Role of nurses
· · · · · · · · · · · · · · · · · · · ·

While historically the role of the psychiatric nurse was as a custodial carer within the institutional setting, in 1984 the philosophy and policy of psychiatric care was altered to embrace the model of community-based care (Department of Health, 1984). The emphasis in this new paradigm has been on 'comprehensive, community-oriented care delivered by a multidisciplinary team' (Cowman *et al.*, 2001). Parallel changes were taking place both within the structure of the psychiatric services and within the profession of nursing. In 1985, a new Nurses Act was enacted establishing a new An Bord Altranais (Irish Nursing Board). Changes in the nature of the apprenticeship model of preregistration nursing education recommended by the various reports over the years were adopted, and implementation began with the introduction of the first registration/diploma programme in 1994 (An Bord Altranais, 2005). Subsequently, the 'Galway model', as it became commonly known, was extended to all preregistration programmes in Ireland by 1998. Under the terms of the registration/diploma programme, student nurses gained supernumerary status as students of universities/third-level institutions. Two new nursing grades – clinical placement coordinator and nurse practice development coordinator – were created to support the implementation of the new programme.

The report which has had the most immediate and far-reaching impact on the profession of nursing in Ireland over the past two decades was the Commission on Nursing (1998). The establishing of this commission in 1997 resulted from a recommendation of the labour court while attempting to resolve a series of issues in dispute between health service employers and the Nursing Alliance (an alliance of all four trade unions representing all branches of Irish nurses), which had been ongoing for a protracted period of time. In total, the commission made 106 recommendations, and while it is not appropriate to outline all of these, some of the key recommendations are summarised below:

- regulation of the profession, including altering the structure and functions of the Nursing Board, and revision of fitness to practice procedures
- preparation for the profession, including the transition of preregistration education into third-level education at degree level
- professional development, including establishment of an independent statutory agency with responsibility for post-registration professional development of nursing
- role of nurses in management of services, including effective internal communication strategies in all organisations, establishment of the post of chief nurse at the Department of Health and Children, establishment of nursing and midwifery planning and development units in each health board with the remit of strategic planning and development including workforce planning, education and quality assurance of nursing services

- nursing in the community, including the development of the role of nurses in the community
- nursing in care of the elderly, including an urgent review of conditions and staffing in care of the elderly services
- issues concerning mental handicap nursing, midwifery and sick children's nursing, including promotion of the distinct identity and unique working environment of mental handicap nursing
- other recommendations – development of formal and informal procedures to deal with bullying in the workplace
- implementation of the report, including establishing a monitoring committee and a timetable for the achieving of key events.

The recommendations of the Commission on Nursing and their subsequent implementation have had a significant impact on both the nature and pace of change within the Irish nursing profession in the years since their publication. However, the implementations of these recommendations have not occurred without difficulties. Initially, the apparent lack of commitment on the part of the Department of Health and Children regarding implementation of key recommendations contributed to the first ever national nurse's strike in October 1999, which lasted 9 days.

The recommendations of the Commission on Nursing regarding changes in preregistration nursing education, namely the introduction of a 4-year honours degree programme for all branches of direct-entry nurse training, commenced in 2002. In 2002, a 4-year honours degree programme, BSc Nursing, based wholly within third-level institutions, along with the associated relocation of all resources, human and financial, into those institutions, commenced. The Nursing Education Forum (Government of Ireland, 1998) also recommended that An Bord Altranais, as the regulatory authority for nursing, should impartially and without prejudice 'undertake further research to examine the rationale for, and impact of, maintaining three points of entry to pre-registration nursing' (p. 38). The review recommended that distinct registration education programmes should be retained in each of the five divisions of the register, including psychiatric nursing. This was based on recognition of the existence of unique client groups with unique needs, and further recognises that there are various aspects of the health of the population, which need to be addressed by nurses with specialist training (An Bord Altranais, 2005, p. 303). The undergraduate degree programmes for psychiatric, general and intellectual disability nursing commenced in 2002. Application to all nursing and midwifery programmes is made through the Central Application Office (CAO), which is the process for entry to all third-level education.

While Ireland lagged behind her international counterparts with regard to the development of psychiatric and mental health services, the past two decades have seen increasing developments in community-based mental health services and in the role of the psychiatric nurse. Psychiatric nurses have expanded their professional role in response to the changing health and social policy and the emerging associated health service demands. Psychiatric nurses function across a range of diverse practice settings, and in 2011 a total of 568 clinical nurse specialist (CNS) and 20 advanced nurse practitioner (ANP) posts were approved in the following areas. Table 6.2 presents a summary of the service areas where clinical nurse specialists and advanced nurse practitioners are currently working.

TABLE 6.2 Clinical nurse specialists and advanced nurse practitioner posts

Clinical nurse specialists	Advanced nurse practitioners
Addiction counselling	Addiction and mental health
Child and adolescent services	Child and adolescent mental health psychotherapy
Anxiety disorders	Cognitive behaviour therapy
Art therapy	Psychotherapy
Assertive outreach	Dementia care
Autism	Eating disorders
Behaviour/cognitive/family therapist	Forensic mental health
Bereavement	Liaison mental health
Intellectual disability	Mental health & psychotherapy in primary care
Community mental health	Recovery and rehabilitation in mental health care and psychosis
Community services for older people	
Counselling and psychotherapy	
Liaison/crisis intervention/self-harm	
Health promotion	
Dementia services	
Rehabilitation services	
Serious and enduring mental illness	
Psychosis	

Source: National Council for the Professional Development of Nursing and Midwifery Personal Communication, 2011

Future plans for mental health care

In 2006, almost a quarter of a century following the publication of *Planning for the Future*, a new national mental health policy, *A Vision for Change*, was published. This policy, which was widely welcomed, envisioned future mental health services in Ireland as comprehensive, fostering positive mental health across the entire community and providing accessible, community-based specialist services for people with mental illness (Department of Health and Children, 2006, p. 8). A central tenet of this policy is the involvement of service users and their carers in every aspect of service development and delivery. The policy makes wide-ranging recommendations addressing the broad scope of mental health services, ranging from their underpinning philosophy of adopting a recovery orientation to the development of a multidisciplinary workforce planning policy linked to projected service plans. Among the key recommendations are:

- the establishment of fully staffed and well-trained multidisciplinary community mental health teams (CMHT) to provide mental health services across the lifespan
- a recovery orientation informing every aspect of service delivery and service users as partners in their own care with care plans that reflect service users' particular needs
- strengthening of links between specialist mental health, primary care services and voluntary groups
- planning to realise closure of all mental hospitals and redirection of released resources into mental health services.

The policy adopts a lifespan approach and details services required for each population group. In addition, special categories of provision which cross-cut age-related boundaries, including service for people with forensic needs, people who are homeless and those with neuropsychiatric needs, are also outlined.

While *A Vision for Change* (Department of Health and Children, 2006) emphasises the importance of independence and recovery for those with persistent mental health problems, unlike its predecessor in 1984, there is little attention or information in the policy about the role of community residences. Given that these community residences constitute a mainstay of existing community mental health service provision, this is an omission which is likely to impact on providing for residents' well-being and independence.

Initial optimism regarding the potential of the policy to initiate profound change in mental health services in Ireland has been short-lived. Although published at the height of the economic boom, as with previous mental health policy, the funding required and promised for implementation has not been realised. The independent monitoring group established to monitor implementation has repeatedly expressed concern regarding the slow pace of implementation. Furthermore, in an analysis of the implementation of *A Vision for Change* in 2009, the Mental Health Commission identified four major themes of concern:

 i) the need for a clear, detailed implementation plan
 ii) the need for accountable, effective leadership
 iii) the provision and use of resources
 iv) the closure of remaining psychiatric hospitals.

In 2007, the inspector of Mental Health Services, reporting on the slow pace of progress towards the provision of a quality national mental health service, commented that the 'wait continues' for adequately staffed community teams, closure of large psychiatric hospitals and the development of even a minimal service for people with intellectual disabilities (MHC, 2008, p. 85).

Conclusions

Over the last four decades, there has been a considerable decline in the number of patients resident in Irish psychiatric units and hospitals, with numbers declining from a high of 19 801 in 1963 to 2812 in 2010. This represents a reduction of 86% in inpatient numbers since 1963 and a reduction of 17% since 2006 (HRB, 2010). While significant advances have been made in community care and in the range of services and therapies available, over-reliance on a medical model of care, psychopharmacology and some physical treatments, including electro-convulsive therapy, remain as part of the mainstay of therapeutic interventions. Significant variability also exists with regard to availability of and access to mental health services in different parts of the country.

Over the past 5 years, many positive developments have occurred in mental health services. The increasing involvement of service users, advocates and carers in the development of services is very positive, as is the commitment of mental health services management and professional groups. However, during the past 5 years, progress in implementing *A Vision for Change* and reforming the mental health services has been slow. As identified by the monitoring group, the continued absence of a national directorate for mental health services and senior executive accountability continues to seriously impede implementation.

Mental health services in Ireland are already disproportionately underfunded, having reduced in real terms from 13% of the health budget in 1986 to 5.4% in 2010. This compares unfavourably with the rates of 12% in England and 18% in Scotland. Though the Government's 2006 strategy, *A Vision for Change*, promised over €21 million each year for a 7-year period, this promise has not been realised.

While there is clear evidence that psychiatric nurses contribute in a significant way to developing new and innovative community-based nursing services, there is also continuing evidence that nurses have developed their clinical career pathways in ways that support, sustain and advance the medical model of care (An Bord Altranais, 2005). Thus, while there is evidence of a broadening of the scope of psychiatric nursing practice over the past decade, there is also evidence that the scope of practice and nurse autonomy in terms of adopting specific therapeutic approaches continues to be contingent upon the type of setting in which nurses undertake their practice (Sheridan, 2005). Moreover, there is evidence that as the scope of practice and autonomy expand, psychiatric nurses provide less direct care to patients and become more involved in patient care management activities at the expense of direct therapeutic interventions.

Case scenario

A 23-year-old unemployed man is reported by his landlord as acting increasingly strangely. He has barricaded his room, talking about being spied upon by the CIA. He can be heard shouting within his room in an angry and incoherent way. He has not been seen by a psychiatrist in the past, although his mother has told the landlord that he has been isolating himself and acting increasingly oddly over the last couple of years.

The most likely way this man will come to the attention of the mental health services is through an application for involuntary admission being made by either his mother or his landlord, or, given that this man has barricaded his room, the intervention of An Garda Siochana (police). This application will require an examination by a registered medical practitioner, e.g. general practitioner, which will be undertaken within 24 hours of receipt of the application. The person must be informed of the purpose of the examination, unless in the view of the medical practitioner such information might be 'prejudicial to the person's mental health, well-being or emotional condition'. The general practitioner will then make a recommendation. If this is for involuntary admission, a copy of the recommendation is sent to the clinical director of the approved centre and a copy is given to the applicant. This recommendation remains in force for 7 days. The person who made the application is responsible for arranging removal of the person to the approved centre. If they are unable to do so, the clinical director of the approved centre acting on the recommendation of the general practitioner will arrange removal of the person to the approved centre by members of staff of the approved centre. If there is a risk of serious harm to self or others, An Garda Siochana may be requested to assist staff of the approved centre, and An Garda Siochana is required to comply with such a request.

As soon as practicable, but not later than 24 hours after arrival on the ward, an examination will be made by a consultant psychiatrist, who will either complete an admission order or refuse to complete an admission order. If the admission order is made, it authorises the reception, detention and treatment of the individual for a period of 21 days, and this period may be extended up to 3 months. The consultant psychiatrist must inform the Mental Health Commission of the completion of an involuntary admission order. Within 21 days, the Mental Health Commission will then:

i) refer the matter to a mental health tribunal,

ii) assign a legal representative to the patient, and

iii) direct an independent psychiatrist to examine the patient, interview the patient's consultant and review the patient's records and either confirm or revoke the order.

Prescribed treatment will most likely include administration of neuroleptic medication aimed at reducing the evident positive symptoms of psychosis, coupled with anxiolytics aimed at minimising anxiety levels associated with admission to an inpatient setting. In addition, the patient will be placed on level 1 observation, which equates to high observation in a secure high-dependency area. This will involve ongoing observation of the patient over the 24-hour period to ensure safety, establish trust, undertake initial assessment and establish evidence of effectiveness of administered medication.

Access to other services, including social work, occupational therapy and to a lesser extent psychological therapy, may be provided, as will access to any physical health care required. As outlined above, the patient will also have access, under law, to an independent mental health tribunal and to a patient advocate to assist him with any issues he may have.

Nursing staff would aim to establish a rapport with this man and undertake an in-depth nursing assessment to identify immediate nursing care priorities, including both psychological and physical health care needs. Priorities for immediate care are likely to focus on ensuring his physical and psychological safety. Information about his detention would be provided and every attempt to respond to his concerns would be made. A nursing care plan spanning the first 72 hours from arrival will be documented. Every effort would be made to include the patient and his family in all aspects of care planning. Nursing staff would also administer prescribed medication and observe for any response to this. Nursing interventions would be directed at establishing a trusting therapeutic relationship with this man.

The average length of stay in an inpatient centre is approximately 3 weeks. Following the acute management of this patient's condition, it is likely that he would continue to receive ongoing care for an extended period of time within community-based services. The following components may be included:

● continuation with prescribed medication
● referral to a community mental health nurse
● referral to acute day hospital to consolidate stabilisation and promote further recovery
● recommendation for specific programmes, e.g. rehabilitation
● outpatient clinic follow-up
● family engagement to support recovery

- liaison with his work or educational institution to re-establish contact and provide support with the aim of re-engagement
- link to patient support groups.

Acknowledgements

I would like to acknowledge Mr Des Williams, HR Management Information, Health Service Executive, for his assistance with the provision of data pertaining to actual whole-time equivalent personnel currently working within mental health services.

References

An Bord Altranais/UCD. *The Five Points Project*. Dublin: An Bord Altranais/UCD School of Nursing, Midwifery & Health Systems; 2005.

Barton R. *Institutional Neurosis*. Bristol: J Wright & Son; 1959.

Byrne M, Onyett S. *Teamwork within Mental Health Services in Ireland* [resource paper]. Dublin: Mental Health Commission; 2010.

Central Statistics Office. *2006 Census of Population Volume 1 – population classified by area*. Dublin: Stationery Office; 2007.

Central Statistics Office. *Population and Labour Force Projection 2011–2041*. Dublin: Stationery Office; 2008a.

Central Statistics Office. *Population and Population Predictions. Section A: health statistics*. Dublin: Stationery Office; 2008b.

Chief Medical Officer. *Better Health for Everyone. Annual Report of the Chief Medical Officer 2001*. Dublin: Department of Health and Children; 2002.

Conrad P. The shifting engines of medicalization. *J Health Soc Behav*. 2005; **46**(1): 3–14.

Cooney J. *John Charles McQuaid: ruler of Catholic Ireland*. Dublin: O'Brien Press; 1999.

Cowman S, Farrelly M, Gilheany P. An examination of the role and function of psychiatric nurses in clinical practice in Ireland. *J Adv Nurs*. 2001; **34**(6): 745–53.

Daly A, Walsh D. *Activities of Irish Psychiatric Units and Hospitals 2008*. HRB Statistics Series 7. Dublin: Health Research Board; 2009.

Department of Health. *Report of the Commission of Inquiry on Mental Illness*. Dublin: The Stationery Office; 1966.

Department of Health. *Psychiatric Nursing Services of Health Boards: report of the working party*. Dublin: The Stationery Office; 1972.

Department of Health. *The Psychiatric Services: planning for the future*. Dublin: The Stationery Office; 1984.

Department of Health and Children. *Report of the Commission on Nursing: a blueprint for the future*. Dublin: The Stationery Office; 1998.

Department of Health and Children. *The Mental Health Act 2001*. Dublin: The Stationery Office; 2001.

Department of Health and Children. *The Nursing and Midwifery Resource Final Report of the Steering Group. Towards Workforce Planning*. Dublin: Department of Health and Children; 2002.

Department of Health and Children. *A Vision for Change. Report of the Expert Group on Mental Health Policy*. Dublin: The Stationery Office; 2006.

Farrell C, McAvoy H, Wilde J, *et al. Tackling Health Inequalities: an all-Ireland approach to social determinants*. Dublin: Combat Poverty Agency/Institute of Public Health in Ireland; 2008.

Finnane M. *Insanity and the Insane in Post-famine Ireland*. London: Croom-Helm; 1981.

General Nursing Council. *Supplementary Register for Mental Nurses, 1921–1944*. Dublin: An Bord Altranais Archives.

Government of Ireland. *Report of the Commission on Nursing: a blueprint for the future*. Dublin: The Stationery Office; 1998.

Harkin AM. *Equity of Access to Health Services: some relevant issues in an Irish context*. Dublin: Institute of Public Health in Ireland; 2001.

Health Information Quality Authority. *Guidance on Developing Key Performance Indicators and Minimum data Sets to Monitor Health care Quality*. Dublin: Health Information Quality Authority, Department of Health; 2005.

Health Research Board. *Irish Psychiatric Units and Hospitals Census 2010*. Dublin: Department of Health; 2010.

Health Services Executive. *National Office for Suicide Prevention Annual Report 2009*. Dublin: Health Services Executive; 2009.

Healy D. Irish psychiatry in the twentieth century. In: Freeman H, Berrios G, editors. *150 Years of British Psychiatry Volume II: the aftermath*. London: Athlone Press; 1996. pp. 268–91.

Johnstone MJ. Stigma, social justice and the rights of the mentally ill: challenging the status quo. *Aust N Z J Men Health Nurs*. 2001; **10**(4): 200–9.

Kelly BD. The Irish Mental Health Act 2001. *Psychiatr Bull*. 2007; **31**: 21–4.

Kelly BD. The Mental Treatment Act 1945 in Ireland: an historical enquiry. *Hist Psychiatry*. 2008; **19**(1): 47–67.

Key R. *Ireland: a history*. London: Abacus; 1982.

Keys M. The Mental Health Act 2001. In: Morrissey J, Keogh B, Doyle L, editors. *Psychiatric/ Mental Health Nursing: an Irish perspective*. Dublin: Gill & Macmillan; 2008. pp. 31–46.

Malcolm E. *Swift's Hospital: a history of St Patrick's Hospital, Dublin, 1746–1989*. Dublin: Gill and Macmillan; 1989.

McDaid D, Wiley M, Maresso A, *et al*. Ireland health system review. *Health Syst Transit*. 2009; **11**(4): 1–268.

Medico-Psychological Association/Royal Medico-Psychological Association. *Registers of Certificate of Proficiency on Attending on and Nursing the Insane, 1895–1951*. London: Royal College of Psychiatrists Archives.

Mental Health Commission. *Community Mental Health Services in Ireland: activity and catchment area characteristics 2004*. Dublin: Mental Health Commission; 2006.

Mental Health Commission. *Annual Report for 2007 Including the Report of the Inspector of Mental Health Services*. Dublin: Mental Health Commission; 2008.

Mental Health Commission. *Annual Report for 2008 Including the Report of the Inspector of Mental Health Services*. Dublin: Mental Health Commission; 2009a.

Mental Health Commission. *From Vision to Action? An Analysis of the Implementation of A Vision for Change*. Dublin: Mental Health Commission; 2009b.

Mental Health Commission. *An Overview of the Evidence on Economic Adversity and Mental Health*. Dublin: Mental Health Commission, Department of Health; 2011.

National Disability Authority. *Public Attitudes to Disability in Ireland*. Disability Research Series 8. Dublin: National Disability Authority; 2007.

National Suicide Research Foundation. *National Registry of Deliberate Self Harm Annual Report 2009*. Cork: National Suicide Research Foundation; 2010.

Oosterhuis H. Insanity and other discomforts: a century of outpatient psychiatry and mental health care in the Netherlands 1900–2000. In: Gijswijt-Hofstra M, Oosterhuis H, Vijselaar J, *et al*., editors. *Psychiatric Cultures Compared: psychiatry and mental health care in the twentieth century*. Amsterdam: Amsterdam University Press; 2005. pp. 72–80.

O'Shea E, Kennelly B. *The Economics of Mental Health Care in Ireland*. NUI Galway: Mental Health Commission; 2008.

Porter R. *Madness: a brief history.* Oxford: Oxford University Press; 2002.

Prince P, Gerber GJ. Subjective well-being and community integration among clients of assertive community treatment. *Qual Life Res.* 2005; **14**(1): 161–9.

Reidpath D, Chan K, Gifford S, *et al.* 'He hath the French pox': stigma, social value and social exclusion. *Sociol Health Illn*. 2005; **27**(4): 468–89.

Repper J, Perkins R. *Social Inclusion and Recovery. A Model for Mental Health Practice.* Edinburgh: Bailliere Tindal; 2003.

Reynolds J. *Grangegorman: psychiatric care in Dublin since 1815*. Dublin: Institute of Public Administration in Association with Eastern Health Board; 1992.

Robbins J. *Fools and Mad: a history of the insane in Ireland.* Dublin: Institute of Public Administration; 1986.

Robins J. *Nursing and Midwifery in Ireland in the Twentieth Century*. Dublin: An Bord Altranais; 2000.

Saris J. Mad kings, proper houses, and an asylum in rural Ireland. *Am Anthropol.* 1996; **98**(3): 539–54.

Sheridan AJ. Letting the past illuminate the future: a focus on Irish psychiatric nursing. In: Ryan D, Jacob A, Kirwan M, editors. *Reflection and Rejuvenation Issues for Irish Psychiatric Nursing into the Millennium.* Kilkenny: Association of Psychiatric Nurse Mangers; 1999. pp. 1–18.

Sheridan AJ. Psychiatric nursing. In: Robins J, editor. *Nursing and Midwifery in Ireland in the Twentieth Century.* Dublin: An Bord Altranais; 2000. pp. 141–61.

Sheridan AJ. An analysis of the activity patterns of psychiatric nurses practicing in Ireland 1950–2000. Unpublished PhD thesis, University of Birmingham; 2003.

Sheridan AJ. An analysis of the activities of psychiatric nurses practicing in Ireland 1950–2000. *Psychiatr Nurs.* 2004; **2**(1): 19–22.

Sheridan AJ. Being a psychiatric nurse in Ireland in the 1950s. In: Fealy GM, editor. *Care to Remember: nursing and midwifery in Ireland.* Cork: Mercier Press; 2005. pp. 172–84.

Sheridan AJ. The impact of political transition on psychiatric nursing – a case study of twentieth-century Ireland. *Nurs Inq.* 2006; **13**(4): 289–99.

Stewart D. Obstacles to the advancement in Ireland of psychological medicine. *J Ment Sci.* 1876; **21**: 383.

Tait L, Lester H. Encouraging user involvement in mental health services. *Advances in Psychiatric Treatment.* 2005; **11**: 168–75.

Tedstone-Doherty D, Walsh D, Moran R. *A Survey and Evaluation of Community Residential Mental Health Services in Ireland.* Dublin: Mental Health Commission; 2007.

US Department of Health and Human Services. *Why Population Aging Matters. A Global Perspective.* Washington: Department of State; 2007.

World Health Organization Europe. *Mental Health in WHO's European Region.* Copenhagen: World Health Organization Regional Office for Europe; 2003.

World Health Organization. *Mental Health Action Plan for Europe.* Copenhagen: Regional Office for Europe; 2004.

Mental health services in Luxembourg

Claude Besenius

Introduction

The current chapter describes the different stages of development that Luxembourg's mental health services have been through, current services and future plans. These developments largely follow the common historical pattern of an initial focus on the hospitalisation of the mentally ill for humanitarian and public order reasons (De Smet and Spautz, 2005) and, later, decentralisation of care into the community.

National profile and context

The Grand Duchy of Luxembourg, a constitutional monarchy, is an independent sovereign state, bordering Belgium, France and Germany. Founded in 963, Luxembourg became a Grand Duchy in 1815 and an independent state. Its independence was confirmed by the 1839 First Treaty of London. The ruling house of Nassau came to the throne of Luxembourg in 1890; the present Grand Duke Henri succeeded his father in 2000. Overrun by Germany in both world wars, it ended its neutrality in 1948 when it entered into the Benelux Customs Union and joined NATO the following year. In 1957, Luxembourg became one of the six founding countries of the European Economic Community (later the European Union), and in 1999 joined the euro currency area.

Population and demographics

Luxembourg is one of the smallest countries in Europe and is about 2,586 km² in size. Of the country's 502 000 inhabitants, some 90 000 live in Luxembourg city and its immediate surroundings. The number of foreign residents in the Grand Duchy exceeds 43% of the population, which constitutes the highest proportion of foreigners of any EU country. This number consists of 80 000 Portuguese, 28 000 French, 19 400 Italian, 16 700 Belgian, 12 000 German, 5300 British and 53 600 other EU and non-EU members. Luxembourg has a population density of 190 inhabitants per square kilometre. In 2001, there was an increase of 2514 foreigners in Luxembourg, but a decrease of 513 Luxembourgers. As of 2000, 87% of the Luxembourg population was Roman Catholic, the other 13% consisting of Protestants, Muslims and Jews.

Gross domestic product per capita in Luxembourg is currently estimated at US\$78 723 (IMF, 2009), which is the third-highest in the world. Allegrezza *et al.* (2004) found that levels of poverty and income inequality in Luxembourg are among the lowest in the world. Four per cent of people living in Luxembourg are considered to be severely affected by a lack of resources, compared to 11% in the UK. Thirteen per cent of people have an equalised disposable income below the risk of poverty threshold. Five per cent of people aged 65 and above have an income below the poverty line, compared to 30% in the UK. All of the foreigners registered in Luxembourg have the same right to health care as Luxembourg people. In 2000, Luxembourg had an unemployment rate of 2.6%, which increased to 6.1% in December 2009. Utilising the Gini coefficient, the Central Intelligence Agency (2008) found that Luxembourg is the fourth-least-unequal out of 134 measured countries, the most equal country being Sweden and the UK ranking 42nd. (The Gini coefficient is a measure of the distribution of wealth within a population. A value of 0 expresses perfect equality and a value of 1 maximal inequality.) The industrial sector, which was dominated until the 1960s by steel, has diversified to include chemicals, rubber and other products. In the past few decades, growth in the financial sector has more than compensated for the decline in steel. Services, especially banking and other financial exports, account for the majority of economic output. The Luxembourg government has also tried to attract Internet start-ups. Skype and eBay are two of the many Internet companies that have shifted their local or global headquarters to Luxembourg. However, the current Europe-wide economic troubles have led to tighter finances in Luxembourg for health services.

Lëtzebuergesch (Luxemburgish) is the everyday spoken language of the people, and the symbol of the Luxembourgers' national identity. Since the creation of a dictionary and a grammar, this former Mosel-Frankish dialect is now recognised as the national language (since 1984), while both French and German remain official languages. Lëtzebuergesch, German and French are used in the press, in political and religious life; however, French is the official language of the administration. In parliament, the three languages are used with a strong tendency towards Lëtzebuergesch, the reports being written in the language the members of parliament used. Public offices, though, are held to answer – wherever possible – in the language they are addressed in. This peculiar language situation is a direct result of the size of the country, and its historical associations with both France and Germany. Luxembourg has a trilingual education system, starting school in Lëtzebuergesch, before changing to German, and while in secondary school, the language of instruction changes to French. This multilingual system has a large impact on health care in Luxembourg, as patients, as well as staff, have to swap between languages when speaking to each other.

General health need

Over a period of 30 years, life expectancy at birth in Luxembourg has increased by 8 years for men and 6 years for women. Today, it stands at about 77 years for men and 83 years for women (WHO, 2008). A clear decline in infant mortality has played a central role in this trend. The number of deaths of infants under the age of five is four per 1000 live births. People aged 65 and over have increased in number from 42 800 in 1970 to 61 000 in 2000 (+42.8%). In 2009, 14% of the Luxembourg population was aged 65 or more. There is an undeniable increase in the absolute number of elderly people, although their relative weight in the total population is increasing much more slowly. This is due to strong net immigration, which continually feeds younger age groups.

The prevalence of chronic illnesses in Luxembourg lies at about 22% (Tchicaya, 2006). There is an increasing correlation with age, where 11% of 16- to 24-year-olds and 47% of those over 74 suffer from chronic illnesses. Women in particular often suffer health problems for longer due to their longer life expectancy (EHEMU, 2005). In Luxembourg, cardiovascular diseases are currently the most common causes of death (39%), and a quarter of mortality is caused by cancer (26%) (STATEC, 2006). Tchicaya (2007) found that 23% of the adult population stated that they smoked on a daily basis. On top of this, there was a relatively high proportion of people consuming alcohol on a daily basis as well as other behaviours detrimental to health (Ministère de la Santé, 2005). A fifth of the population (18.6%) is overweight (OECD, 2007).

Health care funding

The Luxembourg health care system is based on the values of solidarity, universal access and equality of treatment, and is characterised by universal coverage of the population through compulsory health and long-term care insurance.

There is a need for health providers to be approved to practise and a requirement to comply with financial rates set by the National Health Fund. The health system is characterised by medically defined need, with the doctor as the initiator of all services that are covered by health insurance. The health care system is also characterised by government planning of the hospital and pharmaceutical sectors, as well as free choice of provider and equity of treatment for all patients, whatever their status.

The supply of primary care in Luxembourg is dictated by demand, since patients are fee to choose their primary care provider and there is no legal means to limit the volume of medical activity. This includes mainly preventive and less specialised diagnoses and treatment of diseases. Health services, such as hospitals, but also medical practices of physician-specialists, provide secondary care consisting primarily of advice, diagnosis, treatment and specialised care. Numbers of hospitals and minimum standards for hospital services are planned via regulations (the so-called National Hospital Plans) enacted under this law.

The Luxembourg system is not divided by differences in treatment for people dependent on whether they have private insurance or not, as in many other countries. Medical services have relatively high numbers of doctors, particularly specialists, and have high-quality equipment and access to a number of hospital beds that is still above the level aimed for by the government. Consequently, there are no waiting lists (Hartmann-Hirsch and Tchicaya, 2009).

Compulsory health insurance (*assurance maladie-maternité*) for manufacturing and industrial workers was introduced in Luxembourg in 1901, following a similar scheme introduced in Germany by Bismarck in 1883. After the Second World War, Luxembourg retained elements of the German insurance system, which had replaced Luxembourg's Code des Assurances Sociales during the German occupation of 1940–44. Most significant of these elements was the extension of insurance to cover pensioners. By 1973, the working population, their families and all pensioners were covered by compulsory health insurance. Further reform was to follow in 1992. The government originally intended to abolish the nine separate sickness funds, but faced with strong opposition from professional groups, it settled for a compromise. The funds were allowed to continue only as agencies for direct contact with the insured citizen, while all of their responsibilities except the actual administration of reimbursement to members were transferred to the Union of Sickness Funds.

In 1999, long-term care insurance (*assurance dépendance*) was introduced as a compulsory part of insurance. It supports the costs of necessary assistance and care for dependent people. This care insurance is included in the social security side of health insurance and operates on the same principles: everyone pays a fee required and when an insured becomes dependent, he or she has the right to receive dependence benefits.

From 2009, health insurance structures changed profoundly. The fusion of the three health funds from the private sector and the two funds from the unemployment sector led to the creation of the Caisse Nationale de Santé (CNS). The CNS is responsible for three processes: management of health care, management of maternity benefits and management of sickness benefits. The main consequence introduced by the new law is the creation of a single status for employees of the private sector, meaning harmonisation of conditions and levels of reimbursements for sickness leave for workers and employees. The aim of this health insurance is to guarantee the whole of the population, regardless of their social status, equal access to health care and free choice of treating doctor (except in the case of an emergency). In 2008, the CNS had incomings of €8836.7 million and outgoings of €7931.9 million (Ministère de la Sécurité Sociale, 2009).

The Luxembourg health care system is generous: the contributions of the insured are relatively low due to the financial contributions of the state; the average reimbursement rate lies around 95% (OECD, 2008). The resources necessary for financing the health system are provided by contributions from employers and employees (5.6% of gross salaries in 2008) and by the state contributing approximately 40%. The state contributes to the financing of the building of hospitals as well as their large equipment (80%). As to the financing of long-term care insurance, all assets and all pensioners pay a special contribution of 1.4% on all their earned income and all unearned income. This contribution is supplemented by a contribution from the state and by a contribution from the electricity sector.

Mental health need

According to the European Commission (2010), the latest suicide rates available for Luxembourg (15 cases per 100 000 during the 2000–04 period) are above the EU average (10.5 cases per 100 000). The various studies carried out to date are inconclusive as to why this is the case. According to the Eurobarometer (European Commission, 2006), 9% of the population report to have, or have had, chronic anxiety or depression, and 7% say that they are undergoing medical treatment for this reason. The first Health Behaviour in School-Aged Children (HBSC) study (WHO, 2004) reported that during 1999/2000 20% of adolescents regularly suffered from at least one of the specified physical complaints, some of which may have an important psychological aspect (headache, stomach ache, difficulty sleeping). Some 36% of young people said that they are sad every day or at least once a week, 14% complained about isolation and 9.4% suffered from stress.

In 2009, the most common diagnoses for those admitted to the neuropsychiatric hospital (Centre Hospitalier Neuro-Psychiatrique, CHNP) were organic mental health disorders (21 clinical cases), psychoactive substance use (257), schizophrenia, schizotypal and delusional disorders (105), mood disorders (17), nervous system disorders (5), personality and behavioural disorders among adults (8), and behavioural and emotional disorders among adolescents (43) (CHNP, 2010).

Attitudes to mental health problems

In order to understand the stigma towards mental ill health in Luxembourg, one has to understand the history of mental health services. The town that hosts the neuropsychiatric hospital has long been synonymous with mental illness (Roberts in an interview with Dr Joosten, 2008). Ettelbruck has long been seen as a dark place to which mad people are sent for lengthy periods of time. The CHNP, which Ettelbruck is now called, has existed in one form or another for 155 years. It was founded in 1855, and Dr Joosten, the current director of the CHNP, explained in an interview:

> This was a typical asylum where everyone who didn't fit into society was sent. They were hidden away.

Back then, depression was thought to be contagious, and the main priority of the legislators was to 'secure society'; patients were not even treated. Even today, widespread stigma attached to mental health problems jeopardises the development and implementation of mental health policy. There is still a certain taboo attached to the CHNP and the name Ettelbruck, but changes are happening surrounding new infrastructures and the legal framework regarding patient admissions. In the last 20 years, the CHNP has changed and will continue to change in the future with the creation of new decentralised structures, moving from an asylum model to a modern rehabilitation clinic. This change has taken place in an environment which has not always been benevolent in attitude towards people with mental health problems. The distrust that has been shown to the CHNP has been embedded in both public opinion and the media. However, in the last few years, the CHNP has been successful in creating a more favourable opinion in the eye of the public, which has been generally shown by a more benevolent attitude in the media. Nevertheless, this picture is fragile, as was shown by the recent escape of an involuntarily placed patient, who had managed to escape twice. Without money and papers, he was stranded in Switzerland and lived as a homeless person on the street. In Geneva, social workers managed to persuade him to return to Ettelbruck. This incident did expose the degree of public apprehension of the mentally ill that still exists in Luxembourg. However, due to more openness on the part of mental health services, better conditions in which people are treated and cared for and generally better outcomes following treatment, public opinion is noticeably changing for the better.

Expenditure on mental health

The CNS spent €1.3 billion on general health care in Luxembourg in 2008, and €261 million on health care in other countries. Total expenditure on health in Luxembourg represented 7.1% of GDP in 2008 (Ministère de la Sécurité Sociale, 2009). Health care costs per person are the highest among the OECD countries (OECD, 2006), although direct payments by the insured are actually among the lowest (OECD, 2008). General government expenditure on health was 90.9% of total expenditure in 2006. In fact, more than 90% of the costs arising from health claims (Ministère de la Sécurité Sociale, 2008) are taken on by the CNS, which is financed by the state, as well as by employees and employers.

Mental health has been identified as one of the public health priorities in Luxembourg, and 13.4% (approximately €200 million) of the overall health budget is devoted to mental health (with England, one of the highest among all EU countries) (Knapp *et al.*, 2007). In 2006, the cost for one bed was €236,287 per year, illustrating that hospital stays consume by far the largest portion of the budget (Consbruck, 2009).

History of the development of mental health services

The 155-year history of the Centre Hospitalier Neuro Psychiatrique (CHNP) tells a moving story of the treatment of the mentally ill in Luxembourg and its surrounding countries. The history of the CHNP shows how much the treatment of psychiatric patients and institutions has been influenced by culture, by the public and by politics of the era (Häfner *et al.*, 1993; Rössler, 2005). The treatment of mentally ill people in Luxembourg went from social exclusion, in the sense of French social philosopher Michel Foucault (1969), to the provision of a typical large psychiatric hospital and is, nowadays, provided by a specialised clinic working within a network of mental health community care. The evolution of mental health services is in many respects similar to that in other countries.

The founding of the sanatorium (Hospice Central) in Ettelbruck in 1865 was a milestone in the history of health care, especially mental health care, in Luxembourg (Majerus, 2009). However, the history of mental health care goes back much further than that. Dr Adolph Buffet, former director of the Hospice Central, points out that, regrettably, there are few sources detailing the treatment of the mentally ill before the eighteenth century (Buffet, 1889). The first indirect references to the care of the sick in Luxembourg were made during the time of Christianisation in the early Middle Ages, by the Anglo-Saxon preacher, bishop and monastery founder Willibrord (Schroeder, 1999). In the following centuries, the mentally ill were treated similarly in Luxembourg as they were in the rest of Western Europe. Patients were locked away together with other people excluded from society (Geremek, 1976). The situation of the mentally ill got worse after the plague of 1348–49, as people in Western Europe were feeling deeply insecure and wanted to protect themselves from the then inexplicable illnesses. Symptoms were seen as the work of the devil, and mentally ill people were frequently hunted by the Inquisition as witches or magicians (Majerus, 2009). Often such people were confined together with the poor, prostitutes, the homeless, cripples and criminals, all having to endure the burden of stigmatisation. All these were expected to work under the control and guidance of untrained guards or were chained and vegetated in asylums. One of these asylums was situated in Pfaffenthal, a suburb of Luxembourg city (Goerens, 1935).

The enlightenment of the eighteenth century did not bring about improvements: some doctors experimented with brutal therapies, and 'fools' were commonly used as living exhibits for the amusement of high society (Bersani, 1996). Foucault (1969) claimed that the emergence of psychiatry had a covert purpose – that of identifying and excluding from society those who were thought to behave in a disruptive and deviating manner. It was not until the French Revolution and the proclamation of human rights that changes took place, at least on a political and legal level. A new French law introduced medical control and put together a commission of attorneys, administrators and doctors who had to decide on the patient's fate. After the conquest of Luxembourg by French Republican troops, this law was applied in Luxembourg in 1796. Philippe Pinel's release of lunatics from their chains, in the context of the French Revolution, can be seen as the start of a more humanitarian approach to psychiatric care, one no longer dominated by the processes described by Foucault. Pinel (1801) stated that:

> one could even talk with lunatics who had previously been in a state of constant arousal without putting oneself into great danger as before.

It had been noticeable from around that time that a lack of social communication and treating people in an aggressive, authoritarian way caused them to become violent in return. Whilst this experience should have been acknowledged when psychiatric hospitals were built and staff employed and trained, in fact it took more than 200 years until this insight was truly translated into practice.

Foundation of the Hospice Central

After recognition of Luxembourg's independence by King Wilhelm I of the Netherlands in 1839, Luxembourg became an independent country in 1839 and started its history in relative poverty (De Smet and Spautz, 2005). The Grand

Duchy was an underdeveloped country around this time, without a proper economy. In 1847, close to 12.3% of the population were considered indigent. Wars, epidemics and famines created large numbers of people with disabilities, sick people, people in poverty and begging orphans in Europe (Häfner, 2006). This led to a wave of social disciplinary actions that were aimed at locking away unwanted, socially isolated, helpless and lunatic people. In Luxembourg, the poorhouse got the name *Bettlerdepot* ('cleaning'). The 'cleaning' of unwanted people from society caused a huge demand for institutions in which to lock these people away. The founding of a sanatorium, the Hospice Central, was linked to the increase in this demand, which could not be covered by the poorhouse which then existed in the mid-nineteenth century.

In 1855, government buildings situated in Ettelbruck, previously occupied by the military, were made available in order to establish a sanatorium (Hospice Central) for indigent patients and the 'lunatic'. This was decided by Wilhelm III 'through God's Grace King of the Netherlands and Grand Duke of Luxembourg', for 'overriding reasons of humanity and public order' (De Smet and Spautz, 2005). Both of these motives caused the development of hospices, prisons, work institutions and lunatic asylums, which were dedicated to look after unwanted and helpless persons. Until 1867, only 'peaceful mentally ill' patients were admitted to the Hospice Central; the so-called frenetically crazed patients were still in the infirmary in Pfaffenthal. However, this asylum burned down in 1867, and all the patients were sent to Ettelbruck, where new buildings had to be constructed (Spautz, 2005a; Jetter, 1986; De Smet and Spautz, 2005). This was the first step of the Hospice Central turning into a psychiatric hospital. The sick and poor were moved into new buildings in 1893. After 1868, where all categories of lunatics were admitted into the Hospice Central, Majerus (2005) stated:

> one did not know restraints, chains, or dark cells in Ettelbruck and the lunatics were being treated with gentleness and mildness.

Dr Müller, then superintendent, apparently tried early on to implement the British 'non-restraint' approach which challenged force and violence against patients (Conolly, 1830). However, the implementation of this was extremely difficult. The three wardens that worked at the Hospice Central in 1868 had no training for their jobs. Apart from the three wardens, five female wardens and the sisters from the Elisabeth Hospital, one pastor and a maximum of two doctors were available to the 200 and ever-growing number of inpatients.

The Hospice Central after 1880

In 1880, Luxembourg was recovering from the political and social crises of the mid-nineteenth century. However, depressing poverty still existed at the beginning of the industrial era. After the immigration of German mining experts, Luxembourg was slowly transformed into a modern industrial state. Baron Felix Blochausen, Luxembourg prime minister between 1874 and 1885, submitted a new law that fundamentally changed psychiatric services in Luxembourg (Majerus, 2003). This law had been inspired by French and Belgian examples and was the first that focused on the rights of the mentally ill rather than protection of society from the person, thereby allowing improvements in care. Medical understanding of illnesses took over and was promoted by developments in neurology and the disease model of infection (Spautz, 2005b). Dr Adolf Buffet, director of the Hospice Central from 1883 until 1905, when describing the hospice, stated that 'for a long time it stayed a rallying point for an indescribable chaos, where the sick and the old, the widow and the orphan, all in a way worthy of sympathy, had to live together with the punishable tramp and the disgusting drunkard, the unwed mother and the prostitute'. The Hospice Central was now used only for the mentally ill. In 1901, the Hospice Central in Ettelbruck was transformed into the Maison de Santé (nursing home). The chronically ill were able to stay, but healing stayed a euphemism. There did not appear to be an alternative to the locking away tradition of the prisons, and their motto 'Ora et labora' ('To pray and work') was an aspiration rather than a reality. Life in the institution was supposedly to follow this Benedictine principle aligned with Ettelbruck's religious and worldly objectives. Helplessness in the face of chronic illness led to the development of theories that were ultimately harmful (Häfner, 2006). One leading German psychiatrist espoused the belief that the causes of mental illness were the influence of false education, disruptive family life and the environment and that it would therefore be best to isolate the mentally ill from everyone in their surroundings (Roller, 1831). This isolation ideology proved to be powerless to heal patients. Pinel's (1801) observations were rediscovered: isolation and social deprivation of patients in an institution leads to loss of activities and language, self-neglect and social incompetency.

The world wars

The world wars of the twentieth century presented major challenges for Ettelbruck. Doctors and carers were subject to unpredictable events. People with mental health problems, who struggle with their environment in normal times, are burdened even more during crises and war (Majerus, 2005). The effects and consequences of the two wars were, in fact, different, even though the country was occupied by Germany on both occasions (Majerus, 2009). In the First World War, Ettelbruck was under German military administration from 1914 (Melchers, 1991). In general, this administration let the Luxembourg civil administration continue to work, as long as German interests were not affected. However, the Allied economic blockade hit Luxembourg hard, and the government struggled more and more to get food from neutral third countries. The patients of the Maison de Santé became weak and many died from infectious diseases, especially the Spanish flu in 1917, during which 22% of the 500 patients died (Spautz, 2005a).

During the Second World War, the civil administration under NS-Gauleiter Simon tried to Germanise the country, even committing war crimes to achieve this (Dostert, 1985). A number of resistance movements started, the Luxembourg administration was consequently annihilated and Luxembourg became part of Germany (Fletcher, 1970). In Germany, mass killings of psychiatric patients took place. In Luxembourg, because of the enormous courage and resistance of the doctors and other professionals, patients of the Maison de Santé were able to avoid this fate, although they were, sadly, not able to save the Jewish patients (Spautz *et al.*, 2000). Even though most of Luxembourg was freed by American troops on 10 September 1944, the war was not over for Ettelbruck, as it became a front-line town (Melchers, 1982) and the Maison de Santé's patients had to live underground until after the Battle of the Bulge, where a number of buildings were used as prisons for German war captives (De Smet, 2008).

The aftermath of the wars

In the aftermath of the wars, Luxembourg changed into a European capital, and through the industrial and service sectors became one of the richest countries in the world. The change to more open and humanitarian care of psychiatric patients in Luxembourg did not begin with the introduction of psychopharmacology, as it did in the US and UK from 1952 onwards. The improvement of psychiatric services happened before that, even though the first influential antipsychotic was introduced at a symposium in Ettelbruck in 1952.

In the United States, a radical decrease in psychiatric beds started in 1954, due to scandals spread by the media and the influence of an outraged public; the hospital was no longer the centre and the site of a monopoly on psychiatric care. In Luxembourg, this second psychiatric reform did not start until much later. In the State Neuropsychiatric Hospital (HNPE, Hôpital Neuro-Psychiatrique de l'État), the number of beds kept climbing: from 683 in 1950 to 1025 in 1970 and 860 in 1990, one of the highest numbers in the world at the time. The urgent need for reform became irrefutable (Häfner *et al.*, 1993). In the early 1970s, the monopoly of the HNPE in psychiatric treatment was being criticised. In 1974, a new law emphasised that psychiatric patients should receive care through multidisciplinary means. New doctors, psychologists, social workers and trained carers were employed and new therapeutic groups started to be provided as part of a bio-psycho-social model of patient care (Spautz, 2005b). Psychiatric services started entering general hospitals: the first psychiatric service with about 40 beds was offered with the beginning of the Centre Hospitalier Luxembourg

(1976–77). Private clinics and public hospitals followed slowly after this, and there are currently four hospitals that take care of all acute psychiatric admissions. However, according to the 1974 law, the HNPE was still too big. In 1998, the CHNP (Centre Hospitalier Neuro-Psychiatrique), a new statutory public establishment, was founded. A new independent administrative board was put in place, and employees became private employees rather than public servants.

Häfner planning study 1993

This study was carried out at the order of the Luxembourg Ministry of Health as the authorities had become conscious that there was an urgent need to modernise mental health care. The Ministry of Health appointed the Central Institute for Mental Health of Mannheim (Germany) to examine the situation in Luxembourg and make recommendations for organisational models of psychiatric care. The research work was carried out all over the country, and was published in 1993 as *Mental Health Care in Luxembourg, Current State and Recommendations for Future Development* (Häfner *et al.*, 1993). The recommendations referred to results of international research and evaluation studies on psychiatric care, as well as reported experiences in different European countries. This part of the study was submitted to a group of WHO experts, which gave an international dimension to the work and helped local decision-makers to propose solutions, regardless of pressure from local interest groups. The main recommendations were the decentralisation of psychiatric services, the treatment of patients with mental health problems according to the evidence available and the reduction of stigmatisation, including a quick reintegration of patients into society and the avoidance of long-term institutionalisation.

Rössler planning study 2005

The 2005 study recommended a quantitative and qualitative expansion of the general hospitals' specialised psychiatric departments, existing day clinics and specialised departments, as well as the development of outpatient care. The main recommendations concentrated on the restructuring of the CHNP into five national centres: centre for prevention, early detection and rehabilitation; centre for social and community psychiatry; centre for addictions; centre for gerontopsychiatry; and centre for forensics.

The recommendations that had been made by the 1992 study were broadly implemented. This is especially true of the reorganisation of three psychiatric departments in general hospitals around the country. The new, well-equipped departments illustrated the political intention to see psychiatry as part of general health care. However, a clear general plan for further progression of psychiatric care was not identified. This mainly concerned the CHNP, which even after a significant reduction in beds failed to take on the recommended rehabilitation role, and often continued to carry out its previous role of long-term care of patients.

In 2004, one specialised hospital and four psychiatric departments in general hospitals shared the responsibility for the total care of psychiatric patients in Luxembourg. According to the 2001 Hospital Plan, acute care should only be carried out by four general hospitals with psychiatric departments, and the CHNP should only carry out rehabilitation from mid-2005 onwards. Forty-five beds were planned for each of these hospitals, 12 of these being in secure units. Each psychiatric service was to have a psychiatric day clinic, which are now operational. There were structural and staffing differences between the general hospitals and the CHNP. The general hospitals had all, except one, recently been renovated and possessed good staffing levels. The CHNP, however, had poor infrastructure that limited the quality of care for patients, mainly a lack of somatic care due to low general health care resources (i.e. two general practitioners for 257 patients). After the implementation of the 2001 Hospital Plan, the efforts to reform lessened.

Since 2003, there has been a steady growth in the building of day clinics, linked to the general hospitals and working according to European standards. The outpatient sector was covered by 56 psychiatrists, at a ratio of 0.124 psychiatrists per inhabitant. This is consistent with a high relative number of psychiatrists compared to the rest of Europe; although some psychiatrists have a double role as consultants in general hospitals. With a rate of 0.25 supported living spaces per 1000 inhabitants, Luxembourg is below WHO guidelines which suggest 0.3–0.5 spaces per 1000 inhabitants for long-term care of chronically ill patients.

The reasons for the slow transformation of the recommendations from 1992 were largely a result of three factors: politics, the structure of the health care system and a lack of cooperation among different providers. While psychiatry played a marginal role in political agendas, organisational and financial problems caused problems in the transformation of the recommendations on a structural level.

Current mental health care

At the end of 2004, psychiatric care was provided by four specialised psychiatric wards, one specialised hospital and a clinic. The CHNP had 318 beds; the four psychiatric services each had 45 beds. There were a total of 498 beds, i.e. 0.98 beds per 1000 inhabitants. These consisted of 170 beds for short or medium-length treatments in general hospitals, 36 acute beds and 240 beds for long-term care at the CHNP. Generally, the specialised wards tended to treat the 'milder problems' with neurotic disorders, affective disorders and eating disorders, whereas the CHNP tended to treat patients with psychoses and substance use problems. A total of 54 day clinic places were available for adults with mental health problems.

From 1 July 2005, no patients were directly admitted to the CHNP. Finally, after 150 years, the era of the asylum had finished. From this time, all acute admissions were made to the specialised general hospital services; the related law had been changed following European guidelines as well as responding to the views of human rights organisations. Psychiatric patients can finally walk in through the same doors as other patients and their treatment is consistent with evidence-based research, as it is in other branches of health care. Patients are able to choose a self-employed psychiatrist or other specialists to go to for care. However, if an acute admission has to be made, this can only be done in a hospital that accepts new patients on that particular day. From there, appropriate referrals will then be made if necessary.

In 2006, the CHNP presented a strategic plan for 2006–10. This plan focused on five objectives, which were reduction of hospitalisation, decentralisation, development of an outpatient service, development of specialised psychiatric services and the development of an adolescent psychiatric unit. To support the reduction of beds, the CHNP is obligated to adhere to modern principles of care, which means that psychiatric hospitals are not suitable sites for long-term mentally ill people.

The wards in the various facilities include specialist units for people with psychosis and for the rehabilitation of drink- or drug-dependent patients. The closed units mainly consist of beds for: persons under judicial custody (Article 71 of the Criminal Code) to ensure their protection or that of society; people under a medical admission sent by the criminal psychiatric medical service and requiring 24/7 care; people under a medical admission addressed by the acute psychiatric wards in general hospitals on a waiting list and requiring 24/7 care; and adolescents in difficulty. The open units support all psychiatric disorders requiring preparation for specific rehabilitation, as well as patients in relapse or crisis. The services offered are organised within different departments, poly-drug use, alcohol dependency, psychogeriatric department; psychosis, long-term stay, general psychiatric sector and child psychiatry sector. A centre for adolescents with mental health problems has been developed as a growing number of adolescents had been put in prison due to a lack of other services. Since involuntary admissions have been made directly into specialised units, there has been a significant reduction in the length of stay for people. The maximum legally possible observation period is two periods of 2 weeks with a review in between, which is now in most cases not exceeded. The number of involuntary admissions, however, has been increasing (2006, 438; 2007, 473; 2008, 573).

Each of the four general hospitals has a psychiatric home-care service (SPAD). The SPAD provides a range of interventions for patients, including individual contact, information sharing with the patient and the family, patient education, counselling with families, counselling focusing on adaptation to reality, psycho-therapeutic approaches, reintegration, provision of guidance, leadership and company, and support with financial and household management. The duration of treatment varies widely. It can be short-, medium- or long-term, depending on the patient's individual needs.

Quality control

The CHNP is an active member of the European Foundation of Quality Management (EFQM) which aims to promote competence and excellence. This process involves planning, assessment and change which aims to guarantee excellent services for patients/residents, high-quality relationships with partners and staff satisfaction. The Committed to Excellence (C2E) programme is a framework that aims to optimise the process of project management for company projects. The model, based on leadership, on the specification of outcomes and solutions to achieve these objectives, supports the continuous optimisation of internal processes at the CHNP.

The CHNP has already successfully completed the first phase of the certification process of the C2E and has taken a further step in its policy of restructuring started by the reform of psychiatry in Luxembourg. The CHNP's aims for 2010 are to be the centre of excellence in psychiatric rehabilitation, to be one of the centres of excellence in supporting people with mental disabilities and to be one of the centres of excellence in supporting the elderly. Its main objectives are the decentralisation, deinstitutionalisation and destigmatisation of psychiatry. To achieve these objectives, the CHNP has planned a complete renovation of its infrastructure, including a complete renovation of some of the buildings and locations.

The CHNP has taken the initiative to participate in the European Leonardo da Vinci VII project in order to compare processes of care and outcomes with international partners. The overall project objectives are exchange of good practice, observation and comparison of vocational skills, and evaluating quality and skills development. In early September 2009, a systematic customer survey assessed the discharge procedure of each hospitalised client and gave the opportunity to evaluate the release plans of each individual hospital and thus observe the reduction of the population referred to as long-term-care patients.

The Grand Duchy of Luxembourg has achieved a standard of care comparable to other (Western) European countries, and in some areas above average (Rössler, 2009). However, there is a need for continuous efforts to not only keep this level of care, but to dynamically evolve. Rössler rates the qualitative and quantitative provision of acute psychiatric care as good to very good and comparable to the standards in other European countries. Whereas in 2005, there was still a lack of beds in acute psychiatric care, this was resolved by 2008.

The professions

The first existing official document referring to health care in Luxembourg, in 1732, forbids medical practice without licence, and throughout the following century the government would continue to attempt to register and control all those who claimed skills in the provision of health care, via the establishment of medical commissions created in 1818. By 1841, Luxembourg had become a Grand Duchy independent of the Netherlands but under the sovereignty of its king. At his instigation, the medical commissions were supplemented by a body which still exists to this day: the Medical College. Throughout the history of Luxembourg's health care system, the vast majority of medical personnel have not been state employees, but rather self-employed workers. The neuropsychiatric hospital, established in the late nineteenth century, was the last to be run by the state, but was brought into line with all other hospitals by legislation in 1998.

Presently, there is no medical school at the University of Luxembourg. Medical students therefore receive their training abroad, mainly in Belgium, France or Germany. Dentists and graduate nurses are also trained abroad; in short, any health profession requiring more than 3 years' training after secondary school will require a period of training abroad. Following completion of their training, physicians simply need approval of their foreign diploma by the Ministry of Health (if delivered in an EU member state) or by the Ministry of Education (if delivered in other countries) and authorisation from the Ministry of Health to practise in Luxembourg.

Professional qualifications requiring 3 years of training (e.g. the basic nursing qualification and those for paramedics, laboratory technicians and surgical assistants) can be gained in Luxembourg itself. The Ministry of Education takes the lead in determining policy for this training. The first training was organised in 1939, in Ettelbruck, where young people were educated to become psychiatric nurses. Training colleges for nurses in general care were founded in 1945–46, one by the state, others by religious organisations. Nursing schools in Ettelbruck and Esch-sur-Alzette followed later.

Students decide in secondary school after completing year 11 whether they want to become a nurse. Requirements are the successful completion of year 11 at either the technical or classical secondary schools in Luxembourg. From 2010–11 onwards, nursing will require 4 years of training and psychiatric nursing will last an extra 2 years. Psychiatric nursing studies can be carried out either in

Luxembourg or abroad in a public or private psychiatric nursing school recognised by the Ministry of Health in Luxembourg. A candidate who wishes to study abroad has to notify the minister of health in advance, indicating their school of choice. Within 2 months of this notice, the minister of health will inform the applicant whether they meet the conditions for admission to the school and if the school is accredited for studies of psychiatric nursing.

Following the new law of 1992, 20 occupations are now recognised as health professions. Some are older, such as nursing, psychiatric nursing or midwifery, whilst others are newer, such as the three types of assistant medical technicians and the various specialisations of the profession of nursing. Whilst the 1967 act refers to 'paramedical professions', the term now used is 'health professionals'. This change reflects less a quest for autonomy of the professions from the medical profession than an evolution in the philosophy that guides these professions. Previously, the focus was on working with medicine focusing on the cure of disease, but now the focus on disease has been replaced by one which focuses on health.

One distinct feature of the Luxembourg hospital system worthy of note is the affiliated doctor system, i.e. with few exceptions; the hospitals are run by doctors, who are also working as self-employed doctors. There are advantages and disadvantages with this system. One disadvantage is that self-employed doctors cannot fully dedicate their services to the hospital. However, a major advantage is the close link between the outpatient and inpatient areas, where the crisis points that can happen during admission or discharge can be avoided by offering continuous treatment by the same person. This continuity, however, also lowers the threshold for hospital admissions, which can be seen in the relatively high admission rate and short length of stays when compared to other countries.

Staff numbers

As of 31 December 2009, there were 703 professionals working for the CHNP, an equivalent of 611.8 full-time staff: 14 specialists in psychiatry or neuropsychiatry, two child psychiatry specialists, three general practitioners, 518 care staff and medical technicians, 80 administrative staff and 86 technical staff. These staff came from 21 different nationalities, 57% of which were Luxembourg, 19% German, 11% Belgian, 5% Portuguese and 3% French. Sixty-eight per cent were females and 32% males, and they took part in 15 682 hours of personal and professional development training. The general director has to be a doctor; the position cannot be filled by another profession.

Contribution of nursing

Psychiatric nurses provide support and a helping therapeutic relationship for people in psychological crisis or with mental health problems. They contribute to the diagnosis made by the doctor and the application of medical and psychiatric treatment. Psychiatric nurses base their activity on the nursing process, both in their autonomous role and in their actions supporting medical prescription. They are expected to adopt a holistic approach, taking into account the needs of the patient: physiological, psychological, social and cultural. The psychiatric nurse participates in health education and promotes the rehabilitation of the patient. In addition, they can provide mentoring and training of others. Psychiatric nurses are expected to keep up to date with evidence-based practice. Without prejudice to the powers reserved to physicians or other health professionals, psychiatric nurses can carry out the following professional acts: observation, assessing the person in relation to their basic needs and supporting their efforts to meet them, and developing strategies to achieve a healthy life for the person cared for; supporting the patient and keeping a safe environment during admission, calming the patient in a psychological crisis and supporting them by providing information and onwards referral; and finally therapeutic individual or group work.

As part of a protocol for emergency care previously determined, dated and signed by a physician, psychiatric nurses are empowered to care for and take necessary protective measures in relation to a patient until a physician can intervene, provided the behaviour of the patient may endanger their own physical integrity or that of third parties. As psychiatrists are not generally present on the wards during the day, but work from their private practices, nurses are expected to intervene in emergencies awaiting recommendations of the psychiatrists, which often used to be made by phone but now have to be given in writing. Psychiatric nurses can implement measures of isolation or restraint in accordance with the legislation. Nurses have to act according to doctors' prescriptions for care, rather than being allowed to take decisions independently. The starting salary for a psychiatric nurse is €2758 and can go up to €5251.

Mental health law

The compulsory admission and involuntary treatment of mentally ill persons in Luxembourg is governed by a special mental health act (Loi du 26 mai, 1988) that repealed the old law on the insane (Loi du 7 juillet, 1880). The Youth Protection Law regulates the procedures concerning minors (Loi du 10 août, 1992). In order to regulate the judicial procedures of the admission and treatment of mentally ill offenders, a new law was issued in 2009 relating to the hospital admission of people with mental problems without their consent. The respective legal texts are available online at www.legilux.lu (in French). The text of Article 71 of the Penal Code dates back to 1810 and states: 'There is no infraction (of the law) if the accused or the prisoner was in a state of dementia whilst committing the act'. It was introduced in national legislation at the same time as the Penal Code, by the law of 16 June 1879, and for a long time was identical to articles of the French and Belgian penal codes (Salize and Dreßing, 2005). The new Article 71 now includes a clause of penal irresponsibility for persons suffering from mental disorders who do not have the ability to discern and control their actions. The mental disorder is considered to have influence not over the acts themselves, but over the perpetrator of the acts. For this reason, the legislator has introduced the concept of penal irresponsibility. In the case of an offence committed while under the influence of alcohol or drugs, the judge remains the one to decide whether or not the suspect is fully responsible. Another major change in Article 71 is the fact that if the article is applied and if the person continues to represent a danger to himself or to others, the judge then has to order the admission of the offender to a certified institution or ward, thereby introducing the concept of 'judicial admission'. Concerned persons, such as family members or teachers, are informed in the event of an involuntary admission. There is an established special committee dealing with judicial admissions. It is composed of a judge who chairs the commission, a crown magistrate and two members appointed by the minister of health, including a specialist psychiatrist or child psychiatrist. Within 2 months of the judicial admission, the physician reports to the committee on the mental state of the person and on the continued appropriateness of this admission. Discharge cannot be granted unless the court has serious reasons to conclude that the patient no longer presents a danger to themselves or others.

The number of compulsory admissions in 2003 was around 545, which at that time contributed to nearly half of CHNP admissions, as it was the only institution allowed to accept these. This resulted in a rate of about 100 compulsory admissions per 100000 inhabitants. In comparison to other European countries, this put Luxembourg as the highest, together with Germany.

The law of 10 December 2009

This act regulates the admission and residence, without consent, of people with mental disorders in a psychiatric unit. It states categorically that wherever possible, people with mental disorders should be treated in the area in which they live. They may only be subject to an admission if their severe mental health problems render them dangerous to themselves or others or if the admission has been ordered by a court trial or trial under Article 71 of the Penal Code. The decline of mental health abilities due to ageing is not, by itself, sufficient grounds for admission. Lack of congruity with moral, social, political or other societal values cannot be considered, per se, as a mental disorder. Treatment must be based on an individualised care plan, administered by medical personnel and include skilled care. It must be orientated towards the reintegration of patients into society. Treatment should be offered with respect for the freedom of expression and the patient's religious or philosophical beliefs. It should also promote physical health, family and social contacts, as well as their cultural development.

Admission procedure

A person cannot be admitted unless there is a written request for admission submitted by any of the following:
- guardian or trustee of an incapacitated adult
- a member of the family of the person or any other interested person
- mayor of the municipality or the territory in which the person concerned is staying
- heads of intervention centres or police stations near the national police, and in their absence, a police officer
- the state prosecutor for the judicial district in which the person concerned is staying.

In exceptional cases of imminent danger to the health of the person concerned or the safety of others, certified by a medical officer not attached to the psychiatric service, the admission can take place without being in possession of the application described. On the day of admission, information is given in writing to the judge. The judge checks whether the conditions of substance and form of admission are met. After the admission, the person is admitted under observation for a period not to exceed 30 days. The decision to maintain the observation is not appealable.

The decision to terminate the admission of a person is made by a judge. Before making his decision, the judge has a hearing in the treatment facility which the person has been admitted to. The judge may, if deemed advisable, hear the person admitted in the presence of his doctor. Within 48 hours of the hearing, the judge makes an order declaring either the discharge of the person admitted or his admission.

If, after the decision to admit, the attending physician believes that the condition of the person requires a long-term stay, he transfers them to a psychiatric institution. The doctor records the mental health state of the patient at least every month on the register. He also reconsiders the necessity of staying in the establishment at the end of the third month following the decision to admit. On his own initiative, or at the request of the person detained or any interested person, the treating doctor may, on a trial basis, grant the person placed under care permission to leave the facility. If the conditions imposed on the person are not met, or if the condition of the person has changed to the point where it becomes necessary to terminate the trial period, the physician shall inform the state prosecutor of the residence of the placed person, who will take all necessary steps to bring them back to the institution.

Discharge

If the doctor believes that the person's condition has improved to an extent that admission is no longer necessary, he makes the declaration on a register. If the person leaves the institution, the physician may attach discharge conditions of residence and/or medical surveillance. If the person fails to comply with these conditions, the person who had requested the admission may readmit the person to the institution on request without producing a new medical certificate. A year after the date of the admission decision, a panel decides, after obtaining the advice of the treating physician and with necessary supporting information, whether continuing with the admission is justified. The panel consists of a judge, who chairs, a physician specialising in psychiatry or child psychiatry and a social worker unattached to the institution. If the committee finds that the admission is no longer necessary, the person is immediately discharged. If the admission is maintained, then the committee carries out a review of the person placed every 2 years.

Future mental health services (recommendations made by Rössler, 2009)

In Luxembourg, there is still a problem with people who have been institutionalised for many years and, even after attempts to reintegrate into society, have not managed to live independently. The CHNP has now entered into an agreement with the Ministry of Health that other resources for these patients need to have been found by 2012.

Currently, one of the major problems for the CHNP is an inadequate infrastructure for compulsory admissions. This area of treatment is one that attracts most media attention and places psychiatric care in Luxembourg in a negative light. In the long run, it is suggested that the best solution would be the opening of a new institute for forensic psychiatry, separate from the CHNP, but linked to the CHNP on an administrative and structural basis.

As previously mentioned, the development of the different specialised units in the four general hospitals has essentially been completed. Further work is needed to create day clinics, and one possibility is to start up a so-called integrated day hospital. The term 'integrated' refers to the fact that this day clinic should be flexible, in that it can also, if necessary, admit acute patients into inpatient care again. This means that the care would always be undertaken by the same staff. An integrated day clinic treatment comes closer to the ideal of a person-orientated care model than the traditional structures, as it can respond flexibly to the changing needs of patients.

Unlike inpatient care, outpatient treatment by self-employed doctors is not subject to state planning. This leads to self-employed doctors taking on the responsibility of care. Despite the relatively large numbers of doctors working in outpatient settings, there is often a lack of psychotherapy and other forms of psychosocial care available. Recommendations have therefore been made that psychiatrists establish a hotline for available psychotherapy sessions. Rössler (2009) also suggests that the self-employed psychiatrists should keep emergency appointments free according to a plan, and let the media be aware of this. Currently, emergency admissions are usually carried out via the hospitals' emergency outpatient departments; however, this increases the risk of hospitalisation.

The process of mental health reform in Luxembourg provides a good illustration of the fact that money alone does not accomplish successful reform. Luxembourg has, for many years, substantially invested in the psychiatry field without the country following some of the better developments found in other European countries. In addition to funds being available, it is mainly long-term political commitment, jointly agreed objectives and guided cooperation which create desired changes in this area.

The planned structural reforms are soon to be completed. The next step is the improvement of the quality of care in institutions. Patients should be entitled to a transparent, understandable and consistent quality of care throughout the range of facilities and services. This issue currently concerns experts more than politicians, but it will be a combination of both that will see the continued improvement of mental health services.

Case scenario

A 23-year-old unemployed man is reported by his landlord as acting increasingly strangely. He has barricaded his room, talking about being spied upon by the CIA. He can be heard shouting within his room in an angry and incoherent way. He has not been seen by a psychiatrist in the past, although his mother has told the landlord that he has been isolating himself and acting increasingly oddly over the last couple of years.

A person may be brought into psychiatric care against his will. For this to happen, it is necessary for a doctor (there is no need for this to be a psychiatrist) to confirm that the person poses a danger to himself or others. At the same time, there is a need for an admission request, which may be made by a family member or by any other person following legal safeguards. If these two conditions are satisfied, the person would be brought into a psychiatric service. It may be that the police have to intervene, as may be the case for this 23-year-old man. In Luxembourg, psychiatrists do not typically see patients at home; especially not in acute cases. However, in some non-profit organisations or the community psychiatric service (SPAD), it can happen from time to time that a psychiatrist goes to see a patient at home together with a nurse. Once the patient is admitted to a psychiatric ward, the psychiatrist decides on the need to continue with the admission, at least for the first few days. If the psychiatrist believes that the patient is not affected by mental health problems, he may immediately discharge the patient.

Treatment in an inpatient setting would consist primarily of drug treatment. Use of medication is widespread within the different inpatient services. Depending on the diagnosis, the psychiatrist prescribes the drug that is deemed most suitable in his or her view; psychiatrists have a large amount of therapeutic freedom. This freedom is vigorously defended by all physicians. Unfortunately, there are currently no defined clinical pathways, so each doctor is free to do as he or she deems appropriate.

In three of the four psychiatric services which provide acute admissions, doctors are private physicians; whereas doctors at the Centre Hospitalier de Luxembourg have an employee status. All inpatient psychiatric services include psychologists, occupational therapists, social workers and nurses working in a multidisciplinary team. Even though there are multidisciplinary teams, treatment is prescribed by the doctors involved in the patient's care.

Nursing staff carry out close observations of patients over the first few days, depending on the condition of the person. The nurses would provide individual care and offer therapeutic activities, as well as occupational therapy activities. Depending on availability, they also accompany patients to other activities, such as occupational therapy or physiotherapy. There are various options for patients in terms of long-term care following discharge from hospital. They may be seen by a psychiatrist in his practice, they can be enrolled in a psychiatric day hospital or they can be seen at home by the SPAD. There is also a non-profit association (ATP) which provides work therapies in numerous sites. Patients may be taken under the care of a number of different non-profit associations offering outpatient psychiatric services. Though the types of services vary in how they are funded, delivered and what they entail, nevertheless, their aim is similar, i.e. to enable the person to become as independent as possible and resume the life they had before they became ill.

References
• • • • • • • • • • • • • • • • •

Allegrezza S, Heinrich G, Jesuit D. Poverty and income inequality in Luxembourg and the Grande Région in comparative perspective. *Socioecon Rev.* 2004; **2**: 263–83.

Barry M, Jenkins R. *Implementing Mental Health Promotion.* Churchill Livingstone: China; 2007.

Bersani, J. *Encyclopaedia Universalis,* Paris: Enyclopaedia Universalis; 1996.

Bossaert D, Calmes C. *Die Geschichte des Großherzogtums Luxemburg von 1815 bis heute.* Luxembourg; 1994.

Buffet A. *Régime hospitalier et légal des aliénés 1815–1889.* Luxembourg; 1889.

CHNP. Rapport annuel. 2010. Available at: www.chnp.lu/fr/corporate/documentation/rapport_annuel (accessed 8 May 2010).

CIA. Gini Index. 2008. Available at: www.cia.gov/library/publications/the-world-factbook/rankorder/2172rank.html (accessed 8 May 2010).

Code pénal du Grand-Duché de Luxembourg. *Livre Ier, Chapitre VIII.* Ministère de la Justice: Luxembourg; 2000.

Conolly J. *The Indications of Insanity.* London: J Taylor; 1830.

Consbruck R. Saar-Lor-Lux Symposium 'Der Preis der Psychiatrie': Sich kontinuierlich in Frage stellen. *Luxemburger Wort.* 24 November 2009: 15.

De Smet Y. Centre hospitalier neuro-psychiatrique. In: Administration Communale Ettelbruck. *Ettelbruck – 100 Joer Stad 1907–2007.* 2008. pp. 75–9.

De Smet Y, Spautz JM. Création de l'Hospice central d'Ettelbruck. *Die Warte, Luxemburger Wort.* 21 April 2005.

Dostert P. *Luxemburg zwischen Selbstbehauptung und nationaler Selbstaufgabe: deutsche Besatzungspolitik und die Volksdeutsche Bewegung 1940–1945.* Luxembourg: Editions Saint-Paul; 1985.

European Commission. *Special Eurobarometer: mental well-being.* 2006. Available at: http://ec.europa.eu/health/ph_information/documents/ebs_248_en.pdf (accessed 8 May 2010).

European Commission. *Mental Health Briefing Sheets: facts and activities in member states.* 2010. Available at: http://ec.europa.eu/health/ph_determinants/life_style/mental/docs/Luxembourg.pdf (accessed 8 May 2010).

European Health Expectancy Monitoring Unit. Différentes estimations des espérances de santé dans les pays de l'Union européenne en 2002, Calculs réalisés à partir des données d'Eurobaromètre 58. *EHEMU Technical Report 3.* Montpellier; 2005.

European Observatory on Health Care Systems. *Health Care Systems in Transition: Luxembourg.* 1999. Available at: www.euro.who.int/document/e67498.pdf (accessed 8 May 2010).

Fletcher WA. The German administration in Luxembourg 1940–1942; towards a 'de facto' annexation. *The Historical Journal.* 1970; **13**: 533–44.

Foucault M. *Wahnsinn und Gesellschaft.* Frankfurt: Suhrkamp; 1969.

Geremek B. *Les marginaux parisiens aux XIVᵉ et XVᵉ siècles.* Paris: Flammarion; 1976.

Goerens J. L'Hospice civil de Luxembourg. *Cahiers Luxembourgeois.* 1935; **2**.

Häfner H. Dringliche Reformen in der psychiatrischen krankenversorgung der Bundesrepublik. *Helfen und Heilen.* 1965; **4**: 1–8.

Häfner H. 150 ans Centre Hospitalier neuro-Psychiatrique (CHNP): Die Ideengeschichte psychiatrischer Versorgung. *Bulletin de la Société des Sciences Médicales du Grand-Duché de Luxembourg.* 2006; **1**: 87–107.

Häfner H, Rössler W, Salize HJ. *Gemeindepsychiatrie, Grundlagen und Leitlinien: Planungsstudie Luxemburg.* Wien: Verlag Integrative Psychiatrie; 1993.

Hartmann-Hirsch C, Tchicaya A. Politique de la santé. In: Reuter C, Schneider M, Brandhorst K, editors. *Handbuch der sozialen und erzieherischen Arbeit in Luxembourg.* Luxembourg: Editions Saint-Paul; 2009.

IMF. *Luxembourg and the IMF.* 2009. Available at: www.imf.org/external/country/LUX/index.htm. (accessed 8 May 2010).

Jetter D. *Das europäische Hospital – Von der Spätantike bis 1800.* Köln: Du Mont Buchverlag; 1986.

Knapp M, McDaid D, Amaddeo F, *et al.* Financing mental health care in Europe. *J Ment Health.* 2007; **16**(2): 167–80.

Loi du 26 mai 1988 relative au admission des personnes atteintes de troubles mentaux dans des établissements ou services psychiatriques fermés. *Mémorial A (n° 28), 16 juin 1988,* 560–3.

Loi du 31 décembre 2009 a) relative à l'hospitalisation sans leur consentement de personnes atteintes de troubles mentaux, b) modifiant la loi modifiée du 31 mai 1999 sur la Police et l'Inspection générale de la Police et c) modifiant l'article 73 de la loi communale modifiée du 13 décembre 1988. *Mémorial A (n° 263), 31 décembre 2009,* 5489–97.

Loi du 7 juillet 1880 sur le régime des aliénés. *Mémorial 1880,* 445ff.

Loi du 10 août 1992 relative à la protection de la Jeunesse. *Mémorial A (n° 70) 25 septembre 1992,* 2195–202.

Majerus JM. Felix Blochausen. In: Haag E, editor. *400 Joer Kolleisch. L'Athénée et ses grands anciens.* 2003; **3**: 255–418.

Majerus JM. *Discours à l'Occasion de 150 Joer CHNP Ettelbruck 2005.* Unpublished.

Majerus JM. Das Centre hospitalier neuro-psychiatrique. In: Reuter C, Schneider M, Brandhorst K, editors. *Handbuch der sozialen und erzieherischen Arbeit in Luxemburg.* Luxembourg: Editions Saint-Paul; 2009.

Melchers ET. *Kriegsschauplatz Luxemburg August 1914. Mai 1940.* Luxemburg: Editions Saint-Paul; 1991.

Ministère de la Santé. Available at: www.sante.public.lu/fr/index.html (accessed 8 May 2010).

Ministère de la Santé. *Carte Sanitaire, 1998–2005.* Ministère de la Santé: Luxembourg; 2005.

Ministère de la Sécurité Sociale. *Rapport général sur la sécurité sociale.* Luxembourg: Imprimés et fournitures de bureau de l'Etat; 2009.

Ministère de la Sécurité Sociale. *Rapport sur la situation de l'assurance maladie-maternité.* Luxembourg; Imprimés et fournitures de bureau de l'Etat; 2008.

OECD. Statistiques et Indicateurs pour 30 pays. *Eco-Santé OCDE 2007,* Luxembourg; 2007.

OECD. *Etudes économiques de l'OCDE Luxembourg, 12.* 2008.

OECD. *OECD in Figures 2008.* Paris; 2008.

Pinel P. *Traité medico-philosophique sur l'aliénation mentale ou la manie.* Paris: Richard, Caille et Ravier; 1801.

Roberts D. Modernising mental health care in Luxembourg: interview with Dr. Jo Joosten. *Luxembourg News.* 2008; **352**.

Roller CFW. *Die Irrenanstalt in allen ihren Beziehungen.* Karlsruhe: CF Müller; 1831.

Rössler W. *Psychiatrie Luxemburg: Stand der Umsetzung der Empfehlungen der Planungsstudie 2005.* Auftragsbericht, Ministère de la Santé: Luxemburg; 2009.

Rössler W, Koch U. *Psychiatrie Luxemburg, Planungsstudie 2005.* Auftragsbericht, Ministère de la Santé: Luxemburg; 2005.

Salize HJ, Dreßing H. *Admission and Treatment of Mentally Ill Offenders: legislation and practice in EU member states.* European Commission Research Project; 2005.

Schroeder J. Vom Ursprung der Springprozession. In: Ferrari MC, Schroeder J, Trauffler H, editors. *Die Abtei Echternach 698–1998.* Luxembourg; CLUDEM; 1999.

Spautz JM, Graas M, Hentgen P. La psychiatrie au Luxembourg. *L'Information Psychiatrique.* 2000; **9**.

Spautz JM. *Centre hospitalier neuro-psychiatrique 150 Joer 1855–2005.* Broschüre: 2005a.

Spautz JM. *Discours à l'occasion de 150 Joer CHNP Ettelbruck 2005* (unpublished); 2005b.

STATEC. *Statistiques des causes de décès pour l'année 2005*. Luxembourg; 2006. Available at: www.sante.public.lu/fr/catalogue-publications/maladies-traitements/statistiques-causes-deces/index.html (accessed 8 May 2010).

Tchicaya A. État de santé et facteurs de risque: quelques indicateurs pour le Luxembourg en 2005. *Population & Emploi*. 2007; **24**: 1–8.

WHO. Young people's health in context: international report from the HBSC 2001/02 survey, (health policy for children and adolescents, no. 4). Copenhagen: WHO Regional Office for Europe; 2004.

WHO. World Health Statistics 2009. Available at: www.who.int/whosis/whostat/EN_WHS09_Full.pdf (accessed 8 May 2010).

World Health Organization and Wonca. *Integrating Mental Health into Primary Care: a global perspective*. Geneva: WHO and Wonca; 2008.

Mental health care in the Netherlands

Roland van de Sande and Edwin Hellendoorn

Introduction

The Netherlands has a long history of providing high-quality mental health care for its citizens. This chapter describes the political and religious approaches that have given rise to separate and discrete approaches to health care and which are accommodated in today's modern health services. The authors critically discuss the current health needs of the nation and compare these with the types of services available. In addition to responding to the mental health problems common to all countries, the Netherlands has devoted considerable resources towards improving substance abuse and suicide prevention services. The contribution to services by nurses is seen as significant, and it is intended that this role will be extended further in the future.

Profile of the Dutch population

Understanding the political, economic and demographic context of the Netherlands allows an insight into the factors that continue to influence the structure and approach of its mental health services. The Netherlands currently has a population of 16 515 057 inhabitants (CBS, 2010) and is one of the most densely populated countries in Europe (3977 per square kilometre). Approximately 80% of the total population is located in urban areas. The country has a long democratic parliamentary tradition and was an early participant in several international collaborative bodies, such as the EU and the United

Nations. From an economic perspective, the Netherlands is one of the top 20 wealthiest countries in the world, which is the result of decades of low inflation and unemployment rates. According to the Eurostat database (2011), the unemployment rate is the lowest in Europe (4.6%), although there is emerging evidence that unemployment rates are beginning to rise due to the harsh economic climate.

From the early 1970s, there has been a steady flow of economic immigrants from the Mediterranean areas, Asia and the Caribbean to strengthen the workforce and contribute to the rapidly growing economy. In 2008, it was estimated that there were 143 516 new immigrants in the Netherlands, compared to 11 779 citizens who decided to live abroad (CBS, 2010).

At present, cities like Amsterdam and Rotterdam have large immigrant communities. As many as 60% of all urban inhabitants are not descended from Dutch, and are from over 160 nationalities. In fact, Amsterdam is the most multicultural city in the world, followed by Antwerp and New York. The multicultural nature of the society is not reflected in the ethnic mix of existing health care staff, although in some urban acute psychiatric wards the majority of patients have a migrant background. Religion is part of daily life for 58% of the Dutch population, who identify themselves as Roman Catholic (29%), Protestant (19%), Muslim (4%) and other religions (4%).

History of mental health services

Up until 1900, psychiatric patients were normally sent to asylums in remote, isolated areas (Gijswijt-Hofstra and Oosterhuis, 2001), where they were supervised rather than treated, mainly by untrained guards. In 1892, the first formal psychiatric nursing examinations were held, and the first certificates were officially issued in the Netherlands (Boschma, 1997). At that time, religious organisations (both Roman Catholic and Protestant) had acquired considerable expertise, experience and influence in how the care for people with psychiatric problems should be structured and provided. The Roman Catholic influence tended to be more prevalent in the south of the country, in contrast to the Protestant church, which had more influence in the north. Around the beginning of the twentieth century, several serious conflicts arose between religious and medically orientated providers of health care as to the best way to treat and care for those with psychiatric illnesses. Conflicts in approach arose that threatened to be divisive, but eventually agreement was arrived at and both key religious and medical personnel reached a position where they managed to achieve consensus and the best in both approaches could be assimilated so as to provide the best care and treatment possible.

Up until 1950, mental health care was predominantly hospital-based and managed by a distant management board. Despite the absence of adequate pharmacological treatment and the use of restraint, psychiatric hospitals in the Netherlands managed reasonably well in coping with those who presented with multiple problems and difficult behaviour. Before the Second World War, French and German approaches to psychiatry were widely adopted, whereas during the post-war period North American approaches were preferred and eventually prevailed nationally (Ravelli, 2006).

As psychiatric crises were commonly regarded as the climax of a somatic illness, mainly medical interventions were applied to reduce the level of arousal in brain activity. As a result of fostering a medical approach, some patients spent long periods on bed rest for what was regarded as therapeutic reasons, under the supervision of nurses. Gradually, the professional status and identity of nurses was supported and confirmed by specific psychiatric nurse training. Formal and professional psychiatric nursing examinations, which commenced in 1892, have steadily developed since that time (aan den Stegge, 2001). However, the gap between the content and quality of medical training as opposed to nursing training has been and remains considerable. Not only was there a difference in the levels of training but there was also a considerable difference in what nurses and doctors were expected to do in specific situations. The role of the nurse was traditionally more or less regarded as correctional and in helping promote activities of daily living, in contrast to doctors whose role it was to identify, diagnose and combat the somatic consequences of mental suffering (Boschma, 1997). The doctors invariably oversaw the medical management of patients and the work of nurses.

Until 1900, the scientific foundation of most therapies and interventions prescribed by psychiatrists was mainly driven by biological and bacteriological insights. The Dutch Association of Psychiatrists, founded in 1890, had the authority to dictate the form and content of psychiatric nurse training, a duty they exercised for at least the next century. Many psychiatrists viewed training as a means of 'civilising' the nursing staff, many of whom had little or no education and came from families who were unskilled manual workers. Recruiting nurses proved difficult, and almost half of the nurses left nursing in their first year of training. Doctors tended to criticise nurses for this situation and regarded them as poorly motivated, a threat to a stable workforce, rough and often drunk on duty, whilst no attempt was made to examine how the training was delivered nor the conditions in which nurses were expected to work (Boschma, 1997). Against this background, the number of chronic psychiatric patients was increasing and the wards of the asylums were becoming increasingly overcrowded, disorganised and barely manageable. It was no wonder that the confidence of nurses was undermined and compromised by the situation in which they found themselves.

Prominent policy-makers in the early part of the twentieth century were convinced that renaming asylums with the title 'hospital' would improve the standing of psychiatrists and nurses, while at the same time raise the standard of care provided. In bringing about these changes, it was also hoped that recruitment to the psychiatric nursing profession would improve. Treatment modalities at the time were mainly based on the assumption that minimising stimuli would reduce cerebral arousal in patients, and by so doing would lead to improved social functioning. This approach did not meet with the approval of a number of male nursing staff and some felt so uncomfortable that they sought employment elsewhere, in contrast to female nurses, who favoured the approach. As a consequence, the number of females entering psychiatric nursing increased (Boschma, 1997).

Initially, the process of professionalisation in the nursing discipline was strongly influenced by medical knowledge and their practice was diligently supervised by doctors. Academic input from psychiatric nurses was non-existent initially and uncommon until 1980 (Boschma,1997; aan den Stegge, 2001). The in-service training provided by psychiatric hospitals was mainly practice-driven and supported by a limited amount of educational input; however, from 1900 the number of lecture hours increased from 240 to 1320 hours in a 3-year direct entry course for registered nurses in psychiatric care (Koekoek *et al.*, 1990).

Since the introduction of occupational therapy in 1925, there has been greater emphasis in psychiatric care on the acquisition of healthy lifestyle practices and the enhancement of the quality of patients' lives (de Lange, 2001). This relatively new approach also resulted in the development of self-supporting communities in the hospital environment, with patients making use of the facilities available to them to produce their own home-made food.

A more sociological way of thinking was adopted in Dutch psychiatry after the Second World War, giving rise to a number of community psychiatric care initiatives, mainly in the big cities Amsterdam and Rotterdam. Home visiting, which started in 1930, came more to the fore and was seen as having many advantages. Not only did it provide early access to services for those with mental health problems, but it proved less expensive than hospital treatment, permitted patients to be more empowered, involved families more and generally provided a more agreeable means of supporting people undergoing severe mental health crises. Between 1933 and 1988, outreach care was provided to over 200 000 patients (mostly psychotic, suicidal and manic) and their families by the community psychiatric service in Amsterdam (Akkermans, 2001). So successful was this initiative that other parts of the country, over the past three decades, have adopted it and it is proving equally successful there.

Current mental health services

Large psychiatric hospitals have been steadily downsized over the years and substituted by smaller inpatient facilities spread over specific catchment areas. Despite reducing the capacity of the large institutions, ironically the total number of beds remains one of the highest in Europe, slightly above Belgium and Germany (Priebe *et al.*, 2008). In 2006, the Netherlands provided 131.1 conventional psychiatric beds per 100 000 inhabitants, considerably more than, for example, the UK (59.1 beds). In the UK, mental health services have witnessed a depletion of 68% in bed capacity while catering for a similar, vulnerable population's profile. However, when making international comparisons great caution needs to be exercised. For instance, there are issues surrounding the use of acute care services that are not entirely clear and where a number of different perceptions can appear. Some of these questions are: What is an acute service? Could it be that a person receiving acute care is not necessarily allocated a bed? How is an average length of stay calculated? And could a person ever be deemed to be in receipt of services from two sources, e.g. acute care and assertive outreach? Commentators in England argue that the number of acute beds has now gone as low as they can reasonably go and to reduce them further would pose a threat to patients themselves and the community at large (Lelliott, 2006). Even at the level acute beds are at in the Netherlands, there is still considerable demand, and complaints arise from time to time stating that there are insufficient facilities to meet the need.

One major means of finding alternatives to hospital beds is by reducing them, thus forcing mental health and other service personnel to negotiate how services might be reconfigured outside the confines of institutions. In some regions, crisis home teams and assertive community treatment teams have contributed to a shift to providing intensive crisis care in the community.

Community psychiatric services developed rapidly in the last half of the twentieth century and are now much more widely available than in the early eighties (Wolf *et al.*, 1997; Akkermans, 2001). The assumption that the growth of community psychiatric services would inevitably lead to a decrease in psychiatric beds remains highly debatable in the Netherlands. In fact, there is some evidence, coupled with increasing concern, that reinstitutionalisation is on the increase (Priebe *et al.*, 2008). Although community care facilities increased, factors such as social support and risk management strategies have played some part in the increase of beds (Priebe *et al.*, 2008). However, the length of stay has decreased considerably, but on the other hand the number of readmissions has increased and the number of compulsory admissions doubled over the last decade (Mulder *et al.*, 2006).

This phenomenon, which is far from satisfactory, has been influenced by a number of factors, e.g. changes in mental health legislation, more opportunities for psychiatrists to have access to beds, a growing ageing population, assertive outreach teams who identify hidden severe mental health problems in specific regions, and poor informal support for vulnerable people in urban areas. Although some people will require access to inpatient beds and medical treatment for a temporary period, to focus predominantly on these inpatient services to the exclusion of other social and supportive services is to miss the essence of what is contained in recent EU directives on good practice in mental health care. In fact, simply extending services that always existed is short-sighted and ultimately self-defeating.

Substance misuse

The classical approach to separating general psychiatric facilities from addiction services has met with criticism over the last decade, especially as it is now evident that a large number of depressed and psychotic patients use alcohol and street drugs as a form of self-medication, thus giving rise to additional problems (van der Stel, 2001). It is now apparent that the way that services are configured, and the personnel employed there, is as important as the treatments and interventions provided within them. At present, more and more services in both these domains have merged and care teams frequently comprise personnel with a range of skills able to deal with a range of mental health problems.

Current mental health law

The Dutch Mental Health Act has changed considerably since 1992 (Simons *et al.*, 1992) and is now strongly driven by risk assessments on specific dangerousness criteria, rather than best-interest principles and formal assessments of need or individual mental capacity. Compared to several other European countries, the many legal requirements can cause long delays in patients being given medication against their will. According to the Dutch constitution, the integrity of one's body is regarded as one of the most important principles in health law. For example, administering depot medication against an individual's will is regarded as a very intrusive intervention and cannot be used involuntarily during a crisis episode. Nevertheless, rapid tranquilisation can be used to avoid imminent escalations, but may not be repeated systematically if the level of dangerousness declines. Currently, political debates are taking place about when the rights of individuals can be overridden, allowing the administration of medication to take place. Increasingly, politicians are finding themselves caught between safeguarding the rights of individuals and protecting society. Establishing how best to deal with situations that may arise in the management of psychiatric patients continues to exercise the public, the media and individual patients and their families.

If there are no evident signs of imminent danger due to the psychiatric symptoms the person is suffering from, a watchful, waiting approach is adopted. In case of sudden changes in the mental state and loss of control of behaviour observed, an emergency procedure can be activated. These types of urgent mental state evaluations are in most cases initially performed by community psychiatric nurses and/or junior doctors and then re-evaluated by a psychiatrist within 24 hours. This means, in detail, that the person will be immediately assessed, in most cases by a community psychiatric nurse at home or in the police station in the first instance, and if required, by an on-call psychiatrist. It is up to the clinical judgement of an independent psychiatrist whether or not the person is forcefully removed to a psychiatric emergency facility. When the psychiatrist has completed her/his assessments and investigations, a formal written report is produced by him/her which is then taken to the mayor of the city or village in which the emergency assessment was undertaken. Only after the mayor (in his role of head of police) has given his approval can the person can be transported to the psychiatric hospital. Involuntary admissions only be admitted to formally accredited admission wards.

Meanwhile, the psychiatric evaluation report and the mayor's approval will be sent by fax to the law court officials and, within no more than 3 days, a judge will visit the person face to face in the hospital to confirm the compulsory admission or release the person from their involuntary stay. In 2008, the Dutch Psychiatry Association issued new guidelines binding on all those involved in the admission of involuntary patients and on administering coercive treatment (van Tilburg *et al.*, 2008). In addition to the legal procedures being carried out, it is important that a risk assessment is also completed and integrated into the care plan. In other words, harm reduction is imperative, and the least restrictive and intrusive interventions in a crisis situation should be selected in order to respect the autonomy of the patient. In case of lack of progress in using de-escalation interventions, an assessment by an independent psychiatrist is recommended to find alternatives to enable the least restrictive treatment possible.

A study in Rotterdam revealed that 22% of those admitted involuntarily had not actually been seen by a judge within 3 days to assess their situation (Wierdsma, 2003). In this study, it was also revealed that patients without any history of psychotic conditions, or those who did not display psychotic symptoms at the time of admission, were highly likely to be discharged early. Around 25% of those compulsorily admitted patients were discharged after being seen by a judge in the hospital within the first 3 days following admission. This indicates that differences in opinion may arise between legal and medical personnel and where this occurs, legal opinion prevails. It may also suggest that medical staff tend to admit people too readily just in case the condition of the patient is more serious than the assessment revealed. Another possible explanation is that junior doctors are allocated the task of admitting people, and hence their knowledge and experience may not be as robust as their senior colleagues.

If immediate discharge is not granted, a person is detained for a maximum of 21 days, and extensions are only permitted after a thorough reassessment, in which several stakeholders have to provide evidence of likely short- or medium-term potential risk of danger to self or others. If that is so, the patient is placed under formal supervision, in most cases detained in a locked ward for a maximum of 6 months, after which further reports and assessments are legally required.

Even after a person has been involuntarily admitted, they cannot be forced to have medical treatment unless they are deemed to be an immediate danger. When the likelihood of this imminent danger is identified, only rapid tranquilisation is permitted to decrease the prospect of short-term risk. No depot medication can be administered at this stage. Rapid tranquilisation injections are only allowed to prevent a dangerous situation from getting worse and where staff, or the patient, are in danger of getting injured. Once the mental state of the patient is considered to have improved and he or she can make adequate decisions, interventions of this kind cannot be repeated without the permission of the patient. If, however, it appears that the person continues to pose a threat to himself or others and it further appears that deterioration and social breakdown are inevitable and could lead to potential danger, after the validation of various reports from different stakeholders, treatment can be enforced on the person. Even if this procedure takes several weeks, the administrative process must be adhered to.

In the last 20 years, the numbers of compulsory admissions have doubled from 23 to 46 per 100 000 inhabitants (Mulder *et al.*, 2006). Most of the compulsorily admitted patients were identified as suffering from psychosis (50%), manic episodes (17%), depression (11%) and personality disorders (5%). The administration associated with this growth in involuntary admissions means that nurses spend a considerable amount of time ensuring that the paperwork is prepared correctly. As already stated, it is not done to increase the administrative work around admissions, but to ensure that the human rights of individuals are properly considered and treatments are delivered accordingly.

The Dutch Mental Health Act has been undergoing constant change since 2008, particularly in respect of the process of involuntary admission. The main direction of the changing legal situation is to move away from over-reliance on admission as a means of containing people who threaten themselves or others, to one where admission can be avoided. This can only be achieved if sufficient and appropriate resources exist within community settings to provide for the immediate needs of people who appear to be deteriorating. At present, there is a much stronger political resolve to support community-based involuntary outreach care than has previously been the case. Therefore, the court can order far wider packages of compulsory care arrangements in the community to prevent hospi-talisation than it has had the power to do in the past. An independent mental health act committee is soon to be established to act as an advisory board in the supervision and monitoring of the care and treatment of high-risk patients. In order to assist the board in coming to decisions, different parties, including the patient, will be interviewed by the judge in advance of the court decision on the wisdom, or otherwise, of providing involuntary care in the community (www.pvp. nl, www.psy.nl).

Mental health needs and health service provision

Regional psychiatric case registers have been established to capture patterns in care of inpatients and outpatients in specific catchment areas. The findings are rarely described in the English written literature. From a European perspective, most available studies are from Italian, Spanish, Scandinavian and Dutch origin (Jenner, 2008). A database, as such, can be used for mental health policy pur-poses to identify gaps and bottlenecks in care provision for people with mental health problems. In the larger cities, currently such initiatives have helped to enable more tailor-made care arrangements for several vulnerable groups of citi-zens. At a national level, the Dutch Inspectorate of Health has been monitoring all psychiatric facilities systematically since the early 1970s. This governmental agency is involved in a number of thematic and routine audits as well, in case of adverse incidents or complaints relating to the quality of care.

Like other European countries, it is estimated that approximately 25% of the total population will be affected by mental suffering once or more in their lifetime, for which they will need assistance or treatment (Vollenbergh et al., 2003). At present, 1 million inhabitants are provided with individualised mental health care at any one time, which amounts to 6.2% of the total population. The number of people receiving mental health care has rapidly increased since 1980 (Hutschemaekers, 2000), although as many as 30% of people with psychiatric needs are not attending mental health facilities for their care and treatment.

From an international perspective, the number of those who access mental health care is relatively low in the Netherlands (Kovess-Masfety et al., 2007). Reasons identified for this are lack of confidence in health care providers, a reluctance to accept that people were ill or a lack of insight on the part of those who would have benefited from being treated. For example, a Dutch study on care consumption of bipolar patients revealed that around 25% of this group actively avoids contact with treatment services for various reasons (Vollenbergh et al., 2003).

As in other European countries, the population is ageing, and therefore complex mixtures of somatic and mental health issues have to be dealt with by health services. Roughly speaking, current mental health services can be broken down as follows:

- adults (73%)
- children and adolescent (13%)
- older people (12%).

According to the Dutch Health Authorities (Nederlandse Zorgautoriteiten, 2009), the vast majority of people with mental health problems fall into the following categories:

- minor mental health problems dealt with by community mental health services (70%)
- those requiring short-term psychiatric admissions (12%)
- those requiring intensive community psychiatric care including frequent short admissions (9%)
- patients requiring long-stay care in psychiatric hospitals (3%)
- those with frequent involuntary admissions (3%)
- those with first admissions to acute psychiatric wards (1%).

Suicide

Suicide rates have proved to be relatively stable over time. Each year approximately 1500 people commit suicide, around 9% of whom are people in Dutch inpatient services (Dishoeck et al., 2009). In about 90% of all cases analysed retrospectively, previous mental problems were identified in those patients who had committed suicide.

A trend has been emerging whereby suicides among adolescents are on the increase and there is a discernable decrease in the number of adult suicides over the past decade. From a European perspective, the Netherlands is ranked in the mid-range, having an annual suicide rate of 8.1 suicides per 100 000, comparable to that found in Germany and Ireland. However, suicide rate comparisons between European countries can be highly inaccurate because of inbuilt biases relating to registration procedures, criteria for arriving at 'death by suicide verdicts' and the judgements of those who sign death certificates (Chishti et al., 2003).

As community care has improved, it has been found that the amount of suicides in adult psychiatric patients has decreased (Kerkhof, 2008). It is possible that as the population continues to get older and as demands on health services increase, suicides in the older age group may rise. Consequently, there will be greater need for community services for older people close to where they live.

Tholen (2010) identifies the potential conflict that might arise between, on the one hand, central government, whose ambition it is to reduce the suicide rates, and on the other, local psychiatric services which will be held responsible for any that do occur. To avoid this situation, professionals may embark on defensive practices, which could include being overly concerned about people, to the point where compulsory admissions will be seen as a first line of approach.

Forensic services

There are 12 forensic psychiatric hospitals in the Netherlands, which care for 2000 patients who have been convicted of criminal offences directly as a result of their mental health problems. Forensic care facilities commenced in the Netherlands in 1886 (Bakker, 2005), and forensic beds have doubled over the last 15 years (Kaldien and Eggen 2009). Despite this increase, it is estimated that there is still a shortage of beds. According to Dutch law, persons with a psychiatric condition that have been convicted of violent acts and are at high risk of recidivism can be sent directly to forensic psychiatric hospitals for treatment and rehabilitation programmes. Admission to forensic psychiatric hospital is only permitted after long and intensive criminal court procedures. Within the forensic service, around 95% of the patients are male and approximately 90% hold Dutch citizenship. The average stay in forensic settings has increased in the last 15 years from 5 years to 8.2 years (Kaldien and Eggen, 2009). Throughout a person's stay, frequent actuarial and dynamic risk assessments are undertaken and combined with clinical assessments to assist in deciding when discharge planning should commence and when temporary leave would be advantageous. In Dutch forensic psychiatric hospitals, weekend leave is only allowed after highly structured risk assessments have been conducted. Data on unauthorised absences shows that they are rare in forensic clinics in the Netherlands, and if this occurs, 95% of those patients are back in the clinic within a week (Bakker, 2004).

Staff working in mental health services

The Dutch Mental Health Services Association states that upwards of 70 000 mental health professionals are employed, around 35% of whom have had a psychiatric nurse training (3 to 6 years formal psychiatric training). Mental health care professionals are required to be registered on a database of the Ministry of Health. Professionals are only allowed on this register when they have satisfactorily satisfied academic requirements, have conformed with codes of conduct relating to their specific discipline, have undertaken a legal minimum of hours in clinical practice and have shown evidence of being involved in continuous educational development.

The National Psychiatrist Association (NVVP) has a live registration list of 3300 junior psychiatrists and the National Psychologist Association (NIP) reports 12 933 formally recognised members, of whom 5500 psychologists are employed in psychiatric care facilities. Mental health nurses are the largest workforce group in the country, totalling 24 000. All three professional bodies recognise the unique contribution of each professional group, but they also subscribe to the importance of collaborative and multidisciplinary working when it comes to the provision of mental health services.

Attitudes to mental health problems and service user involvement

In common with other countries, the Netherlands has always had to contend with stigma and social inequality when it comes to those with mental health problems (van Weeghel *et al.*, 2005). Currently there are several nationwide projects under way with the aim of assisting people with mental health problems to integrate socially following discharge from inpatient services. These include studies on individual placements and support at work and assisting people to undertake specific educational programmes geared towards permanent employment (Michon and van Weeghel, 2010).

The media has always taken a keen interest in reporting and informing people regarding issues and concerns relating to mental illness in general. The public seems to appreciate it when public figures, such as prominent politicians, artists and athletes, have something to say about mental health, particularly if they are talking about their own and what they do to remain mentally healthy. Real-life documentaries on mental health services are popular and mental health issues are often covered in a wide range of newspapers and magazines. Relatives and former service users contribute to media presentations and they are also becoming involved in the work of mental health service teams. There exists a degree-level training course for this group at several universities that provide education in applied social science. Involvement of former service users in assertive community treatment teams is now well established.

Service user movements in mental health care have been active since 1970 and have been involved in the promotion of patient rights and the improvement of the quality of psychiatric services. Since the early eighties, every psychiatric facility has employed patient advocacy officers to be available when conflicts arise between patients and mental health care staff. More recently, some service users have applied for and obtained formal training in various aspects of mental health care so that they are now involved in the provision of specific community and inpatient treatments. However, although growing, the number of these patient-experts remains low.

Despite several anti-stigma campaigns, European research reveals that more than half the population of people with mental health problems do not wish to engage with mental health services (Codony *et al.*, 2009). This study shows that shame and feelings of fear are not just directed at individuals, but can be directed equally at services and institutions. Consequently, there remains much work to be done in minimising the negative perceptions held by society towards enabling services and those that provide them. As this problem is not confined to the Netherlands alone, it could be adopted as an EU project and assistance could be provided to enhance the standing of mental health services across all European countries.

National expenditure on mental health care

There exists a new system of health care insurance, which has been in place since 2006. The traditional involvement of governmental control in a broad spectrum of health care services has loosened, and as a result more commercial initiatives are now taking place. It is now mandatory for all citizens to pay a health insurance premium to the commercial health insurance company of their choice, and in the last decade we have seen a growth in competiveness between insurers in the health care market. What is now beginning to emerge is that various health care insurance companies are linking with and commissioning services from different health care providers. Although insurers and providers may vary on a number of issues, there are certain criteria that they agree on, e.g. cost-effectiveness, stepped care and the abolition of long waiting lists. A major consequence of this is that enormous mergers have taken place among service providers in order to ensure the safety of health care facilities, cost effectiveness, the minimisation of competition and the clustering of clinical and research expertise.

In both somatic and mental health care facilities, developments have shown that hospitals and community-based services have catchment areas ranging from 500 000 to 2 million inhabitants. In some of the larger merged mental health service trusts, there are as many as 100–150 different service provision locations, allowing patients to find most care facilities within the area in which they live. The extent of those changes currently taking place is challenging, but the opportunities for practice development and research have increased. On the other hand, there is a tendency to establish structured evidence-informed care programmes for specific diagnostic groups, whereas in reality most patients suffer from other co-morbid disorders.

Several professionals argue that the DSM-IV-driven health-care cost-control approach, which was introduced by the government, can also cause fragmentation and may impede the continuity of care and does little to improve the complexity of mental health care provision. It raises the question: What about those who have poor mental health and do not satisfy the criteria for DSM-IV diagnosis? Therefore, currently many debates are taking place about the consequences of disorder-driven care versus needs-driven care (Zwartekot, 2008). At present, a specific psychiatric diagnosis is often needed to get access to specific treatment modalities and the system is getting more and more time-limited. This type of health care financing is distinct from primary prevention activities. Concern is currently being expressed regarding the financial provision that is directed towards diagnostics and treatments, while less resources are directed towards people in need of psychological and social support (van den Berg, 2010).

Meijer and van 't Land (2008) have pointed out that the indirect costs of mental health disorders are much higher than the allocated mental health budget, which then stood at €5 billion. Only 6% of the total health care budget is spent directly on mental health care, whereas government estimates suggest that mental disorders command four times more public financing than any other somatic illness. Most costs will be related to unemployment, subsistence allowances and individual debt. This picture is confirmed by similar findings published by Bosmans et al. (2010). In the Netherlands, around 10% of the total health care budget is available for specific mental health care provision. General practitioners identify psychiatric problems in around 11%–13% of their patients; however, what types of interventions they provide are influenced by the time available to GPs, their expertise in dealing with and managing mental health problems, their ability to carry out thorough mental health assessments and their interest in treating mental health problems generally. Another difficulty is that most patients tend only to present somatic problems to their GP, fearing the stigma that might result if they mentioned their mental health concerns (De Graaf et al., 2010). Over the past decade, more and more GPs have come to rely on part-time community psychiatric nurses and around 25% of all GPs are supported by CPNs (Hansen et al., 2007). There is a need to utilise the expertise in assessment competencies of other professionals; however, despite the workforce shortages this does not appear to have happened yet (Zwaanswijk and Verhaak, 2009). It is interesting to note that just as the mental health workforce has grown by 5% over the past few years, so too have the number of citizens requiring mental health services, currently estimated at 12% more (GGZ Nederland, 2009). However, those figures should be appraised with caution, because many patients can be referred to mental health services more than once in the same calendar year.

Contribution of psychiatric nurses to mental health care

In the Netherlands, independent university-based formal psychiatric nursing training did not exist before 1975. Currently, 10% of the total number of nurses in the Dutch health care system (240 000) are employed in psychiatric care facilities. Recent estimates indicate that 60% of mental health nurses are educated to diploma level and the remaining 40% are prepared to bachelor's or master's level.

Hoekstra *et al.* (2010) found that most nursing students have negative perceptions of and attitudes towards psychiatric patients, not unlike those held by the general public. The majority of nursing students hold that most psychiatric patients tend to be aggressive and unpredictable, are difficult to manage and don't respond to treatments. Therefore, much better education of the public is required in the form of anti-stigma campaigns, more realistic and better-informed information programmes about the number of people who actually do recover from mental illness, and that in the majority of cases interventions are effective. Without this, negativity towards the mentally ill will persist and in the future it will prove difficult to recruit nurses that have appropriate attitudes and insights to mental health care.

Increasingly, criticisms have been levelled at both the form and content of psychiatric nursing courses, stating that they are too closely based on medical training and their content is far too medically orientated (Eliens, 1997). For years, debates and discussions about the training of psychiatric nurses have taken place in the Netherlands, and general agreement has only been reached recently regarding developing more generic curricula for nurses in all health care domains. One of the main reasons for this situation was the wishes of employers, who wanted to see their nurses fitting into different care types, and secondly, the ongoing need for somatic-focused interventions in mental health care settings.

Direct entry into mental health nursing (3-year course) in-service training at diploma level was abolished nationwide in 1996 and replaced by 4-year generic nursing training at diploma or bachelor level. This training is based in universities where departments of applied health science already existed. Since 1998, a 3-year post-bachelor clinical nurse specialist course has been available, and since 2007, a 2-year master's degree in advanced nursing practice in mental health care has been available. At present, those who have completed this master's degree (including pharmacotherapy and physical examination) are allowed on the national health care specialist register. The master's degree allows nurses to undertake specific medical and psychiatric assessments and prescribe medication. Those issues are formally incorporated in the curricula of advanced nursing practice courses at master's level; however, in reality there are a variety of definitions as to what constitutes the extended roles for those specialist nurses. Evidence-based practice and involvement in research projects is highly valued and encouraged by the Dutch Nurse Practitioners Association.

In the past, the emphasis was focused entirely on preparing specialist nurses for work in inpatient psychiatric settings. However, the new approach, once ratified, will allow nurses who trained under the old scheme to undertake a 3-year part-time degree which is geared towards preparing nurses to work in different community settings and in different mental health teams. Most of them have also completed an additional 2-year, part-time postgraduate advanced course in community psychiatric nursing, which conferred on them the title of community psychiatric nurse (CPN). Koekoek *et al.* (2009) found that despite the growing mass of postgraduate trained nurses (almost 3000 CPNs), few scientific findings about their work was actually published, nor was there any evidence that they were applying what they learned in their work. It is possible, as happened in the past, that because the clinical work of nurses is both determined and controlled by doctors, nurses have little opportunity to implement the ideas and skills they have acquired.

It is known, however, that this group of professionals can potentially utilise a variety of interventions and are able to adopt a holistic and eclectic way of caring for patients. The mean caseload of full-time community psychiatric nurses is around 48 patients, according to Koekoek *et al.* (2009). The CPNs do not seem to use evidence-based protocols frequently in their day-to-day practice. Therefore, as would be expected, they are frequently criticised by other professional groups for continuing hospital-based approaches in community settings. Nevertheless, CPNs are highly respected by many stakeholders because of their ability to respond speedily and appropriately to different situations, while managing to ensure that care is coordinated to the benefit of service users.

During the 1980s and 1990s, many CPNs undertook advanced training in various psychosocial interventions, such as family counselling, psycho-education and various types of psychotherapy. Because of their elective approach, the work of CPNs was hard to capture from a research perspective, and consequently what studies were undertaken were largely descriptive. Another factor in holding back the development of psychiatric nursing is the small number of academic centres in which nursing science is offered. At present, only the universities of Utrecht, Maastricht and Nijmegen have professors in psychiatric nursing and academic facilities where nurses can study at PhD level. This undoubtedly has affected the amount of research undertaken and the formation of an evidence base upon which nurses can design their work. There is striking evidence from the last decade that formal training courses are now rapidly expanding and stimulating students to contribute actively to the development of evidence-directed practice (van Meijel, 2008). This has seen the rise of greater multidisciplinary research, the production of evidence-based guidelines and a plethora of working groups focusing on specific aspects of mental health care.

Since 2005, changes in governmental funding have led to considerable curriculum modifications. Currently, there is a 2-year generic nursing training (for all branches of nursing) followed by specific mental health training in the final 2 years of the programme. This course is provided at diploma and bachelor levels. The contents of both courses are such as to meet the requirements of inpatient and community-based care. It would appear that many mental health organisations send their nurses to do advanced study programmes in order to assist in the promotion and development of high-quality care standards.

Future of mental health services

The last decade has seen an enormous increase in the growth of primary mental health services. Most regions now have community psychiatric nurses available in general health care facilities for psychiatric screening and to provide brief solution-focused therapy. This service has now developed to an extent that very few inappropriate psychiatric referrals are made to what are termed polyclinics. The existence of these clinics has been instrumental in reducing the number of crisis episodes, while at the same time speeding up access to services. This approach has not resulted in less hospital admissions, but has enabled more tailored and individualised care to be provided, which has in turn reduced the long waiting lists that once existed. By being able to recognise the early symptoms of mental illnesses and offering brief therapeutic interventions, patients' outcomes can be improved considerably. Hopefully, empirical evaluation of these services will show even more promising results in the future when services have had time to mature and consolidate.

As research methods get more sophisticated and outcome measurement becomes more standardised, Dutch mental health care should show signs of general improvement nationally. The importance of routine measurements and service evaluations are set to become much more prominent than they have been. The findings as to which treatments and services are shown to be effective in these services will be significant. More standardised, validated and rigorous measurements should be undertaken in every service, using instruments that have been validated. Leading Dutch psychiatric academics have recently published a consensus document on the importance of routine outcome measurements as a means of establishing best treatment (Mulder *et al.*, 2010).

As a result of the amount of investment in training and education for mental health professionals, a number of new services have been introduced, including assertive community treatment, which is now widely available across the country. This approach is characterised by multidisciplinary outreach services providing care for those patients who are difficult to engage. In the past few years, a national assertive community treatment organisation has been established with the aim of linking all research and educational activities to services. For this to happen, the national organisation links closely with regional teams, so that 'best practice' is made instantly available and shared across all regions and disciplines (Dijk *et al.*, 2004). This is yet another way of utilising measurement results, not just to improve the care of each patient, but to improve the overall services provided to all service users and their carers.

The issues of early recognition of alarming symptoms and problematic living conditions, crisis home treatment and avoiding duplicated assessments are becoming more prominent in health care policy. Timely interventions in serious mentally ill patients with a lack of insight are now systematically monitored with respect to patient outcomes (van der Plas *et al.*, 2010). On the other hand, Jenner (2008) argues that in case of acute escalations, the so-called shared caseloads in assertive care treatment (ACT) teams can also lead to confusion as to how and when to intervene. With this in mind, Jenner (2008) argued that it takes time for various teams to orientate to new standards and practices and recommends that a periodic review of crisis management standards should be undertaken within ACT teams. The implications of this finding is that the best way of ensuring the continuous improvement of mental health services is to periodically subject them to review and audit, and for areas for improvement to be identified and acted upon.

Case scenario

A 23-year-old unemployed man is reported by his landlord as acting increasingly strangely. He has barricaded his room, talking about being spied upon by the CIA. He can be heard shouting within his room in an angry and incoherent way. He has not been seen by a psychiatrist in the past, although his mother has told the landlord that he has been isolating himself and acting increasingly oddly over the last couple of years.

Most commonly, this person would be brought to the attention of the assertive outreach team by the general practitioner. These teams work closely with housing cooperations, local authorities, public health care professionals and police officers. Where patients have lost track with their own general practitioners, those individuals would be detected by the council mental health agencies. Larger cities have such bodies in which housing cooperations, social services, the police and public (mental) health officers are involved. These bodies can be consulted by any individual who is concerned about the mental well-being of a specific person in their neighbourhood. In most cases, the primary focus will be to enhance the living conditions of high-risk citizens. This can be achieved by the utilisation of outreach community care teams. If there are indications of mental illness, a case manager (in most areas a community psychiatric nurse) will conduct an enquiry among all involved, informal and formal stakeholders, and will go through global (psychiatric) risk assessment procedures in conjunction with a psychiatrist. Normally, the first steps would be that staff of an assertive community outreach team would try to do several home visits to get a more refined impression of the current mental health state and the living conditions of the identified patient.

In this particular case, mental health nurses will try to get in touch with the patient by repeatedly doing home visits. If this is unsuccessful, they will raise concerns with significant people within the social network of the patients. Due to privacy legislation, they will not be able to provide specific information, but they will try to give global psycho-education about managing a psychiatric crisis as such. If the danger levels change rapidly, nurses will be alerted to get in contact with the patient directly. In many occasions, the police will intervene first for safety reasons and will directly communicate with the community crisis nurse on duty to do an assessment within 1 hour. These assessments are always performed in collaboration with a psychiatrist on call. The nurse will monitor the patient's safety and observe the mental and somatic state of the patient during this period. If the outcome of the assessment indicates intensive community-based surveillance is advisable, the nurse will coordinate the care planning in collaboration with key persons in the patient's network. In those circumstances, the patient may benefit from an assertive community treatment team which can assist with living conditions, financial issues and the provision of psychiatric monitoring and symptom management. Again, this holistic type of care will be mainly nurse-driven.

Specific assessment

The seeming presence of a number of problems will influence the approach taken in this case. The following aspects will probably be assessed in standard practice:
1. Potential danger of poor hygiene, fire and risk of being victimised by others.
2. Present mental state and relationship with the identified behavioural problems. In addition to this, the course of the illness will be reviewed and risk of sudden (risky) changes in the mental state will be taken into consideration.

The presence of adequate resources for safe and healthy conditions of living will also be taken into account. In addition to this, the financial resources of the person and possible debts and risk of becoming homeless will be reviewed as far as possible and within legal boundaries. The prevention of homelessness will be of the highest priority in this stage.

From a legal point of view, if there are no evident signs of imminent danger due to the psychiatric symptoms the person is suffering from, a watchful waiting approach will be observed. In the case of sudden changes in mental state and loss of control, an emergency procedure will be started. In detail, this means that the person will be immediately assessed by a community psychiatric nurse at home or in the police station in the first place and, if required, by a psychiatrist on call. Only the clinical judgement of an independent psychiatrist is required to finalise an involuntary emergency admission. When the psychiatrist has completed his written psychiatric evaluation, the police or ambulance service will bring the report immediately to the mayor of the city or village in which the emergency assessment was undertaken. Only after approval by the mayor (head of the local police), can the person be transported to the psychiatric hospital by an ambulance. Involuntary admitted patients can only be transported to formally accredited locked regional admission wards. Meanwhile, the psychiatric evaluation report and the mayor's approval will be sent by fax to the law court officials and within no more than 3 days a judge will visit the person and conduct a face-to-face interview in the hospital to validate the compulsory admission or release the person from involuntary stay in the hospital. This emergency measure can last for a maximum of 21 days and extension is only permitted after a thorough, new legal procedure in which several stakeholders have to provide evidence of short- or mid-term potential risk of danger in relation to the present mental state. In that case, the patient can be detained or monitored in the community under strict conditions for a maximum of 6 months, and after that new reports and evaluations are legally required.

In the case of emergency involuntary admission, the person can be deprived of their liberty, but cannot be forced to accept medical treatment unless they appear to be in immediate danger, or it is deemed that they will benefit from immediate medical intervention. More concretely, this would mean that if a person were suffering from a severe psychosis, a depot medication is not permitted to be given against their will even in situations which are deemed to be an emergency. However, staff will work on the stabilisation process by reducing crisis-provoking risk factors, try to establish therapeutic engagement in day programmes and offer psycho-education tailored to the current mental state, and taking into account recovery possibilities and future community support.

Nurses on the wards will take care of frequent and structured risk assessments and mental state evaluations, health and Activities of Daily Living promotion, medication management, social skill training and psycho-education.

The nature of long-term follow-up after discharge will strongly depend on the degree of insight that the patient has into his condition and his level of motivation to accept long-term engagement with mental health services. Assuming that this is a first psychotic episode, the person would be also referred to the early psychosis intervention team, which are available in most large cities. This team will conduct more detailed assessments and will guide the further diagnostic process to enable a tailor-made treatment plan. In general, evidence-based guidelines for psychosis treatment will be followed. In most cases, this will involve medication management, psycho-education, cognitive behavioural therapy, early warning and crisis plans, individual placements and support for work and education and various sorts of recovery-based programmes. If this person is difficult to engage in formal care programmes, an assertive community treatment team will provide outreach care, while providing support for family members and significant others.

References

Akkermans C. [Local council mental health care. The social psychiatric service as part of the Amsterdam gg& gd (Amsterdam District Health Authority)] [Dutch]. *Maandblad Geestelijke Volksgezondheid*. 2001; **56**: 644–58.

Bakker B. TBS, weg ermee!? *Maandblad Geestelijke volksgezondheid*. 2005; **60**: 138–40.

Berg van den R. DBC's nader ontleed. Falend systeem moet worden afgebouwd, *Maandblad Geestelijke Volksgezondheid*. 2010; **65**: 336–48.

Boschma G. Psychiatrische verpleegkunde, een historisch perspectief. *Maandblad Geestelijke Volksgezondheid*. 1997; **52**: 59–76.

Bosmans J, Bruine de M, Hout van H, *et al*. Healthcare costs in primary care patients in the Netherlands. *Fam Pract*. 2010; **27**(5): 542–8.

CBS. *Bevolkingstrends, statistisch kwartaalblad over de demografie van Nederland*. Jaargang 50, 2 e kwartaal, 2010, Centraal Bureau voor de Statistiek, Den Haag; 2010. Available at: http://statline. cbs.nl/StatWeb/publication/?VW=T&DM=SLNL&PA=71090ned (accessed 26 January 2011).

CBS. *Gezondheid en zorg in cijfers 2008*. Centraal Bureau van de Statistiek, Den Haag/ Heerlen; 2008. Available at: www.cbs.nl/NR/rdonlyres/516BE7D7-B35E-4CFA-BF66-9B48ADF6995F/0/2008c156pub.pdf (accessed 26 January 2011).

Chishti P, Stone P, Corcoran E, *et al*. Suicide mortality in the European Union. *Eur J Public Health*. 2003; **13**(2), 108–14.

Codony M, Alonso J, Almansa J, *et al*. Perceived need for mental health care and service use among adults in Western Europe: results of the ESEMeD project. *Psychiatr Serv*. 2009; **60**: 1051–8.

Dishoeck A, Lingsma H, Kolk van der M. *Haalbaarheidsstudie naar de kwantificering van gezondheidseffecten van toezicht gehouden door de Inspectie voor de Gezondheidszorg*. Rotterdam: Erasmus MC Afdeling Maatschappelijke Gezondheidszorg; 2009.

Dijk van B, Roosenboom B, Kroon H, *et al*. [Assertive community treatment in the Netherlands] [Dutch]. *Maandblad Geestelijke Gezondheidszorg*. 2004; **59**(11): 931–43.

Duren van P. Van gestichtsarts tot psychiater, kleine historische demografie van een beroepsgroep. *Maandblad Geestelijke Volksgezondheid*. 2008; **63**(9): 704–17.

Eliens A. Psychiatrische verpleegkunde, nu en straks. *Maandblad Geestelijke Volksgezondheid*. 1997; **52**: 943–58.

Eurostat database. Available at: http://epp.eurostat.ec.europa.eu/portal/page/portal/eurostat/home (accessed 25 February 2011).

GGZ Nederland. *Zorg op waarde geschat*. Amersfoort: GGZ Nederland; 2009.

GGZ Nederland. *Zorg op waarde geschat. Sectorrapport GGZ 2009*. Amersfoort: GGZ Nederland; 2009. Available at: www.ggznederland.nl/scrivo/asset.php?id=293117 (accessed 23 January 2011).

Gijswijt-Hofsta M, Oosterhuis H. Leeswijzer voor het psychiatrisch verleden. *Maandblad Geestelijke Volksgezondheid*. 2001; **56**: 627–43.

Graaf De R, Have ten M, Dorsselaer van S. *De psychische gezondheid van de Nederlandse bevolking. NEMESIS-2: Opzet en eerste resultaten*. Utrecht: Trimbos-instituut; 2010.

Hansen J, Nuijen T, Hingstman L. *Monitormultidisciplinairesamenwerkingsverbanden in de eerste lijn*. Utrecht: NIVEL; 2007.

Have ten M, Graaf de R, Ormel J, *et al*. Attituden aangaande zoeken van professionele hulp voor psychische problemen en werkelijk hulpzoekgedrag: verschillen in Europa. *Tijdschr Psychiatr.* 2010; **52**: 205–17.

Have ten M, Land van t' H, Graaf de R. *Voorspellers van zorggebruik in de eerste en tweede lijn GGZ.* Utrecht: Trimbos Instituut; 2009.

Hoekstra H, Meijel van B, Hooft van der-Leemans T. A nursing career in mental health care: choices and motives of nursing students. *Nurse Educ Today.* 2010; **30**(1): 4–8.

Hutschemaekers G. [Is The Netherlands becoming increasingly unhealthy? Indicators and background analyses of mental health.] [Dutch]. *Maandblad Geestelijke Volksgezondheid.* 2000; **55**: 314–35.

Jenner J. Heeft ACT de toekomst? *Maandblad Geestelijke Volksgezondheid.* 2008; **63**(3): 207–16.

Kaldien S, Eggen A. *Criminaliteit en rechtshandhaving 2008, ontwikkelingen en samenhangen.* The Hague: Centraal Bureau voor de Statistiek & Wetenschappelijk Onderzoek & Wetenschappelijk Onderzoek en Documentatiecentrum, Ministerie van Justitie; 2008.

Kerkhof A. Behandelen van chronische suicidaliteit vraagt vooral om continuïteit van zorg. *Tijdschr Psychiatr.* 2008; **505**(5): 289–91.

Koekoek B, Meijel van B, Schene A, *et al.* Community psychiatric nursing in the Netherlands, a survey of a thriving but threatened profession. *J Psychiatr Ment Health Nurs.* 2009; **16**(9): 822–8.

Kovess-Masfety V, Alonso J, Brugha TS, *et al.* Differences in lifetime use of services for mental health problems in six European countries. *Psychiatr Serv.* 2007; **58**: 213–20.

Lange de J. De vroege bewegingstherapie in het psychiatrisch ziekenhuis, 1926–1954. *Maandblad Geestelijke Volksgezondheid.* 2001; **56**: 676–90.

Lelliott P. Acute inpatient psychiatry in England: an old problem and a new priority. *Epidemiol Psichiatr Soc.* 2006; **15**(2): 91–4.

Meijel B van. Naar verdere professionalisering van de psychiatrisch verpleegkundige zorg. Verpleegkundige. *Nederlands-Vlaams wetenschappelijk tijdschrift voor verpleegkundigen.* 2008; **23**(2): 139–42.

Meijer S, Land van 't H. Aan welke ziekten en aandoeningen wordt het geld besteed? In: *Volksgezondheid Toekomst Verkenning, Nationaal Kompas Volksgezondheid.* Bilthoven: RIVM; 2010.

Michon H, Weeghel van J. [Rehabilitation research in the Netherlands: research review and synthesis of recent findings] [Dutch]. *Tijdschr Psychiatr.* 2010; **52**(10): 683–94.

Mulder CL, Broer J, Uitenbroek D, *et al.* Versnelde stijging van het aantal inbewaringstellingen na de invoering van de Wet BOPZ. *Ned Tijdschr Geneeskd.* 2006; **150**: 319–22.

Mulder CL, Gaag van der N, Bruggeman R, *et al.* [Routine outcome monitoring for patients with severe mental illness] [Dutch]. *Tijdschr Psychiatr.* 2010; **52**(3): 169–79.

Mulder CL, Tielens J. [Views on social decay influences decisions on involuntary admissions] [Dutch]. *Tijdschr Psychiatr.* 2008; **50**(4): 229–33.

Nederlandse zorgautoriteit. *Uitvoering toets Geneeskundige. GGZ.* Nederlandse Zorg Autoriteit, Utrecht; 2009. Available at: www.nza.nl/organisatie/Contact/webportaal/ (accessed 26 January 2011).

Nijman H, à Campo J, Ravelli D. [Increase in the number of involuntary admissions] [Dutch]. *Tijdschr Psychiatr.* 1998; **40**(11): 715.

Plas van der A, Abdoelbasier S, Hemert van B. [Engaging patients with serious mental illness in care services by critical time intervention] [Dutch]. *Ned Tijdschr Geneeskd.* 2010; **154**: A1791.

Priebe S, Badesconyi A, Fioritti A. Reinstitutionalisation in mental health care: comparison of data on service provision from six European countries. *BMJ.* 2005; **330**: 123–6.

Priebe S, Frottier P, Gaddini A, *et al.* Mental health care institutions in nine European countries, 2002 to 2006. *Psychiatr Serv.* 2008; **59**: 570–3.

Ravelli D. Deinstitutionalization of mental healthcare in the Netherlands, towards an integrative approach. *Int J Integr Care.* 2006; Jan–Mar; **6**: e04.

Sande van de R. Beoordelen en bewaken van acute gezondheidsbedreigende risico's. In: Kuiper de M, Jansen M, Ettema R, *et al.*, editors. *Basis principes voor Advanced Nursing Practice.* Houten: Bohn Stafleu van Loghum; 2007.

Sande van de R. Risicomanagement,voorbeelden uit de psychiatrische ketenzorg. In: Kuiper de M, editor. *Ontwerp van zorg-trajecten/zorgketens.* Houten: Bohn Stafleu van Loghum; 2009.

Simons H, Hirsch Ballin E. *Wet Bijzondere Opnemingen Psychiatrische Ziekenhuizen.* The Hague: Ministerie Volksgezondheid en Minister van Justitie; 1992.

Stegge aan den G. Debat en beleid in Nederland gedurende de twintigste eeuw. *Maandblad Geestelijke Volksgezondheid.* 2001; **56**: 691–708.

Stel van der J. De positie van verslavinszorg en ggz. *Maandblad Geestelijke Volksgezondheid.* 2001; **56**: 331–41.

Tholen F. Suïcidegevaar en onvrijwillige opname. Beoordeling en afweging van risico en noodzaak. *Maandblad Geestelijke Volksgezondheid.* 2010; **65**(6): 454–65.

Tilburg van W, Veldhuizen van JR, Beijaert WMV, *et al.* [Guideline decision-making on coercion, admission and treatment, Dutch Psychiatry Association] [Dutch]. Utrecht: Tijdstroom; 2008.

Vollenbergh W, Graaf R, Have ten R, *et al.* [Mental disorders in the Netherlands, overview of the NEMESIS project results] [Dutch]. Utrecht: Trimbos Instituut; 2003.

Wahlbeck K, Makinen M. *Consensus Paper: prevention of depression and suicide.* 2008. Available at: www.ec-mental health-process.net (accessed 26 January 2011).

Weeghel van J, Audenhove van C, Colucci M, *et al.* The components of good community care for people with severe mental illnesses: views of stakeholders in five European countries. *Psychiatr Rehabil J.* 2005; **28**(3): 274–81.

Weert van Oene de GH, Schrijvers A. [Care needs and care demands in mental health care in the region of Mid West Utrecht: an assessment over the period 1990–2010] [Dutch]. Utrecht: Julius Centrum voor Gezondheidswetenschappen en Eerstelijnsgeneeskunde; 2010.

Wierdsma A. Inbewaringstelling . . . en dan? Een Rotterdams onderzoek naar de motieven van Justitie om gedwongen opnemingen niet voort te zetten. *Maandblad Geestelijke Volksgezondheid.* 2003; **58**: 337–49.

Wolf J, Hoof van F, Neijmeijer L. Sociaal psychiatrisch verpleegkundigen en psychiatrisch verpleegkundigen. *Maanblad Geestelijke Gezondheidszorg.* 1997; **52**: 1007–20.

Zwaanswijk M, Verhaak PFM. *Effectieve kortdurende interventies voor psychische problemen: een kennissynthese over hun toepasbaarheid in de huisartsenvoorziening.* Utrecht: NIVEL; 2009.

Zwartekot F. DBC's in de GGZ, een schijnvertoning, waarom marktwerking met DBC's in de ambulante GGZ niet werkt. *Tijdschr Psychother.* 2008; **34**(1): 58–81.

Mental health services in Portugal

José Carlos Pereira Santos, Cândida Rosalinda Loureiro and Aida Cruz Mendes

Introduction

In this chapter, a detailed portrayal of the evolution of Portugese mental health services is presented. Against growing economic problems, those charged with providing mental health care are seeking to meet the needs of sufferers living in both urban and rural areas. While the statutory services provide a considerable amount of care and support, many service users are partially or wholly dependent on their familes, friends or neighbours. An insightful commentary is provided as to the structure of current services and the range of agencies involved. While resources continue to be a persistent obstacle to service improvement, the stigmatisation of the mentally ill is an even greater obstacle. Mental health nursing has developed over time and is currently making a significant contribution to the Portuguese mental health care system. A critique of modern mental health care is provided, as is a discussion on the future of such services.

National profile and context

To understand the nature and development of mental health services in Portugal, it is first important to understand the nature of Portugal and its population. Aside from the mainland, Portugal comprises the Azores and Madeira islands, together amounting to 92 090 km². It is located in Southern Europe (it is the westernmost country of Europe) and it shares with Spain the Iberian Peninsula.

Lisbon, the capital city, is an Atlantic city on the banks of the Tagus River estuary with a population of 2.8 million inhabitants, by far the largest conurbation on the coastline. Approximately 70% of the total population live in coastal areas, leaving the remainder to reside in dispersed areas of the countryside. Portugal became an independent country in 1143, and its modern-day borders have been in place since 1249, resulting in a strong national identity. The official language of Portugal is Portuguese, a Latin language that has more than 210 million native speakers worldwide, making it the fifth-most-spoken language in the world and third in the Western world. The large majority of the population is white and Catholic. The adult literacy rate is 95.8% for men and 92.0% for women (UNESCO, 2006). Portugal has been part of the EU since 1986 and adopted the euro as the official currency in 1999. The aim of this chapter is to characterise and describe the evolution of mental health services in Portugal.

Population and demographics

Portugal has a population of 10 627 250 inhabitants. With both a birth rate and a mortality rate of 9.8 per 100 000 inhabitants, the country is currently facing serious problems with respect to population renewal. The population growth rate is approximately 0.305%, with a birth rate of 10.45/1000 inhabitants and a death rate of 10.62/1000 population. The fertility rate of 1.49% poses a direct threat to maintaining the constancy of the population. An interesting and related factor is that the infant mortality rate has decreased sharply since 1980, a time when 24 per 1000 newborns died during their first year of life. Today, the rate is three deaths per 1000 newborns. In addition, Portugal has an increasing ageing population, with a ratio of 115 people over the age of 65 to 100 younger people (INE, 2010).

The life expectancy at birth is 75.49 years for males and 81.74 for females (INE, 2010). This trend towards a progressively ageing population has been partially mitigated by migration flows. According to Portugal's Foreign Nationals and Borders Service (SEF, 2008), the largest foreign communities come from Brazil, Ukraine and Cape Verde. By 2010, more than 900 000 immigrants are expected to be working in Portugal, despite the current unemployment rate (9.5%), which has been increasing during the last 3 years. In Portugal, immigrants have access to education and health services, the right to vote, rights at work and social assistance for their families, all provided for and protected in legislation. As for immigrant integration, Portugal is almost always referred to as an example of good multicultural integration, and the United Nations' Human Development Report (2009) praised Portugal's actions for the ways in which immigrants are respected, treated and provided for. The Portuguese GDP per capita is €22 865 and it is worth $243 billion or 0.39% of the world economy, according to the World Bank (2010).

Changing health needs

Portugal, like other Western countries, is facing several challenges with respect to identifying and meeting the health needs of the population. These include the development of scientific knowledge, demographic changes and those resulting from political and cultural changes. Table 9.1 summarises the extent of these changes.

TABLE 9.1 Systemic transformations

Dimensions	Progress	Related consequences
Geographic	Decrease of child mortality and increase of life expectancy	Increase of the impact of chronic diseases
Political	Political commitment to promote the health and well-being of the population	Economic and political crisis of the National Health Service due to social and demographic pressures
Medical-scientific	Development of medical-scientific knowledge and health care increase	Depreciation of the factors which are not part of the biomedical model of illness explanation, prevention and treatment
Social-cultural	Improvement of life conditions	Individualisation of health issues through 'lifestyles'

Source: Amendoeira, 2006

These changes, and their consequences, also have an impact on the creation of new mental health needs. The WHO report *Portugal Country Summary: Effective and Humane Mental Health Treatment and Care for All* (2010) described what the likely effects of these developments might be in the following areas:

- **Ageing population:** The increase in the percentage of people over 65 years old and the decrease of the population under 15 years of age will result in a 'double ageing' effect. Portugal may expect an increase of psychogeriatric problems among the older population in the near future, as well as the need to develop appropriate services for them.
- **Urbanisation:** While in 1970, only 25.9% of the population lived in urban areas, this rose to 29.4% in 1980, 46.7% in 1990, 53.0% by 2000, and 55.1% by 2004. Though this is noticeably below the mean compared with other EU member states (approximately 70%), it has, nevertheless, resulted in some difficulties in terms of access to mental health services for people living in rural areas.
- **Migration:** The migration of the population from the interior to the coastal cities has been steadily on the increase over the last 20 years. Large suburban areas were built to hold the influx of internal and external immigrants. The fast expansion of these suburban neighbourhoods is changing the traditional

family/social networks that prevailed in the rural settings, thus increasing the sense of isolation and non-integration. The Portuguese mental health care system is still struggling to address some of the specific challenges presented by recent legal and illegal immigration from Brazil and central and Eastern Europe, as well as the more traditional immigration from Africa.

- **Poor economic growth and unemployment:** Over the past decade, the Portuguese economy has faced a period of very low growth, with the most visible effect being the increase in the government budget deficit, as well as a rise in unemployment levels. This has had a direct impact on the rise of psychiatric morbidity, as demonstrated by the results of the Eurobarometer (2003).

- **Health disparities and inequality:** In the last three decades, the health status of the Portuguese population has improved significantly on a number of indicators. Improvements in health status seems to be associated with increases in human, material and financial assets devoted to health care, as well as to a general improvement in socio-economic conditions. However, there is still some concern over regional disparities, particularly between urban-coastal and rural-interior regions. The latter has, and continues to have, the worst health conditions. Rural regions are also the poorest in the country. Health inequalities are associated with economic and social factors, such as income, living conditions, unemployment and health care (coverage, utilisation rates, among others). Probably due to these factors, disability-adjusted life expectancy (DALE) levels in Portugal are worse than the average for EU15 members, both for men and for women.

The National Health Service

In Portugal, there is a mixed approach to the provision of health care. The state provides most health care through the National Health Service, but it is complemented by a private health care sector which provides varying types of services. However, the public sector is the most important provider, representing about 70% of total health care. The state has an enormous investment in the health sector, both as insurer and service provider. As an insurer, the state collects taxes so as to, in return, take on the financial responsibility for medical care expenses. As a provider, the state offers and produces different goods and services for all the population. In order to ensure high-quality standards of care, the Regulation State Entity, although part of the Health Department, exists in order to determine that the state, as insurer and provider, relates to other departments of state and with other economic agencies (Barros, 2009). According to Ferreira (2009), from 2000 to 2005, the total health expenditure, per source of revenue, was classified as follows: NHS, 57.2%; public subsystems, 6.7%; other public funding, 6.9%;

social security, 0.8%; private subsystems, 2.2%; private health insurance 2.4%; out of pocket, 22.5%; and other private entities, 1.3%. A variety of means is used to fund the NHS, including family taxation, other general taxation schemes, private insurance and social insurance (Simões *et al.*, 2007).

In Portugal, in 1980, the percentage of health expenditure of GDP was 5.6%, whereas in 2004 it was 10%, then higher than the mean cost in other EU countries, which was 9% and OECD 8.9%. From 1980 to 2004, public expenditure on health in relation to GDP doubled (3.6% in 1980, 7.2% in 2004) (Simões *et al.*, 2007). Today, the per capita total expenditure on health is 1618 international dollars and the per capita government expenditure on health is 1116 international dollars (WHO, 2006).

Explaining the increase in expenditure is complex and there are multiple explanations offered, including:

● The increase reflects the rising costs of providing a national health care service.
● It reflects the costs of providing for an increasing ageing population.
● Innovation and technological developments in the medical and therapeutic fields are responsible for increasing the level of expenditure.
● A growing workforce contributes to the rising costs of health care services.
● Designing services that meet the newly emerging needs of people can be costly.

The challenge for health care provision is to continue to provide good services within existing budgets while ensuring that people with health care needs have access to good-quality care and treatment. That is not always achievable, as some services are more expensive than others, e.g. cancer care, care of the elderly and various forms of community care (Simões *et al.*, 2007).

Mental health needs and demographics

Preliminary data from a study recently conducted by the WHO and Harvard University, coordinated in Portugal by Almeida (2010), indicates that, in the last year, one in five Portuguese citizens were suffering from a psychiatric illness (23%) at any given time and almost half (43%) already had an ongoing disorder, for which some were being treated. According to this study, the most common disorders are anxiety disorders (16.5%), with 3.2% of these being regarded as severe disorders. Other common disorders were found to be phobias towards specific situations (8.6%), followed by obsessive-compulsive disorder (4.4%). Depression was observed in 7.9% of the population, with a prevalence of 6.3% of severe mental illnesses, which include bipolar disorder, disorders that lead to disability and disorders which result in suicide attempts. As for access to specialised care, this study showed that a significant number of people with a severe mental disorder did not receive any type of treatment in the last year (33.6%), and that only 35% of people with depression were treated in the same year as the symptoms first appeared. The median shows a period of 5 years between first complaints and attaining access to treatment. The findings of this study (Almeida, 2010) show that the data confirms that there is a huge gap between Portugal and other European countries with respect to the time it takes between identifying mental health need and initiating treatment. While Portugal has a prevalence rate of 23% for mental health problems, other countries are much less, e.g. Spain (9.2%), Italy (8.2%) and Belgium (12%). It would appear that Ukraine is in a similar situation to Portugal, with a prevalence rate of 20.5%. Severe illnesses in Portugal have been estimated to be above 6%, while in other southern countries their prevalence is 1%, a most serious situation that requires attention. These differences were arrived at by utilising the same instruments but at different times, which may have distorted the results. Further thought and analysis need to be given to these differences in order to confirm whether or not they are valid or whether there are confounding variables that may explain them.

In the past, the existing data showed that 1 557 054 people (16.07% of the adult population, 18 to 65 years) at some time in their lives suffer from a mental disorder in Portugal. These disorders present as follows: 981 766 people (9.46%) suffer from anxiety disorders, 528 122 (5.09%) from affective disorders (including mild depression) and 54 166 (0.52%) from psychotic disorders (European Brain Council, 2005). Though data is collected using different methods and sources, nevertheless, it would appear that anxiety remains the most common disorder, closely followed by affective disorders.

There is evidence that some progress has been made on assisting people to gain access to treatment earlier than in the past. For instance, in 2005, the estimated prevalence of people with mental disorders was 1 555 054, while the number of people receiving treatment in psychiatric mental health services was estimated to be 168 389 (1.7%) (National Mental Health Report, 2005). Survey data from 2010 shows that 33% of the patients were being treated in various mental health services. The result of more people accessing services is that the use of anxiolytics, hypnotics, sedatives and antidepressants has significantly increased in outpatient care (National Coordination for Mental Health, 2009). The use of antidepressants also increased by 76% between 2000 and 2006. Providing better access to services, as has been shown in other countries, inevitably means that prescribing will increase, resulting in an increased cost for medications. It is also possible that the more people who access services, the more unnecessary prescriptions there may be issued.

Portugal has one of the lowest suicide rates in Europe: 9.8/100 000 inhabitants in 2008. The national suicide rate has remained stable over the past 5 years, with a higher prevalence in the population over 65 years old and a lower prevalence in younger populations (Sociedade Portuguesa de Suicidologia, 2010). Suicide and attempted suicide behaviour is more prevalent in the southern region of the country. Ageing, social isolation, low social class, low educational attainment and family history of suicide appear to be some of the contributing factors. This is in contrast to the usual profile of the parasuicidal patient presented in the literature; namely, a young, single female, enrolled in higher education, with depressive symptoms, low self-esteem, problem-solving difficulties and a family environment with high expressed emotion (Santos *et al.*, 2009). As in other contexts, the existence of previous suicidal behaviours increases the risk of death by suicide, as well as of psychiatric disorders: depression, schizophrenia, borderline personality and drug abuse, in particular alcohol consumption.

Alcohol abuse, once an enormous problem in Portugal, has been decreasing in recent years, most noticeably between 1985 and 2003. This decrease results from a public health intervention and cultural changes comprising changes in alcohol-related norms, marketing and values. However, despite this decline it still remains an important public health issue. It is estimated that there are around 600 000 alcoholics and 750 000 excessive drinkers in Portugal (APEF, 2010). The data relating to young people's consumption is also giving cause for concern. Research has shown that young Portuguese people start experimenting with alcohol at a very early age, (mean age, 12.5 years), and the consumption patterns appear to take the form of binge drinking (Matos *et al.*, 2003; Mendes and Barroso, 2006). The most recent data from ESPAD (2007) shows a significant increase of intensive consumption patterns among students, from 25% in 2003 to 56% in 2007.

Over the last few years, some innovative legislative changes have been enacted concerning drug use. Since 2001, a nationwide law in Portugal took effect, decriminalising all drugs, including cocaine and heroin. Thus, drug possession for personal use and drug usage itself are still legally prohibited, but violations of those prohibitions are deemed to be exclusively administrative violations and are completely removed from the criminal realm. Drug trafficking continues to be prosecuted as a criminal offense. While other states in the European Union have developed various forms of actual decriminalisation – whereby substances perceived to be less serious (such as cannabis) rarely lead to criminal prosecution – Portugal remains the only EU member state with a law explicitly declaring drugs to be 'decriminalised' (Greenwald, 2009). This means that consumption is forbidden, but it is not considered to be a crime if a person has consumed a drug; however, trafficking in drugs is still a crime for which people can be penalised.

An evaluation following the implementation of the law showed that drug use was significantly reduced throughout the population (15–64 year olds) (Balsa *et al.*, 2008). Furthermore, a significant reduction of health and social risks related to drug use, such as intravenous practices, were also observed. Drug use among prisoners and ex-prisoners was also found to be reduced, as was a reduction in the number of people with HIV using drugs (Torres *et al.*, 2008).

It is known that immigrants in any country are at risk of becoming mentally ill, and although little information on this topic exists in Portugal, nevertheless there are indications that this may be a growing problem (Muijen, 2008). In this survey, about a third of the immigrant population reported having psychological problems. Approximately 32% of immigrants were estimated to have poor mental health in comparison to Portuguese citizens, 27% of whom reported having some form of mental health problem. Although better methodologies are called for in future studies, it would appear that immigrants are a vulnerable group and may be more prone to mental illness than the indigenous population as the economic situation worsens. It may be that it is the most vulnerable people who immigrate in search of a better life, and find that in new and strange surroundings they are unable to cope. Monteiro (2009) found that immigrants had particular problems in relation to their psychological well-being. Those from Eastern Europe living in Portugal, for instance, encountered a number of economic and social problems, including lack of financial resources, family uprooting, unemployment difficulties and language barriers. These combined to have a negative impact on social and psychological well-being. The lack of social support was found to be significantly correlated to mental health status, the prevalence of psychiatric morbidity and the vulnerability to stress of this population.

History of mental health services

In Portugal, there is reference to the existence of differentiated (specialised) wards for 'patients who lost their mind' in the sixteenth century (Barahona-Fernandes, 1998). The influence of the work of Pinel had an effect in Portugal, and shortly after he implemented improved working practices in Paris, the introduction of medical practices, sustained observation and record-keeping were adopted in some parts of Portugal. Bizarro (1835) was the first to collect data relating to diagnoses of hospitalised patients, care practices and how they responded to treatments. As well as taking a close interest in the practice of psychiatry, the cultural, social, economic and political conditions also influenced the direction that this new branch of medicine took. In 1848, the first Hospital de Loucos de Rilhafoles was founded after the triumph of the liberal campaigns and the Maria da Fonte and Patuleia revolutions, resulting from the implementation of liberalism in Portugal inspired by the ideals of the French Revolution.

At this time, however, there were in existence no more than a few limited attempts at creating specialist provision, and, according to Barahona-Fernandes (1998), most people with mental disorders 'wandered all over the country, filling prisons, subjected to the public's mockery and warders' physical abuse'. Therefore, the founding of this hospital and the Hospital Conde de Ferreira in Porto, in 1883, was considered to be progressive in meeting the needs of people who were psychiatric patients with various disorders. Perhaps the greatest influence in the creation of this provision was the eighteenth-century Enlightenment, with its emphasis on humane approaches towards the weakest members of society. This, in addition to the political will that prevailed at that time in Portugal, resulted in the consideration of humane institutions, similar to that which had taken place at the University of Coimbra, where the experimental method of natural sciences was introduced into the medical curriculum. A number of innovations took place shortly after this, including the discharge and recovery of insane people, adopting the term 'patients', the ending of both slavery and the death penalty, and the reiteration of human rights. Also significant was the attribution of legal irresponsibility to alienated criminals, as can be seen in the Criminal Code of 1852, explicitly stating that these criminals cannot be held accountable for their crimes. However, the progress of reform was constantly slowed down, sometimes due to the disproportion between the number of inpatients and the lack of budget and staff, and at other times because resources were directed towards other social and cultural developments. These circumstances are especially significant in relation to mental patients, because the 'asylum-type' accumulation and treatment was thought by some to contribute to an aggravation of the diseases. Throughout the years, the evolution of mental health policies managed to align two major strands of thought, which at times appeared contradictory, namely: Which was worth investing in, the building of hospitals or the creation of community facilities?

As far as provision is concerned, four different legislative and organisational stages can be seen in the history of Portuguese mental health services:

- **Psychiatric hospitalisation** (1848–1945), from the year of the foundation of the first institution aimed at psychiatric inpatients.
- **The law on psychiatric assistance**, published in 1945, which gave rise to the first services open to the community.
- **Regionalisation and decentralisation** of mental health services (1945–70).
- **The integration of mental health into public health** and the primary health care subsystem (1971–92), coupled with the integration of mental health in the general health care system and the new community model for the provision of mental health services (since 1998).

However, this division is misleading, as we will see later, because of the huge gap that existed between the creation of laws and their implementation. There were instances where previous laws continued to be enacted regardless of the fact that they had been superseded by newer ones.

On 4 July 1889, the 'Law of assistance to madness' was approved, being the first nationwide law to assist alienated people, as they were then called in Portugal at that time, making the distinction between hospitals and asylums. This law was named after the first Portuguese psychiatrist, António Maria de Sena (1845–90), a teacher in Coimbra, and it was created based on his awareness of the need for assistance to alienated people, described in *Os Alienados em Portugal – História e Estatística* (Alienated People in Portugal – History and Statistics) in 1884. He is considered one of the major pioneers of psychiatric assistance and mental health in Portugal. This law foresaw the need for the construction of four hospitals, which were built 50 years later. The law also allowed for the provision of psychiatric wards in prisons, made it compulsory that all psychiatric patients had a medical examination and created a public charity fund that only psychiatric patients could access. It is commonly held that the Sena law was truly the first mental health law in Portugal. However, it was not fully implemented due to a lack of financial and administrative resources.

In 1941, the Hospital Júlio de Matos (Lisbon), and in 1945, the Hospital Sobral Cid (Coimbra), were founded, and they were both considered ideal hospitals at the time. Both symbolised the superiority of institutional care over community care and it was not until the end of 1970 that an attempt was made to regionalise and decentralise mental health services so that a greater emphasis was given to the creation of community-based support structures. On 30 May 1945, another law relating to psychiatric assistance was approved, covering prophylactic, therapeutic and pedagogical interventions. In accordance with this law, prophylactic interventions consisted of a set of individual and collective measures relating to prevention and the promotion of mental hygiene. Therapeutic interventions consisted of the treatment and correction of mental illnesses and disorders, in outpatient care, emergency care and home treatment. Finally, pedagogical interventions consisted of educational approaches using the medico-psychological techniques. At this time, the country was divided into three areas (north, centre and south), with head offices in Porto, Coimbra and Lisbon, respectively, and the services in each area were conducted by a psychiatric assistance centre.

On 25 July 1958, the Institute for Psychiatric Assistance (IAP) was created. This institute took on the direct responsibility to coordinate the institutions/facilities in the different areas of the country. Mobile units were created, composed of 'medical staff or other personnel considered necessary' (Boschma, 1997). On 3 April 1963, the Basic Mental Health Law was approved, based on the French 'sector psychiatry'. With the creation of the Institute for Mental Health and the mobile units, psychiatric assistance changed from the traditional model, based on psychiatric hospitals with asylum and custodial features, to the community model, in which services were closer to the populations' residential areas and, in particular, to primary health care. The creation of mental health centres was promoted all over the country, with the exception of Lisbon, Porto and Coimbra, aiming at a rational organisation of a joint system of mental health care, focused on therapeutic teams and providing assistance to populations living in certain geographical areas. Assistance continued to be mostly provided in the major psychiatric hospitals. This law provided for the creation of mental health centres which comprised, in addition to hospital and dispensary services, day hospitals, night hospitals, post-treatment homes and protected workshops, as well as in-home visits (Ferreira, 1987). Initiating these services proved difficult, until eventually the first centres were created in 1965, with 21 more created before 1980, covering about 60% of the population.

In 1970, Portugal implemented a hospital-centred system, and in 1971 there was an attempt to integrate mental health into public health by passing new legislation. This resulted in the creation of the first health centres, with new competencies, such as basic medical care, education and mental health and, in 1976, family planning. The creation of these services and diplomas aimed at developing cooperation between mental health services and other health services, from a public health perspective, which is the basis of any community psychiatry intervention. Once again, the difficulties of transforming policy into practice stalled because of limited resources, the lack of professionals in rural areas, and the over-reliance on some asylum-type institutions, resulting only in partial implementation of this reform. However, the care provision scene was still significantly changed. The public health issue also shifted as a result of the social and political changes which occurred in 1974, and this was given greater impetus with the introduction of the National Health Service in 1979. However, it was not until the 1990s that mental health was finally integrated into the national health system, despite frequent attempts since 1971.

From 1985 to 1990, the main reform lines foresaw the revision of the Law on Mental Health, namely the creation of a community service network, the restructuration and expansion of district mental health centres, the development of rehabilitation and deinstitutionalisation programmes for chronic patients, and the establishment of cooperation with private institutions. This was a period characterised by consecutive laws which, once again, brought psychiatry closer to the community. However, as has been suggested above, the passing of multiple laws was an indicator that they were not being implemented in practice. With the publication of Decree-Law no. 127 in 1992, mental health centres were closed down, and their functions were transferred to the psychiatry and mental health departments of general hospitals and those of the three infantile-juvenile centres to the paediatric hospitals of Lisbon, Porto and Coimbra. This decision was somewhat imposed as there was no previous discussion, which prompted conflicts among the supporters of different organisational and assistance models, as well as the creation of a resistance movement composed of the supporters of the community perspective.

During 1994, a national conference on mental health was organised, composed of four working groups with members from different ideological perspectives, who debated the way forward. This resulted in the ministerial order of 23 August 1995 that gave rise to the creation of the Portuguese Mental Health Commission. The conclusions of these groups were published in the report 'Organisation Principles of Mental Health Services – Mental Health: A Proposal for Change', which recommended the following:

- sectorisation – ensuring accountability for care provided in each geodemographic area
- greater emphasis on continuity of care
- the development of a community care philosophy and practices
- diversification and coordination of the service networks both between and within each sector
- functional cooperation between specialised mental health services and other health services
- restructuring of psychiatric hospitalisation aiming at the hospitalisation of acute patients in general hospitals and the creation of mechanisms that contribute to the rehabilitation and deinstitutionalisation of chronic patients
- participation of patients, families and other community institutions in mental health care.

The Law on Mental Health, passed on 24 July 1998, stressed the importance of having a diverse network of interconnected services that would require the cooperation of various government ministries and local community organisations. In this law, 44 of the 49 articles are devoted to the regulation of patients compulsorily detained in hospital. This type of hospitalisation is used in cases where a request or complaint by the family or community is submitted to the sanitary or police authorities. At this point, the Public Prosecution Office is asked to intervene, and the final decision to admit is made by a judge. This is an important law in the history of mental health care because it is the first time that the rights and duties of mental health service users were established.

In 1999, a decree-law established the guidelines for the organisation, management and assessment of mental health services, with a special emphasis on the National Council for Mental Health and the competencies of psychiatric hospitals. The legislation resulting from the new Law on Mental Health (1998) offered the possibility of establishing several partnerships through cooperation agreements between health structures, regional social security centres, social solidarity institutions, NGOs and other institutions (employment centres, public and private companies, among others). It was intended that these partnerships would allow the development of interventions which would meet the rehabilitation and social integration needs of patients and their families. According to Guterres and Frasquilho (2004), up to the end of 2001 only 754 people benefited from this range of services, provided by 44 structures (most of them were socio-occupational forums, followed by self-help groups, protected life units, autonomous life units and, finally, supported life units). As happened with previous services, these were unevenly distributed across the country, making it difficult for some people to access. There is a greater concentration of these services in Lisbon and Tagus Valley (72%), followed by Algarve (23%), Centre Region (10%), Northern Region (4%) and Alentejo (1%).

As can be seen from the above, politicians tend to see the passing of new laws and the devising of new policies as the main drivers for change in mental health services. However, two major issues continue to jeopardise this approach. First, the lack of appropriately skilled people to deliver services, and second, the inappropriate location of many of these services. It would appear that up until now, initiatives are largely driven by politicians and interested professionals. If more appropriate improvements and developments are to take place, then a much greater involvement of local people, patients and their families is needed. Their involvement, if properly carried out, should result in better consultation, better decision-making with regard to what treatments should be provided and where services should be sited. Educating people about the valuable contribution they could make to the development of mental health services should be a priority for the foreseeable future.

Attitudes towards mental health problems

Psychological and behavioural disorders can have a large impact on individuals, families and communities. It is estimated that one in four families in Portugal has at least one member currently suffering from a disabling mental or behavioural disorder. In these circumstances, families have to reorganise themselves in order to provide support to these patients. In most cases, there is an increased burden because of financial costs and changes in routines, and high physical and emotional burnout rates are seen in relatives. Families also have to bear the negative impact of stigma and discrimination. In Portugal, families play a key role in the provision of care to their mentally ill family members and are, in many ways, the primary care providers, often because of the lack of other types of support. Today, with the current reform of mental health services in Portugal, including the progressive winding down of psychiatric hospitals, families have to take on many more responsibilities. The effectiveness of family support is dependent on such factors as the level of understanding they have of the problem from which the person is suffering, the depth of knowledge they possess and the skills and abilities they have to care for relatives suffering from mental disorders. For these reasons, an important community-based strategy is being devised to help families understand illnesses, promote therapeutic adherence, recognise the first signs of recurrence, ensure timely solutions to address mental health crises and support their members by developing functional coping mechanisms.

In addition to every patient having a right to appropriate services and good care, continuity of care is considered by far to be the most important objective. Where there is a lack of social/family resource, and deficient cooperation between services, this can lead to a lack of support and an inappropriate use of hospital resources. This problem requires the adoption of measures to promote cooperation between everyone involved in the care process and the improvement of patient care. We believe that the recent reform of mental health services in Portugal is an important and urgent improvement in this direction and to a general improvement of the mental health of the Portuguese population. However, some less positive aspects must be pointed out that are essentially related to health care access, equity and quality.

In Portugal, the number of people with mental disorders who use public services was expected to be higher than it actually is, because according to the National Plan for Mental Health (National Coordination for Mental Health, 2009), only 1.7% of the population use mental health services, while approximately 5%–8% of the population suffer from a mental disorder at any one time. Rodrigues (2004) reported that existing services do not address the needs of the population, in that it is known that approximately 20% of people with psychiatric problems present in primary care, whereas upwards of 32% of people with psychiatric conditions remain unidentified. A number of reasons may be advanced for this, e.g. services are inappropriately located, services are insufficient or inadequately staffed, professionals fail to recognise mental health problems, or people themselves, for various reasons, do not make contact with services. Equally, the results of these studies confirm Goldberg and Huxley's model (1980) that those who find their way to specialist mental health services are considerably fewer than those who experience mental health problems in the population at large. Despite these observations, Portugal continues to concentrate its services and resources in large urban areas, thus limiting the availability of services in rural areas and making it difficult for collaboration between health and social services. Thus, most of the financial resources are spent on inpatient care (83%), and judging by the number of readmissions to hospital it would indicate that there are major problems with the discharge process and the quality of care available following discharge (PNSM, 2008).

The National Coordination for Mental Health (2009), in *Structure and Functions of Community Mental Health Teams*, pointed out deficits in the composition of some mental health teams and recommended that they should be multidisciplinary, encompassing such disciplines as psychiatrists, nurses, social service technicians, occupational therapists, educational psychologists and psychomotor skills specialists. Not only should individuals be skilled in their relevant discipline, they should also be able to work productively with other disciplines. However, many existing teams are composed only of some of these disciplines and not all of them are skilled in the delivery of therapeutic services. Consequently, not all patients derive the benefits they should from contact with these services. The PNSM (2008) concluded that the quality of community services is inferior to that which exists within inpatient services.

Despite the encouragement of the European Pact for Mental Health and Well-Being (2008) to achieve greater involvement of people, their families and carers with mental health issues, especially those relating to policy formation, decision-making and service provision, it is now evident that this degree of involvement will take time. There are only a few associations of patients and relatives and friends of psychiatric patients, thus they are still unable to influence policies and welfare organisations.

The financial and human resources allocated to mental health care in Portugal have always been seen as below that which is required. In Portugal, mental health expenditure represents 3.1% of the general health budget. The PNSM (2008) mentions that these resources are poorly distributed in mental health services throughout the different regions, directly affecting the quality of care provided and the difficulty of implementing new models of care. Of even greater concern are the systems and models of allocating financial resources to mental health services that are outdated and in urgent need of revision. Addressing this issue directly, the PNSM (2008) stated that funding arrangements are:

> A completely anachronistic model, which promotes the system's dysfunctionality and prevents any attempt to develop the services according to the goals that have been set.

The generation of psychiatric and mental health scientific knowledge, especially in the area of health promotion and illness-prevention programmes, is still underdeveloped. Better systems of data collection are required, and more needs to be known about the determinants of mental health problems, the efficacy of interventions and the types of services where epidemiological research can be carried out, if mental health care is to advance and be available to all (European Pact for Mental Health and Well-Being, 2008). Despite these difficulties, there is an optimistic air in the country that problems can be addressed and targets reached. New policy directions, legislation and additional resources suggest that the current difficulties in mental health services are being taken seriously. Further evidence that there is a national determination to assist individuals is the development of new family health units and the creation of psychiatric and mental health units in the new general hospitals under construction and those being planned. Not only will these provide better services for people in the community, but they will provide the conditions where improved collaboration can take place between those delivering services. Also pointed out in the PNSM (2008) was that those who provide services have an obligation to provide evidence of what works and what helps people in order to inform the government of the predictors that are likely to promote positive change. It stated:

> . . . to invest in psychiatric and mental health research, especially in epidemiology and health service research, is an extremely efficient factor for the development of a public health and assessment culture, as well as for the creation of a critical mass which is vital for the improvement of mental health care.

As influential as the EU is in advocating change in mental health care, the influence of the WHO cannot be underestimated, particularly with respect to Portugal. The EU directives, WHO reports and the Helsinki Declaration all combine to signify that the improvement of mental health care is a fundamental means of recognising the human rights of people, modernising mental health services in Portugal and harmonising good practice throughout the EU.

Stigma

Despite the increase in information and awareness about issues relating to mental illness, there are still myths and stereotypes that abound in the population about people with mental health disorders. The deeply rooted perceptions of dangerousness and unpredictability are not only held by members of the public, but by some of the health professionals as well (Ferreira, 2006). The fact that some health professionals hold negative attitudes towards mentally ill people may be one of the reasons treatments and interventions are not as effective as they should be. According to Corrigan (2004), stigma is the societal embodiment of disempowerment, as it promotes expectations in both the public at large and individual consumers that people with mental disorders are incapable of the responsibilities commensurate with living independently. Those who hold strong prejudices about mentally ill people tend to regard them with fear and revulsion and claim that the best way of dealing with them is to isolate them socially. Furthermore, they tend to believe that people with mental disorders should be treated as if they were children, requiring permanent care and protection from their families and the community in general.

In Portugal, Loureiro *et al.* (2008) undertook a study of 843 people in the general population on their 'beliefs and attitudes about mental illnesses and patients' and found that most saw mental illness as being a medical condition susceptible to treatment. The study showed that certain attitudes about the mentally ill, such as stigma and discrimination, incurability and dangerousness, and ability to accept individual responsibility, were still prevalent, although not as strongly held as they once were. As for attitudes, the results indicated low mean scores in authoritarian attitudes, especially with respect to aetiology and irreversibility, authoritarianism and restriction of personal, social rights and hostile and stigmatising separatism. Based on these results, they concluded that despite the development of information and knowledge about these types of illnesses, beliefs are still deeply rooted in the social and cultural context, especially dangerousness and incurability. However, they observed positive attitudes in relation to mental illnesses, which indicated that people with mental health problems were prepared to seek professional help and comply with prescribed treatments. This suggests that some progress has been made in regard to the destigmatising of services. According to these authors, at least in their sample, we are facing a change 'for the better' in attitudes and beliefs, a finding which shows that Portuguese society is becoming more tolerant towards people and families with mental illnesses.

Overall, however, although information and public awareness have increased, these issues are still misunderstood, as society continues to randomly present distorted images of people suffering from mental disorders. Abusive, ridiculing and offensive images sustain the myths, which are both negative and counterproductive to what public information and awareness campaigns seek to do. Because most of the information on mental disorders is presented in the media, it is also important, as Jorge-Monteiro and Madeira (2007) found, that public opinion with respect to mental illness is changing and could be assisted more so if the media were more responsible in how they reported issues relating to mental health problems. Many journalists and editors state that they rarely include articles or features on people who suffer from a mental disorder. There are even those who acknowledge that they would never consider contacting a person with mental illness or any organisation that represents the interests of mentally ill people. Generally, journalists believe that the public are not interested in issues relating to mental illness. There are some in the media who agree that attitudes towards mental disorders and psychiatric patients are not as negative as they once were, and the sooner people with mental illnesses are accepted in society, the better it will be for society at large. Other impressions emerging in the media suggest that the mentally ill should not be restricted in their movements, and should be permitted to marry, have children and be able to live a normal life. More help should be available to people after leaving hospital in order to help them recover and make the appropriate social adjustments. It is also difficult for some to accept the fact they are capable of integrating into their communities following recovery. Only about a third of journalists report positively about those with mental health problems; the rest adopt a highly irresponsible attitude towards those with mental health problems, maintaining that they should remain apart from the community due to them being dangerous, violent and unpredictable.

For a more tolerant attitude to prevail, leaders in the fields of the media, politics, education, health and social care should be seen to protect the rights of all people, especially psychiatric patients, so that communities can be helped to abandon negative stereotypes and treat all people with respect, regardless of physical, behavioural and intellectual differences. The media has an important part to play, and the fact that some influential journalists believe that the mentally ill should not be stigmatised, should not be locked away and should be assisted to live a normal life, bodes well for the future of mental health care in Portugal.

Mental health expenditure

In Portugal, mental health expenditure represents 3.1% of the general health budget for 2008 (Eurotrials, 2009). A total of 83% of that budget was allocated to psychiatric hospitals, even though the scientific evidence shows that community interventions, closer to the people, are more efficient and more appreciated by patients and their families. An inevitable consequence of this resource alloca- tion is the lack of new developments in community services in Portugal. Many local mental health services are still limited to inpatient and outpatient care, and sometimes day hospitals, lacking community mental health teams with pro- grammes of integrated case management, crisis intervention and family support (PNSM, 2008). Portugal has one of the lowest expenditures on mental health in the EU of just less than 5% of GDP (Mental Health Economics, 2004). In the National Mental Health Plan (PNSM, 2008), the establishment of a funding model based on contracting principles has been identified as a priority. To this end, a cost centre for the psychiatry and mental health departments will ensure the protection of the allocated funding. In the future, it is hoped that funding will take into account the various specificities of mental health care and no longer be led by what happens in general hospitals, e.g. inpatient care, outpatient care, day hospital and emergency rooms, which is insufficient to build responsive mental health services.

Nursing in Portugal

In recent decades, nursing in Portugal has been undergoing a significant and rapid transformation in terms of both its assertion as a scientific discipline and a differentiated profession. Nursing in Portugal is as old as the nation itself; the first references to the existence of nurses in Portugal actually go back to 23 years before the formation of the country in 1143. Nursing care was essentially provided by monks and nuns. In 1741, the first Portuguese nursing handbook was published, *A Postilla Religiosa e arte de enfermeiros*, by Frei Diogo de Santiago, who belonged to the religious order of São João de Deus, thus confirming the strong connection between the profession and religious orders (National Mental Health Report, 2005).

In 1860, Florence Nightingale founded modern nursing at St Thomas's Hospital in London, and although she did not consider asylum nurses to be part of what she termed 'general nursing', nevertheless she did exercise some influence on psychiatric nursing as a movement. In that time, there was already a group of people who, together with religious orders, worked in hospitals and asylums. The first nursing courses in Portugal were devised in the second half of the ninteenth century. In 1881, the University of Coimbra Hospital offered the first course to train assistant nurses and the country's first nursing school was founded on 17 October 1881 by Professor António AC Simões. Initially, it was called the School of Nurses of Coimbra, and in 1919 its name was changed to that of the Nursing School of University of Coimbra Hospital. Today, it is known as the Nursing School of Coimbra. As a result of the hospital's legislation reform in 1918, the Professional Nursing School, which could only be approved by a decree-law passed on 25 November 1922, came into existence. Courses run at the university consisted of a nursing general course (lasting 2 years and on completion allowed qualified nursing staff to work in hospitals, but not in senior positions) and a complementary nursing course. The latter lasted for 1 year and permitted successful candidates to apply for jobs in leading positions in hospitals. This only applied to nurses working in general hospitals. Nunes (2003) observed that the establishment of these courses signified the first steps in nursing as a profession enshrined in law. During the 1940s, various specialist courses were created in specific nursing areas, such as psychiatry, paediatrics and public health. The law stated categorically that only single women or widows could provide nursing care and the possession of a diploma was obligatory in order to perform nursing functions.

In the 1950s, nurses' training was restructured; the nursing general course was lengthened to 3 years and the schools were given complete autonomy over curricular content and how the courses were administered. At that time, as many as 75% of nursing students failed to complete their course, choosing instead to perform the functions of nursing assistants because of the low social recognition of nursing and the poor salaries of nurses (Portuguese Nurses Association, 2008). In the early twenty-first century, there were a total of 7006 nursing professionals, including graduates, assistant nurses and those without training. There was one graduate nurse for every 3275 inhabitants in comparison to the US (1 nurse/300 inhabitants), and the United Kingdom (1 nurse/500 inhabitants) (Nunes, 2003). International guidelines suggest that the ideal number of qualified nurses should be one nurse to 500 inhabitants. These figures clearly show that there is a distinct lack of nursing professionals.

During the 1960s, two important developments took place within Portuguese nursing. First, the restriction on married women entering nursing was lifted, and second, experienced nurses were eligible to assume lecturing posts in schools of nursing. In 1965, all courses became 3-year courses, coinciding with the introduction of the first 3-year course in psychiatric nursing. In 1973, the first National Nursing Congress was organised in order to integrate nursing into the national education system and higher education, as well as seeking to protect the professional standing of nursing. It was at that congress that the possibility of creating a nurses' association was first discussed (Ordem dos Enfermeiros, 2008). In the following year, on 25 April, it was decided to terminate the running of all nursing auxiliary courses. A course for the promotion of nursing assistants to nurses was created, thus opening the way for the existence of a single level of training.

The 1980s and 1990s saw further reforms both in nursing as a career and in the way nursing education and training were delivered. Opportunities were created to enable the scope of nursing practice to be better defined and extended, while nurses were encouraged to assume higher posts in health care management. In 1996, the Regulation for Nurses' Professional Practice was approved, and on 4 September 1998, the Portuguese Nurses Association came into existence. Today, discussions are taking place within the Ministry of Health with the aim of extending the nursing role and increasing nurses' involvement in the organisation and administration of services and organisations. Nursing education is now fully integrated into Portuguese higher education: the first master's degrees in nursing were offered in 1991, and the first doctoral degree in nursing was achieved in 2001.

Psychiatric nursing in Portugal

The beginning of psychiatric nursing in Portugal coincided with the foundation of the major psychiatric hospitals in the eighteenth century, more specifically in 1848, with the foundation of Hospital de Rilhafoles in Lisbon. As in other countries, nurses did not have any training. The provision of health care consisted of 'supervising and treating alienated people, being gentle with them, helping and guiding them, teaching them order and hygiene habits, keeping the front doors locked, welcoming visitors while maintaining the necessary silence'. Nursing records consisted of daily notes in a specific notebook – the nurse's journal – about 'everything that the nurse observed in the patient, during and subsequent to admission, as well as the treatment prescribed for the patient. The Head of Nurses would check the records, correct them or add more information, if necessary' (Botelho, 1996, quoted by Ferreira, 2009, pp. 67–8). Despite the very important role that nurses played in caring for patients, the need for training was becoming evident. In the nineteenth century, psychiatric nurse education began to be implemented in some psychiatric hospitals, most notably the Conde de Ferreira Hospital and Miguel Bombarda Hospital (formerly Hospital de Rilhafoles). This training was formalised by a law passed in 1911 which made provision for a course that could be attended by the guards, auxiliary staff and nurses. It consisted of two classes per week over two semesters, and attendance was at the discretion of those who wished to attend. Successful students received a 'diploma of nurses of alienated people and neuropaths' (Ferreira, 2006, p. 69).

The year of 1942 was definitely an important one for mental health and psychiatric nursing in Portugal, with the founding of the Hospital Júlio de Matos, in Lisbon, which recruited a group of Swiss nurses to organise the ergotherapy service and a training centre for psychiatric nurses created 2 years before. In Coimbra, the Hospital Sobral Cid (HSC) was founded on 26 May 1946, and again the contribution of the Swiss nurses was vital to the development of psychiatric nursing there. During its initial operating period, this hospital had only 11 nurses: seven had training in psychiatry (six Swiss nurses and one Portuguese nurse, from Lisbon) and four had the general nursing course qualification. In 1947, the Psychiatric Nursing School was founded in HSC, offering the first course of general and psychiatric nursing. This course lasted 1 year and was aimed at nursing students who had already been working for 1 year at HSC (already with work experience) and they had to pass an entrance exam which included Portuguese language and mathematics. This course was managed by psychiatric physicians and psychiatric nurses. As the course developed, it extended to 2 years, and as more trained Portuguese nurses worked in mental health services, so the Swiss nurses began to diminish (Redondo and Sequeira, 2005).

As psychiatric nurse education became more developed and nursing lecturers became more skilled, nursing education was transferred from psychiatric hospitals to training centres, most notably in Porto and Coimbra. In 1962, the Nursing School of Irmãs Hospitaleiras do Sagrado Coração de Jesus was founded with the sole purpose of training psychiatric nurses and psychiatric nursing assistants. This training model continued until 1968, when the Psychiatric Nursing School of Lisbon was created. There, the management and teaching staff were exclusively composed of nurses, and for the first time psychiatric nurses had responsibility for their selection, training and monitoring of all trained nursing personnel. All courses run there lasted 2 years.

Since 1974, there has been only one level of nursing education, and in 1978 the first specialisation course in mental health and psychiatric nursing was created, aimed at those who already had general nursing training. From 1992 to 1999, the courses of specialised higher education studies in nursing (also in mental health and psychiatry) were created and they were equivalent to a graduate degree. Today, there are postgraduate specialisation courses in nursing lasting three semesters, which offer a specialisation certificate. After completing this course, students can obtain a master's degree by completing an additional curricular semester and developing a thesis in their area of expertise.

Nurses in mental health care

Those seeking to enter nursing can do so by applying to a nursing school in the same way that students in other disciplines do. Those entering psychiatric nursing come from a wide variety of backgrounds and experiences and all are eligible to work in mental health services. Currently, the organisation of the profession comprises different levels of competence, e.g. nurse, graduate nurse, specialist nurse, chief nurse and supervisor of nursing. However, this organisation is about to be restructured. Today (2011) the remuneration for nurses in Portugal ranges from €1020 to €2845 a month. Based on the information provided in the Reference Network for Psychiatry and Mental Health (Directorate General for Health, 2004), there are around 1727 nurses practising in mental health and psychiatry; more specifically, 1166 in adult hospitals, 516 in social solidarity institutions and 45 in child and adolescent psychiatry and mental health. It is estimated that there is a shortage of 159 nurses if the level of service defined by the government is to be delivered effectively.

The health regions of Lisbon and Tagus Valley have the largest number of nurses providing hospital-based interventions in adult services (413), followed by the Centre Region (378), Northern Region (209), Alentejo (46) and Algarve (39) (Eurotrials, 2009). If the data from the Portuguese Nurses Association (Ordem dos Enfermeiros, 2010) in 2009 is taken into account, there were 59 601 nurses (5.6/1000 inhabitants), a ratio below that stated by the OECD of 9.7. Of this total, 1173 are specialised in mental health and psychiatric nursing (797 women and 376 men), which corresponds to a slight increase in relation to 2000 (983 nurses). The nurses' scope of activity in mental health is divided between health care provision and management.

Current mental health care

The current National Plan for Mental Health (2008) is focused on closer collaboration between hospital and community care provision, providing services closer to where people live, based on four goals:
- integrated programme for those with severe psychiatric conditions, with case management overseen by appropriate therapists

- programme of connection with family health and support for common mental disorders
- programme of support for older patients
- programme of prevention in the areas of depression and suicide.

The current reorganisation of institutions being undertaken is essential in order to:

- complete the national network of local mental health services and promote the type of health care provided by these services
- develop services and programmes for the rehabilitation and deinstitutionalisation of patients with severe psychiatric conditions
- develop the regional mental health services necessary to complement local services in specific areas
- coordinate the restructuring of the work of psychiatric hospitals, as what they have traditionally done is being transferred to other services.

Hospitalisation rates and common treatments

The third psychiatric census was conducted at a national level in 2001, in 66 health institutions: 45 (68.2%) public institutions, 18 (27.3%) religious institutes and three (4.5%) private institutions. Of a total of 17 902 individuals, 9768 (55%) were women, 7942 (44%) were men and 192 (1%) did not mention their gender. There were 9414 outpatient appointments, 6839 hospitalisations and 1649 emergencies. Overall, schizophrenia was the most frequent disorder, with 3556 patients (21.2%), followed by depressive disorders, with 2499 (14.9%), mental retardation, with 2247 (13.4%), alcohol-associated disorders, with 1494 (8.9%), and neurosis, with 1436 (8.6%). Although these figures were collected over a decade ago, it can be assumed that they reflect the current position in the country.

TABLE 9.2 Disorders in inpatient units (2001)

Disorder	Number	%
Schizophrenia	2378	36.5
Mental retardation	1846	28.3
Alcohol-associated disorders	460	7.1
Affective disorders (without depression)	350	54
Dementia syndrome	349	5.3
Other psychosis	235	3.6
Neurosis	172	2.6
Personality disorders	92	1.4
Others	253	3.9

Source: Third Psychiatric Census, 2001

TABLE 9.3 Disorders in outpatient appointments (2001)

Disorder	Number	%
Depression	1844	21.5
Neurosis	1085	12.4
Schizophrenia	1083	12.4
Adjustment reactions	914	10.4
Affective psychosis (without depression)	819	9.3
Alcohol-associated disorders	720	8.2
Mental retardation	370	4.2
Other psychosis	333	3.8
Personality disorders	274	3.1
Dementia syndrome	230	2.6
Drug-associated disorders	171	2.0
Diseases of the nervous system and sense organs	88	1
Others	789	9.0

Source: Third Psychiatric Census, 2001

TABLE 9.4 Disorders in emergency services (2001)

Disorder	Number	%
Alcohol-associated disorders	314	21.3
Depression	295	20.0
Neurosis	179	12.1
Adjustment reactions	136	9.2
Affective psychosis (without depression)	104	7.0
Drug-associated disorders	99	6.7
Schizophrenia	95	6.4
Dementia syndrome	51	3.5
Personality disorders	51	3.5
Other psychosis	51	2.1
Mental retardation	31	4.2
Others	71	4.8

Source: Third Psychiatric Census, 2001

According to these tables, schizophrenia is the most common disorder in inpatient units, depression in outpatient units and alcohol-associated problems in emergency services. The average waiting time for a psychiatric hospitalisation in 2002 was 20 days. Those with schizophrenia continue to have the longest waiting time for admission to hospital (35 days).

Quality monitoring and effectiveness of MHS

With only a few quality indicators, the National Plan for Mental Health (2008) foresees the development and implementation of a quality assessment process for psychiatric and mental health services by:

- developing new ways of managing services so as to allow more participation and the sharing of responsibility between different professional groups and non-governmental organisations
- identifying policies that impact on quality improvement
- better use of information and policy documents
- developing accreditation processes (evaluation by external organisations)
- monitoring mental health services (evaluation by internal organisations)
- integrating quality assessments and assurance procedures
- analysing quality mechanisms regularly
- disseminating good practices.

Specific needs and staffing

There is an uneven distribution of specialised psychiatric human resources, especially physicians (including interns). The districts of Porto, Coimbra and Lisbon have 2.0, 4.5 and 2.2 psychiatrists per 25 000 inhabitants, respectively, while the national average is 1 : 5.

The number of child and adolescent psychiatrists and other mental health technicians is clearly below the ratio recommended by the Directorate-General for Health (1995). In 2006, there were 74 child and adolescent psychiatrists in the public sector, a ratio of only 0.74/100 000 inhabitants. According to the above ratios, there should be 150 child and adolescent psychiatrists in the public sector. As for psychiatrists, there is a concentration of child psychiatrists in the specialised hospitals of Lisbon, Porto and Coimbra, with a ratio of two specialists per 66 000 inhabitants, while in the other hospitals this ratio is below 0.3.

Mental health teams continue to have only a few psychologists, nurses, social service technicians, occupational therapists and other non-medical staff. Most teams maintain the traditional model of psychiatric inpatient services, instead of the model which is being used in modern mental health services (Report from the National Commission for the Restructuring of Mental Health Services, 2007). Some of these professions have self-regulation bodies (physicians, nurses and psychologists). Some interventions are specifically assigned to a professional group (e.g. pharmacological prescription to physicians), whereas several other psychological and psycho-educational interventions can be performed by different technicians after specific training. These interventions are partially regulated by different professional associations organised around a specific paradigm and/ or model of intervention (e.g. Portuguese Society of Brief Psychotherapies,

Portuguese Society of Family Therapy, Portuguese Association of Behavioral and Cognitive Therapies).

Hospital-based services

The total number of public mental health service users (168 369) comprises 1.7% of the mainland population, suggesting a low uptake of services. Of the total number of these service users, 24% were treated in psychiatric hospitals. On average, each user attended three medical appointments annually and less than one session took place in a day hospital. In 2005, in all day hospitals, including rehabilitation structures, 4972 patients attended sessions. Of these, 72% were treated in services and departments in general hospitals (on average each patient had 13 consultations with mental health personnel). In contrast, those who were admitted to a psychiatric hospital had on average a total of 56 consultations with mental health staff (Report from the National Commission for the Restructuring of Mental Health Services, 2007).

Mental health law

In accordance with Decree-Law no. 35/99, based on the recommendations from the United Nations and the World Health Organization, a number of factors have emerged as good practice including:
● more emphasis on the promotion of health care in the community
● service settings should be as restrictive as possible
● the general principles of mental health policies included in the new Mental Health Law, Law no. 36/98 of 24 July, should be adhered to
● a radical new organisational system of service delivery should be devised so as to enhance better service delivery.

This system should be established by means of:
● more effective cooperation between the areas of education, employment and social services
● the participation of professionals, families and service users' associations, as well as private institutions, such as religious orders, and advisory bodies
● integration and improved provision of care services in general hospitals, in collaboration with health centres and other institutions within the National Health Service.

As for psychosocial rehabilitation, the guidelines that regulate the interventions of social support and continued health care aimed at people in a situation of dependence should be underlined. These guidelines are included in the joint order of the

Ministries of Health, Labour and Welfare, Order no. 407/98 – II Series *Diário da República* (Portuguese Official Journal), no. 138 of 8 June. This document foresaw the creation of the first residential facilities and social-occupational units until the end of 1999. According to the Directorate-General for Health, all these conclusions have been slowly adopted as mental health policy. This slow and gradual change has been taking place, following the example of other European countries and the United States. According to the recommendations of the Council of Europe, there are four key points that are part of the general principles for restructuring:

1. the creation of an external services network in the community to facilitate users' access and provide a range of support adapted to people's needs
2. the functional cooperation between these services and the other health structures, in particular health centres and general hospitals
3. the reorganisation of traditional psychiatric hospitals, which are still important, although much less than in the past
4. the creation of technical conditions, in the form of an institutional network, which allow for the development of unity and continuity in health care provision.

More recently, the Network of Continued Health Care was approved by Decree-Law no. 281/2003 of 8 November. It was essentially designed to create a network of continued health care composed of all public, social and private institutions, qualified to provide care aimed at the promotion, reestablishment and maintenance of the quality of life, comfort and well-being of citizens. The health care network is based on a set of services which provide recovery care in cooperation with the network of health care provision. This network aims to prevent dependence on the part of patients, in the form of an individual care plan of complementary interventions and total recovery, not traditionally included in health care services.

The Hospital Reference Network for Psychiatry and Mental Health was also created, aiming at a planned development of resources and their optimisation and cooperation, and is supported by Operational Program Health XXI, funded by the European Union and the Portuguese Government under the 3rd Community Support Framework. This framework aimed to modernise health services, develop information systems and promote the intervention of the social and private sectors in the most deprived areas. From 2000 to 2006, this programme aimed at obtaining health gains and guaranteeing access to quality health care. To this end, the organisation of psychiatric and mental health services, programmes and health care was carefully planned, managed and assessed.

The reform of the health sector may offer opportunities to reinforce the position of mental health and begin the process of integration in policies, health services and in the community. Some well-planned changes are called for if reducing the extent of mental health problems amongst the population is to take place (Panter-Brick, 2002). A completely efficient solution for chronic psychiatric patients is still lacking, and better ways of involving communities should be devised. Institutions are not able to meet immediate needs or provide early intervention. Technical, organisational and institutional changes are urgent, as psychiatric services can no longer continue to provide total mental health care as they did in the past.

In Portugal, the National Council for Mental Health (2002) analysed some mental health aspects and issued proposals and recommendations at the three levels of prevention. In primary prevention, we underline the general and specific measures of prevention, such as the development of health, in general, preventing vulnerability and promoting resistance to illness. At the secondary level of prevention, it is important to develop interventions adapted to the needs of the child and adolescent populations, especially through mental health services aimed at well-defined populations and with community-based integrated care. As for tertiary prevention, there should be cooperation and commitment between health, social and community sectors, promoting the rehabilitation of patients with chronic disorders. After analysing rehabilitation resources in Portugal, we observed that psychiatry services and units have:

> . . . occupational therapy, day hospitals or units, and also sometimes self-help and family groups. In-home support is also mentioned, but only as an occasional intervention and not as an organized service aimed at the acquisition of daily life competences. (National Council for Mental Health, 2002, p. 31)

As for private social solidarity institutions, they provide an adequate response to almost every situation. Thus, in-home support services should be developed and adapted to meet actual needs. On 26 April 2006, the National Commission for the Restructuring of Mental Health Services was created by an order of the Ministry of Health. This commission was expected to study the situation of mental health care provision in Portugal, propose an action plan to restructure and develop mental health services and make recommendations about its implementation based on the guidelines of the World Health Organization on the reform of mental health care. This resulted in the report of the National Commission for the Restructuring of Mental Health Services.

This commission identified the different strategies (such as service reorganisation, promotion of research and cooperation between sectors) which, according to current scientific knowledge, are essential to guarantee an effective improvement of mental health care quality, promote the mental health of the population and elaborate a plan for the successful implementation of these strategies.

On 6 March 2008, the National Plan for Mental Health (2007–2010) was created by the resolution of the Council of Ministers no. 49/2008, with the following main goals:

- Ensure equal access to quality care for everyone with mental disorders in the country, including those belonging to especially vulnerable groups.
- Promote and protect the human rights of people with mental disorders.
- Reduce the impact of mental disorders and contribute to the promotion of mental health of the population.
- Promote the decentralisation of mental health services, so as to enable care provision closer to people's homes and to facilitate greater participation by communities, people with mental disorders and their families.
- Promote the integration of mental health care into the general health system, at the primary care level as well as in general hospitals, so as to ensure continuity of care and facilitate access and reduce institutionalisation.

Current role of nursing in mental health care

Today, the nursing profession is based on a legal framework supported by a number of regulatory documents which include the following:

- REPE – Regulation of Nurses' Professional Practice (Decree-Law no. 161/96 of 4 September, with the changes made by Decree-Law no. 104/98 of 21 April).
- The creation of the Portuguese Nurses Association (Decree-Law no. 104/98 of 21 April).
- The Statutes of the Portuguese Nurses Association (republished in Law no. 111/2009 of 16 September and resulting from the first amendment to the Statutes of the Portuguese Nurses Association, approved by Decree-Law no. 104/98 of 21 April).
- The Nurses' Code of Conduct (included in the Statutes of the Portuguese Nurses Association as an appendix to Law no. 111/2009 of 16 September).
- The establishment of Nursing Care Quality Standards (Nursing Council of the Portuguese Nurses Association in 2001).
- The establishment of the Competences of General Nurses (Nursing Council of the Portuguese Nurses Association in October 2003).

The new Model for Professional Development integrated in the System of Certification of Competences and the System of Individualisation of Specialties is currently being implemented. The specific competences of the nurse specialist in mental health and psychiatric nursing have been defined (Ordem dos Enfermeiros, 2010). The competences suggested are the following:

- Possess a high level of self-knowledge and self-awareness both as a person and a nurse.
- Is able to assist the person throughout the life cycle, family, groups and community in the promotion and optimisation of mental health.
- Helps the person throughout the lifespan, within the family, groups and community to recover mental health, mobilising the resources specific to each setting.
- Provides psychotherapeutic, social-therapeutic, psychosocial and psycho-educational care to the person throughout the lifespan, mobilising the individual, family, group or community dynamics and setting, so as to maintain, improve and recover health.

In Portugal, in addition to professional councils, there are also scientific societies that try to provide credibility and regulations to the various psychotherapeutic interventions. There is nothing preventing a nurse from using these therapeutic techniques. However, nurses' competence is only recognised if they are enrolled in the society and meet the necessary requirements, such as those of the Brief Therapy Association, the Cognitive-Behavioural Therapy Association, the Client-Focused Therapy Association and the Family Therapy Association, among others. This reality is the same for all professional groups (e.g. psychologists, social workers), perhaps with the exception of psychiatrists, to whom this recognition is implicitly given.

Future plans for mental health care

The challenges include the capacity to prevent mental illness, increase access to mental health care, improve mental health indicators and implement reforms without jeopardising the universal right to health. According to the Portugal country summary *Effective and Humane Mental Health Treatment and Care for All* (WHO, 2010), the priority tasks are:
- Continue the implementation of the mental health policy and plan.
- Establish a national mental health budget.
- Strengthen human resources in local mental health services, especially in remote areas.
- Establish a more robust training programme for key professionals working in community settings.
- Develop guidelines for community mental health teams.
- Create new child and adolescent mental health teams.
- Develop a new quality assurance policy for services.
- Implement accredited guidelines in routine practice.

- Devise and implement a new mental health training programme for general practitioners in primary health care.
- Establish educational promotional programmes that aim to reduce stigma, suicide, depression and direct better support of vulnerable groups.

As can be seen from the above, Portugal considers the production of policies, guidelines and directives to be important, which they are, but by themselves, they are insufficient. Other countries have come to realise that other factors, such as adequate financing, informed policy-making, skilled leadership, a competent psychiatric profession, workforce reform, involvement of the general population, and empowerment of families and service users, are equally important, if not more so. Despite efforts to provide adequate resources to deliver good mental health services in Portugal, it is to be hoped that the commitment expressed over the past few years to address stigma and discrimination will remain a central part of the policy agenda. The involvement of patients, families, professionals and the general public is vital if mental health is to continue to be viewed as a genuine public health priority in Europe (Muijen, 2008).

Case scenario

A 23-year-old unemployed man is reported by his landlord as acting increasingly strangely. He has barricaded his room, talking about being spied upon by the CIA. He can be heard shouting within his room in an angry and incoherent way. He has not been seen by a psychiatrist in the past, although his mother has told the landlord that he has been isolating himself and acting increasingly oddly over the last couple of years.

Based on the data available, under this scenario, this situation will require an initial approach from the national emergency department, composed of health technicians (without any specific training in mental health), to ensure the individual's adherence. When all attempts for a voluntary collaboration fail, a legal intervention will take place, led by the police, to allow access to the bedroom, and the health technicians to accompany the patient to the emergency department. This is referred to as compulsory admission, i.e. a special permission from a judge in a situation of danger to self or others.

In the nearest emergency department of a general hospital with psychiatric services, according to the hospital referral network, the patient will be seen by a triage nurse, using the Manchester protocol, and referred to a psychiatrist, who will analyse the situation, prescribe medication and, if necessary, hospitalise the patient. In a compulsory admission, the psychiatrist must write a considered report on the facts that supported this decision, and add other clinical, psychiatric and psychosocial reports, whenever possible. The final decision for compulsory admission must be approved by a judge, after consultation with the patient's advocate.

In this situation, antipsychotics will be prescribed and there is a high possibility of hospitalisation, though the prescription of medication is not a nursing intervention in Portugal. In this first stage, the intervention will be mainly pharmacological, gradually including psychosocial interventions as the positive symptoms subside.

Within the scope of hospitalisation, nursing interventions will occur at two levels: individual and familial. At the individual level, a health care plan will be defined to meet the identified needs, following the model in force and using International Classification for Nursing Practice (ICNP) terminology. Intervention programmes will gradually be established to maintain the psychosocial skills and the adherence to and management of the therapeutic regimen. At the familial level, the intervention will aim to reinforce the patient's network of support. To that end, the family will be included in a psycho-educational programme led by psychiatric nurse specialists, according to Falloon's model (1986).

In compulsory admission, the production of a report 5 days after hospitalisation is mandatory, and if hospitalisation continues after this period, a new report should be written every 2 months. Compulsory hospitalisation ends with discharge or the patient's acceptance of hospitalisation.

After discharge, as there are no clear criteria, the psychiatrist will choose one of the two ways to conduct follow-up: the patient will continue to attend outpatient consultation in the psychiatric hospital, maintaining the institutional connection with the hospital and the psychiatrist of reference; or the patient will be referred to primary health care and followed by a general practitioner and a mental health and psychiatric nurse from the health centre, whenever possible.

References

Almeida C. Organization principles of mental health services – mental health: a proposal for change. Lisbon: Ministry of Health; 1995.

Almeida C. Reforma dos CSP: uma janela. *Jornal Médico de Família*. 2009 Setembro; **175**: 30–1.

Almeida C. *Portugal é o país da Europa com mais doenças mentais*. Lisboa: Entrevista conduzida por Rute Araújo; 2010.

Alta Comissária para a Saúde. *Avaliação do plano nacional de saúde 2004–2010*. Lisboa: 3° Fórum Nacional de Saúde: para um futuro com saúde; 2010.

Amendoeira J. *Uma biografia partilhada da Enfermagem*. Coimbra: Formasau; 2006.

APEF. Associação Portuguesa para o Estudo do Fígado. 2010. Available at: www.apef.com.pt/noticias/?im r=8 (accessed 5 January 2010).

Balsa C. *Inquérito Nacional ao Consumo de Substâncias Psicoactivas na População Geral, Portugal 2007*. Lisboa: CEOS/FCSH/UNL; 2008.

Banco de Portugal. *Relatório do Conselho de Administração, Relatório e Contas, Gerência de 2009.* Lisboa: Departamento de Estudos Económicos, Departamento de Contabilidade e Controlo; 2010.

Barahona-Fernandes J. *Antropociências da Psiquiatria e da Saúde Mental. O Homem perturbado.* Lisboa: Fundação Calouste Gulbenkian; 1998.

Barros PP. *Economia da Saúde: Conceitos e Comportamentos.* 2nd ed. Coimbra: Almedina; 2009.

Coordenação Nacional para a Saúde Mental. Documento de Consenso para a Estrutura e Funções das Equipas de Saúde Mental Comunitária (ESMC). Ministério da Saúde, Lisboa; 2009.

Corrigan P. *Enhancing Personal Empowerment of People with Psychiatric Disabilities.* Chicago, IL: University of Chicago Center for Psychiatric Rehabilitation; 2004.

Decreto-Lei nº 104/98 de 21 de Abril. Ministério da saúde. In: DR I Série – A, nº 93. 1998: 1739–56, Lisboa: Imprensa Nacional.

Decreto-Lei nº 161/96 de 4 de Setembro. Regulamento do Exercício Profissional (REPE). In: DR I Série – A, nº 205, 4/09/1996. Lisboa: Imprensa Nacional.

Decreto-Lei nº 437/91 de 8 de Novembro. Ministério da Saúde. In: DR I Série – A, nº 257, 8/11/1991: 5723–41, 1991. Lisboa: Imprensa Nacional.

Decreto-Lei nº 127/92. Extinção e integração nos Hospitais Gerais os Centros de Saúde Mental. In: DR I Série – A 92/07/03, 1992. Lisboa: Imprensa Nacional.

Decreto-Lei nº 281/03. Rede de cuidados continuados de saúde. In: DR I Série – A nº 259, 03/11/08: 7492–9, 2003. Lisboa: Imprensa Nacional.

Decreto-Lei nº 35/99. Princípios orientadores da organização, gestão e avaliação dos serviços de psiquiatria e saúde mental. In: DR I Série – A nº 30, 99/02/05: 676–81, 1999. Lisboa: Imprensa Nacional.

Decreto-Lei nº 413/71. Organização do Ministério da Saúde e Assistência. In: DR I Série A, nº 288, 71/09/27: 1406–34, 1971. Lisboa: Imprensa Nacional.

Decreto-Lei nº 41759. Criação do Instituto de Assistência Psiquiátrica. In: DR I Série nº 698, 25/06/58: 161–4, 1958. Lisboa: Imprensa Nacional.

Despacho Conjunto nº 407/98. Orientações reguladoras da intervenção articulada do apoio social e dos cuidados de saúde continuados dirigidos às pessoas em situação de dependência. In: DR II Série nº 138, 98/06/18: 8328–32, 1998. Lisboa: Imprensa Nacional.

Despacho Conjunto nº 638/99. Criação da comissão para o acompanhamento da execução do regime de internamento compulsivo. In: DR II Série nº 181, 99/08/05: 11557, 1999. Lisboa: Imprensa Nacional.

Direcção-Geral da Saúde. Conferência sobre Saúde Mental. Saúde Mental. Proposta para a mudança – Direcção-Geral da Saúde. Lisboa; 1995.

Direcção Geral da Saúde. Psiquiatria e Saúde Mental, Rede de Referenciação Hospitalar, Direcção dos Serviços de Psiquiatria e Saúde Mental. Lisboa; 2001.

Direcção Geral da Saúde. Rede de Referenciação de Psiquiatria e Saúde Mental. Lisboa; 2004.

Direcção Geral da Saúde. Plano Nacional de Saúde Mental 2007–2016, Resumo Executivo, Coordenação Nacional para a Saúde mental. Alto Comissariado da Saúde. Ministério da Saúde. Lisboa; 2008.

Eurobarometer. *Public Health.* 2003. Available at: http://ec.europa.eu/health/index_en.htm (accessed 20 April 2010).

European Brain Council. *Costs of Disorders of the Brain in Europe.* 2005. Available at: www.european braincouncil.org/publications (accessed 22 April 2010).

European Pact for Mental Health and Well-Being. *Together for Mental Health and Well-Being.* Brussels; 2008.

Eurotrials, Consultores Científicos. Saúde em Mapas e Números. *Boletim Informativo.* 2009 Setembro; **28**.

Ferreira G. Evolução das instituições psiquiátricas e cuidados de saúde mental em Portugal. *Saúde Mental Hoje.* 1987; **1**(1): 3–7.

Mental health services in Europe

Ferreira G. Perspectiva histórica dos cuidados de enfermagem ao doente mental. *Psilogos – Revista do Serviço de Psiquiatria do Hospital Fernando Fonseca*. 2006,3, nº1: 61–70.

Ferreira G. *Concorrência Público-Privado no Sistema de Saúde Português: Uma análise exploratória*. Dissertação para obtenção do Grau de Mestre em Engenharia Biomédica, Instituto Superior Técnico, Universidade de Lisboa; 2009.

Goldberg D. Epidemiology of mental disorders in primary care settings. *Epidemiol Rev*. 1995; **17**: 182–90.

Goldberg D, Huxley P. *Mental Illness in the Community: the pathway to psychiatric care*. London: Tavistock; 1980.

Greenwald G. *Drug Decriminalization in Portugal: lessons for creating fair and successful drug policies*. Washington, DC: CATO Institute; 2009.

Guterres MC, Frasquilho MA. Prevenção terciária em saúde mental: novas respostas em Portugal. *Revista Portuguesa de Saúde Pública*. 2004; **22**(2): 69–77.

Hibell B. *The 2007 ESPAD Report. Substance Use among Students in 35 European Countries*. Stockholm: CAN/Pompidou Group/Council of Europe; 2007.

INE. *Homens e Mulheres em Portugal*. Lisboa: Instituto Nacional de Estatística; 2010.

Instituto da Droga e da Toxicodependência I.P. *Relatório Anual 2007: A Situação do País em Matéria de Drogas e Toxicodependências*. Lisboa: IDT, I.P; 2008.

Jorge-Monteiro F, Madeira T. Considerações sobre doença mental e comunicação social. *Análise Psicológica*. 2007; **1**(25): 97–109.

Lei nº 2006. Bases reguladoras da assistência psiquiátrica. In: DR I Série nº 118, 45/05/30. Lisboa: Imprensa Nacional.

Lei nº 2118. Bases para a promoção da saúde mental. In: DR I Série nº 79, 63/04/03. Lisboa: Imprensa Nacional. pp. 327–32.

Lei nº 36/98. Lei da Saúde Mental. In: DR I Série nº 169, 98/07/24. Lisboa: Imprensa Nacional. pp. 3544–50.

Lei nº 56/79. Lei do Serviço Nacional de Saúde. In: DR I Série nº 15. Lisboa: Imprensa Nacional. p. 2357.

Loureiro L, Dias C, Aragão R. Crenças e Atitudes acerca das doenças e dos doentes mentais – Contributos para o estudo das representações sociais da loucura. *Referência*. 2008; **2**(8): 33–44.

Matos MG, Equipa do Projecto Aventura Social e Saúde. *A saúde dos adolescentes portugueses (quatro anos depois)*. Relatório Português Estudo HBSC. Lisboa: FMH; 2003.

Mendes A, Barroso T. 'Consumo de álcool por jovens adolescentes: comparação entre dois concelhos', Os novos velhos desafios da saúde mental. 1ª Edição, Universidade de S. Paulo, Ribeirão Preto; 2006. p. 251.

Mental Health Economics European Network I. Executive summary of the outcomes of the Mental Health Economics Project, 2004. Brussels: Mental Health Europe; 2004.

Ministério da Saúde. *Proposta de Plano de acção para a Reestruturação e Desenvolvimento dos Serviços de saúde Mental em Portugal, 2007–2016*. Lisboa: Relatório da Comissão Nacional para a Reestruturação dos Serviços de Saúde Mental; 2007.

Monteiro A. Percepção de apoio social e saúde mental em contextos migratórios: imigrantes russófonos a residir em Portugal. *Revista Referência*. 2009; **2**(10): 35–46.

Muijen M. Mental Health Services in Europe: an overview. *Psychiatr Serv*. 2008; **59**(5): 479–82.

National Coordination for Mental Health. *Documento de consenso para a Estrutura e Funções das Equipas de Saúde Mental Comunitária (ESMC)*. 2009. Available at: www.acs.min-saude.pt/wp-content/blogs.dir/1/files/2009/07/consenso-curia-2009-vfinal.pdf (accessed 24 April 2010).

National Council for Mental Health. *Proposals and Recommendations*. Lisbon: Ministry of Health; 2002.

National Mental Health Report. 2005. Caldas de Almeida (coordinator). Available at: www.acs.

min-saude.pt/wp-content/uploads/2008/01/relatorioplanoaccaoservicossaudemental.pdf (accessed 22 April 2010).

Nunes L. *Um olhar sobre o ombro, Enfermagem em Portugal (1881–1998)*. Lisboa: Lusodidacta; 2003.

Ordem dos Enfermeiros. *10 anos 1998–2008*. Lisboa: Enfermagem em Portugal; 2008.

Ordem dos Enfermeiros. *Caderno Temático – Modelo de Desenvolvimento Profissional*. Lisboa; 2009.

Ordem dos Enfermeiros. *Dados estatísticos*. 2010. Available at: www.ordemenfermeiros.pt/membros/Documents/OE_Dados_Estatisticos_2000_2009_VFinal.pdf (accessed 5 May 2010).

Organização Mundial da Saúde. *Relatório Mundial da Saúde, saúde mental: nova concepção, nova esperança*. Lisboa: Direcção Geral da Saúde; 2002.

Panter-Brick C. Street children, human rights and public health: a critique and future direction. *Annu Rev Anthropol*. 2002; **31**: 147–71.

Portugal, Ministério da Saúde, Alto Comissariado da Saúde, Coordenação Nacional para a Saúde Mental. *Plano Nacional de Saúde Mental 2007–2016 – Resumo Executivo*. Lisboa: Coordenação Nacional para a Saúde Mental; 2008.

Portugal, Ministério da Saúde, Comissão Nacional para a Reestruturação dos Serviços de Saúde Mental. *Relatório Reestruturação e Desenvolvimento dos Serviços de Saúde Mental em Portugal*. Lisboa: Ministério da Saúde; 2007.

Redondo J, Sequeira D. *Registos para a memória da história do Hospital Sobral Cid: os primeiros anos*. Porto: Multitema; 2005.

Relatório do Desenvolvimento Humano. *Ultrapassar Barreiras: mobilidade e desenvolvimento humanos*. Coimbra: Programa das Nações Unidas para o Desenvolvimento (PNUD); 2009.

Resolução do Conselho de Ministros nº 49/2008 – Plano Nacional de Saúde Mental. In: DR I Série nº 47, 06/03/08, pp. 1395–409. Lisboa: Imprensa Nacional.

Rodrigues FP. *Articulação entre os cuidados de saúde primários e a saúde mental*. Lisboa: Climepsi; 2004.

Santos J, Saraiva C, Sousa L. The role of expressed emotion, self-concept, coping, and depression in parasuicidal behavior. A follow-up study. *Arch Suicide Res*. 2009; **13**(4): 358–67.

Serviço de Estrangeiros e Fronteiras. *Relatório de Imigração Fronteiras e Asilo*. Lisboa: Departamento de Planeamento e Formação; 2008.

Simões J, Teixeira M, Barros PP, *et al*. *Comissão para a Sustentabilidade do Financiamento do Serviço Nacional de Saúde – Relatório final*. Lisboa: Ministério da Saúde; 2007.

Sociedade Portuguesa de Suicidologia. *Estatísticas*. 2010. Available at: www.spsuicidologia.pt/index.php?option=com_content&view=article&id=5&Itemid=30 (acessed 25 April 2010).

UNESCO. *Country Profile: Portugal*. Montreal: UNESCO Institute for Statistics; 2006. Available at: http://stats.uis.unesco.org/unesco/TableViewer/document.aspx?ReportId=124&IF_Language=eng&BR_Country=6200&BR_Region=40500 (accessed 22 April 2010).

WHO (2010). *Portugal Country Summary: Effective and Humane Mental Health Treatment and Care for All*. Geneva: WHO; 2010.

World Bank. *World Development Indicators 2006*. 2010. Available at: http://devdata.worldbank.org/wdi2006/contents/index2.htm (accessed 26 April 2010).

10

Mental health services in the United Kingdom

Peter Nolan and Neil Brimblecombe

Introduction

The UK has a long history of providing services for people with what are currently referred to as mental health problems. Though the types of services have changed radically over the centuries, the aims have largely remained the same; namely, to provide protection to individuals and to ensure the safety of the wider society. Particularly significant changes have taken place in the structure of mental health services in the last few years and the roles of, and relationships between, the mental health professions. Major challenges remain in relation to an ageing population, inequalities related to ethnicity and continuing stigmatisation of those with mental health problems. The authors describe what has been achieved to date and what the future may hold.

National profile and context

To understand mental health services, it is useful first to understand the context in which those services have developed and in which they continue to exist. The nature of the population and the history, economics and politics of a country, all potentially have a significant impact.

The UK (including England) joined the European Union in 1973, along with Ireland and Denmark. In contrast to other member countries, the UK has elected not to adopt the euro currency, preferring instead to stay with sterling, which has been its traditional currency. Apart from this anomaly, it is a full member of the

EU. This chapter principally describes the evolution of and existing mental health services in England, as this country is by far the largest in the UK. Occasionally, data relating to mental health services in England is presented, combined with that for other countries in the United Kingdom. Where this occurs, it will be pointed out. The differences between UK countries in terms of approaches to service delivery are relatively small, but there are some differences in the structure of organisations planning and delivering health care, the range and precise functions of services in the community and details of mental health law.

Population and demographics

England has a population of 51.1 million and is one of the most densely populated countries in the world, with more than treble the European average of 117 people per square kilometre. It is approximately twice as densely populated as France (106 people per square kilometre), nine times that of the US (27 people per square kilometre) and 100 times that of Australia (two people per square kilometre). As would be expected, the most densely populated areas of England are the major cities of Manchester, Birmingham, Liverpool and London. London has by far the densest population of any of the English regions (4,700 people per square kilometre). According to the Office for National Statistics (2009), the population of England has grown steadily since the Second World War. In 1948, the population was 48 million, and current estimates predict that it will reach 71 million by 2031. This projected growth takes into account the natural increase in population and presumes that there will be more immigration than emigration. The population is diverse culturally, economically and ethnically, and becoming more so. The largest groups by ethnic and religious background are shown in Table 10.1. The main spoken language is English, but where there are large immigrant populations, other languages are spoken. All government departments ensure that information is provided in several languages so that people are informed and involved. It is estimated that as many as 300 languages are spoken in London.

TABLE 10.1 England: ethnic and religious backgrounds of the population

Ethnic background	%	Religion	%
White British	87	Christian	70
Indian	2	Muslim	3.1
Mixed origin	2	Hindu	1.1
Chinese	1.3	Sikh	0.7
Black Caribbean	1	Jewish	0.5
Black African	0.9	Buddhist	0.3
Bangladeshi	0.5	Muslim	–

Source: Howarth *et al.*, 2008

Gross domestic product per capita in the UK is currently estimated at US$44 729 (IMF, 2009), which is well above the European average, although this figure conceals regional variations. Taking the period from 1996–97 to 2009–10 as a whole, median personal income grew by about 1.6% per year while mean income grew by 1.9% per year. After adjusting for regional differences in the cost of living, relative poverty is highest in the West Midlands and lowest in the South East of England. Since the three-year period beginning in 1996–97, poverty has fallen most in the North East of England and has risen only in the West Midlands (Wenchao *et al.*, 2011).

According to Roberts and Coid (2010), England is now the fourth-most socially unequal country in the world, and huge income differences make it one of the least socially mobile countries in the EU. This situation has many implications for the mental health of the nation and how services are designed and delivered. Class differences, for instance, are closely related to housing quality, type of work, health status and length of life. Parts of England are characterised by high levels of unemployment over many decades, resulting in intergenerational low self-esteem and poverty of ambition. Reduced life chances are set for individuals at a very young age, with consequences not only for their own mental health but also for that of whole communities.

The National Health Service

In the United Kingdom, the National Health Service (NHS) provides the majority of health care for the population, with less than 10% being provided by the private sector. The NHS was established by the then health minister Aneurin Bevan in 1948, immediately after the Second World War. Bevan visited and reviewed the health systems in several European countries before designing a comprehensive health care service, available to the entire population, free at the point of delivery and paid for by individual contributions. Today it is one if the biggest employers in the world, with approximately 1.3 million employees. It functions at primary care level (front-line care involving GPs, pharmacists, dentists, etc.), secondary care level (hospital-based, accessed via GP referral) and tertiary care level (involving highly specialised doctors dealing with particularly difficult or rare conditions) (Webster, 2002). Mental health services are provided across all three levels. The Department of Health is responsible for organising, running and improving public health and social care in England. It sets national standards, provides strategic direction and allocates resources. General practitioners are set to manage £80 billion of health care resources and it will be up to them decide what services and resources are required to meet the needs of the population. Specialist mental health services, such as forensics and eating disorders, are commissioned on a regional basis. Three 'special hospitals' in mental health care, Broadmoor, Rampton and Ashworth (together containing approximately 1260 patients), are commissioned nationally, providing high-security services for people with mental health problems who have either been convicted of serious crimes or been found unfit to plead on such crimes.

NHS trusts employ the majority of the health service workforce. They obtain most of their income via contracts with local GP consortia. NHS trusts deliver national priorities and work in partnership with other NHS organisations, local authorities and the voluntary sector. Trusts are largely self-governing. They are accountable either to the strategic health authorities or, if designated as 'foundation trusts', to a national body called Monitor and to groups of local 'governors'. Several monitoring bodies and agencies exist to ensure the overall quality of services provided. The most recent of these bodies is the Care Quality Commission, which was inaugurated in 2009.

General health need

In common with most other countries, the United Kingdom has an increasing ageing population. There are currently 1.3 million people over the age of 85 in the UK, and that number is set to double in the next 20 years (Office for National Statistics, 2010). Life expectancy is higher for women (81 years) than for men (76.6), and although women can expect to live longer, their health in later years is generally poorer than that of men. Health estimates in England now show that people over the age of 65 consume as much as 80% of physical and mental health services. One in five people over the age of 50 years attend an outpatient or casualty department every 3 months, while one in 10 are treated in hospital every year.

In 2005, the leading cause of deaths was diseases of the circulatory system, followed by cancer and then diseases of the respiratory system (Office for National Statistics, 2010). These diseases are all correlated with increasing age. As in all Western countries, whilst previous generations would frequently die from infectious disease, this is now relatively rare.

Advances in medical knowledge and practice also mean that disabled people can live longer and can lead healthier lives. This will impact on both the health and social care systems in the future, with a prediction that over 1.7 million more people will have a need for care and support in 20 years' time (HM Government, 2008).

There is increasing concern about the effects of lifestyle on health, particularly the effects of drug and alcohol abuse and obesity. In England in 2008, there were 6769 deaths directly related to alcohol, an increase of 24% from 2001, whilst many more deaths relate indirectly to alcohol use (Information Centre for Health and Social Care, 2011a). It was also found that almost a quarter of adults (22% of men and 24% of women aged 16 or over) in England were classified as obese in 2009 (Information Centre for Health and Social Care, 2011b).

Current mental health profile

Policy-makers and service providers have come to accept that improving the mental health of the nation requires the best possible information upon which to make decisions. This recognition gave rise to the establishment of the National Mental Health Developmental Unit (NMHDU) in 2009 within the Department of Health, whose main functions are achieved by commissioning or providing:

- specialist expertise in priority areas of policy and delivery
- effective knowledge transfer on research, evidence and good practice
- translation of national policies into practical deliverables that achieve outcomes
- coordination of national activity to help regional and local implementation.

In June 2010, the NMHDU published a series of 'factfiles' containing detailed information about the prevalence of mental health problems and what services are deemed to be required and effective. Mental illness, *Factfile* 3 (NMHDU, 2010) stated, represents the single largest cause of disability in England, and financial costs of the adverse effects of mental illness on people's quality of life are estimated at £41.8 billion per annum, and wider costs to the national economy in terms of welfare benefits and lost productivity at work amount to upwards of £77 billion a year (McCrone *et al.*, 2008). This amounts to 13.8% of England's health budget being spent on mental health care. The extent of mental health problems requiring assistance is summarised in Table 10.2.

TABLE 10.2 Prevalence of mental health conditions in England

- One in six adults have a mental health problem at any one time
- 17.6% of adults have at least one common mental health problem
- 0.4% of adults have a psychotic disorder, 80% of whom are receiving treatment
- 0.3% of adults have an antisocial personality disorder
- 0.4% of adults have a borderline personality
- 10% of children have a diagnosable mental health condition
- 13%–16% of older people have severe depression, and up to 50% are in residential care
- One in 20 people over 65 have some form of dementia, rising to one in five over 80
- One third of all mental health services in England is concerned with the care and treatment of people over 65.

Source: NMHDU *Factfile 3*, 2010

Surveys tend to select data that is easily available, and as such may not reveal the whole story. However, it is estimated that as many as 76% of homeless people and those who sleep rough have mental health problems and are less likely to access mainstream services for help (HM Government, 2011). Equally alarming is the high proportion of people in custody who have severe mental health problems.

Within the prison system, 72% of male and 70% of female prisoners have two or more mental health conditions, and two thirds have a personality disorder (Fazel and Danesh, 2009).

Having established, to some extent, the prevalence of mental health problems in England, *Factfile* 5 (NMHDU, 2010) addresses the evidence that has been amassed to date that attempts to explain why this is so. Much of the explanation, the data suggests, is to be found in the nature and structure of English society, the social divisions that exist and the opportunities for social mobility that are available to people. A major contributing factor is inequality in all its forms, and the opening sentences in *Factfile* 5 (NMHDU, 2010) make this obvious:

> Inequalities are a matter of life and death, of health and sickness, of well-being and misery. Creating a fairer society is fundamental to improving the health of the whole population and ensuring a fairer distribution of good health.

So where are inequalities to be found? A number of groups were identified as being particularly vulnerable to poor mental health because of where they are located within society. These are briefly described under the following headings.

Race

Rates of severe mental illness are much higher among ethnic minorities, and people from the African-Caribbean communities stand a ninefold greater risk of developing a psychosis, being admitted to hospital, feeling more coerced into accepting treatment and being prescribed more than one drug than the indigenous population. Factors that explain raised rates of poor mental health in immigrants and their descendants include stressful life events, discrimination, urban living and socio-economic deprivation. South Asian women have the highest rates of common mental disorders amongst all ethnic groups. Higher rates of suicide, self-harm and eating disorders are found among Asian adolescent girls, and female refugees and asylum seekers have higher rates of post-traumatic stress disorder and other mental illnesses than the indigenous population.

Age

Mental health problems in older people often accompany long-term illnesses. Depression and dementia are common and have a worse outcome than illnesses in younger age groups. Approximately 700 000 people have dementias, and this is predicted to rise to over 1 million by the year 2025. One in four older people living in the community have symptoms of depression that are severe enough to warrant help, but only half of these are diagnosed or treated. Older people do not typically have the same access as working-age adults to assertive outreach, crisis home treatment and early intervention services, or to rehabilitation, psychotherapy and general hospital liaison services. There is evidence of ageism in relation to:

- exclusion of older people from mental health services that are available to younger adults
- very low levels of referrals from GPs to specialist units for older mental health sufferers
- a general lack of age-appropriate service provision

Stigma

Approximately 87% of those with mental health problems have encountered some form of discrimination and stigma, resulting in various negative consequences for them. Stigma and discrimination, people report, cause difficulties in all aspects of their lives, including work, education, friendships, community participation, socialising and talking to people about their mental health problems. As many as 53% of carers say that they feel unable to do things because of fear of stigma and discrimination, and such fear prevents many people from black and ethnic minorities from seeking help in the first place. Two thirds of people with mental health problems live alone, four times more than the general population. More than 50% of people with mental health problems have poor social skills, have fewer friends and participate in fewer social occasions than those with good mental health (NMHDU *Factfile 6*, 2010).

Inequalities and mental health

Upwards of 3.7 million people suffer from multiple disadvantages in England, and it is known that poor mental health is closely related to poor housing, unemployment, low levels of education and income poverty, which are all indicators of multiples of disadvantage. *Factfile 2* (NMHDU, 2010) states that having a secure home is one of the most important components in ensuring mental health and well-being. It states:

> Good quality, affordable, safe housing is essential to our well-being. Mental health and housing are closely interlinked. Mental ill health can lead to homelessness. Homelessness, poor quality housing and housing insecurity can lead to mental health issues. Mental health can also make it difficult for people to find and maintain good quality housing.

Recorded rates of anxiety and depression are twice as high in women than men, and rates of self-harming (cutting, burning and overdose) are three times higher in women than men. Women are also more vulnerable to mental ill health because of poverty, social isolation, violence and abuse, domestic violence, sexual violence and rape. Older women have to cope with many factors that are closely linked to mental health, such as:

- likelihood of experiencing bereavement in old age
- likelihood of experiencing institutional care with its accompanying loss of independence and role
- likelihood of suffering from physical ill health and long-term disability, resulting in restriction of mobility and inability to care for themselves.

Other minority groups

Another group of people who are particularly prone to poor mental health are lesbians, gays, bisexuals and transgendered people. Many experience psychological turmoil in the form of anxiety, depression, self-harm and suicidal feelings, which are made worse by having to cope with stigma and discrimination. Approximately a quarter of people with learning disabilities have some form of mental health problem, which goes largely unrecognised. In fact, many aspects of mental illness are wrongly regarded as challenging behaviour and so do not receive appropriate treatment. It is a salient and significant fact that people with schizophrenia and bipolar disorder die on average 25 years earlier than the general population, mainly due to physical health problems. It is now established that long-term physical illness increases the risks of poor mental health:

- There is a higher risk of depressive disorder for a wider range of physical illnesses, including hypertension, asthma, arthritis and rheumatism, back pain, diabetes, heart disease and chronic bronchitis.
- Physical illness and two or more recent adverse life events increase risk of mental illness sixfold compared to those without physical illness.
- There is a 20% rate of new onset of depression or anxiety within 1 year of diagnosis of cancer or first hospitalisation with a heart attack (Green et al., 2005).

Children and young people with emotional disorders are almost five times more likely to report self-harm and suicide attempts, four times more likely to rate themselves as being in poor health and over four times more likely to have long periods of time off school. Comorbidity of disorders is common, and children and young people with emotional behavioural problems are also more likely to have physical health problems.

Suicide

Despite determined efforts to improve mental health services, 5000 people kill themselves each year, although this is the lowest recorded suicide rate since records began and towards the lower end of rates across Europe (Chishti et al., 2003). Attempted suicide is estimated to be as high as 10 times that of suicide, causing untold distress for people themselves and their carers and relatives (Sainsbury Centre for Mental Health, 2007; Appleby and Butterworth, 2009).

History of mental health services in the UK

Providing a brief overview of the history of mental health services in the UK presents several problems. Shorter (1997) considers that mental health care has developed in a uniformly benign manner, while Jones (1991) thinks that whatever has been achieved for the mentally ill is due more to the legal system and human rights than to clinicians and institutional care. Barham and Hayward (1995) also downplay the interventions of the medical profession, and attribute improvements in the care of people with mental health problems in Britain to social and economic conditions. Scull (1999) is equally critical of psychiatrists and of their 'evangelical' commitment to a biological model of mental illness which dismisses the possibility that there might be other ways of understanding people and their problems.

Pre-asylum period

By the eighth century, in Britain as in other parts of Europe, monastic foundations provided several services for meeting the needs of people, e.g. employment, education, spiritual services and physical care (Clarke, 1975). Itinerant monks, known as 'soul friends', ministered to people with mental health problems in their own homes, providing an early form of outreach service (Hunter and Macalpine, 1974; Philo, 2004). Monastic principles of care were adopted to varying degrees down the centuries by Poor Law institutions, private madhouses, asylums, psychiatric hospitals and modern mental health services (Micale and Porter, 1994). In the mid-sixteenth century, a conflict arose between the king, Henry VIII, and the church, resulting in four fifths of the monasteries being destroyed by 1580, and with them all the services that people had come to rely on, including mental health care. Subsequent to the dissolution, people with mental disturbance had to rely on the kindness of strangers or on members of their families. Many received no assistance and joined the ranks of the destitute that wandered from town to town.

In the late seventeenth century, the need for additional provision for the insane was apparent and business entrepreneurs started to move into the field (Parry-Jones, 1971). Few owners had any medical knowledge and opened houses solely to make money, while others were outstanding. One of these was run by Dr Nathaniel Cotton, a trained doctor who suffered mental health problems himself and experienced the most heart-rending exclusion. Cotton believed that the quality of his servants (nurses) was the key to success with residents, and he took great care in appointing persons who were kind, intelligent, industrious and imaginative.

The growth of the asylum system

Without question, the most famous and influential of all the private madhouses was the York Retreat, founded in 1796 by a Quaker called William Tuke. Tuke was inspired by the wretched death in 1790 of another Quaker, Hannah Mills, a few weeks after she had been admitted to the publicly provided York Asylum. During her time in the asylum, she had been allowed no visits from friends or family, was treated worse than an animal and died alone, lying in her own filth. The York Retreat challenged commonly held beliefs that the mentally ill were akin to wild beasts and were best treated by purging, induced vomiting, bleeding, painful blistering, manacling and sudden immersion in cold baths. Tuke's approach was known as 'moral treatment', a translation of the French *traitement morale*, used to describe the work of the great French reformers Pussin and Pinel (Digby, 1985).

The York Retreat strongly influenced such reformers as Lord Shaftesbury (Digby, 1985), who wished to apply its principles within publicly funded asylums. Working with John Conolly, a doctor, who had initiated a humane regime at the Hanwell Asylum in London that was partly modeled on the Retreat, Shaftesbury persuaded the government to pass the 1845 Lunacy Act, making it compulsory for every county to make provision for the insane. Once separate provision was available, both men believed that the science of psychiatry would be able to develop and that people with mental health conditions would be able to receive the same standard of treatment and care as those suffering from physical conditions.

The asylum period

The 1845 act initiated a building programme which led to approximately 100 asylums being established over the next 50 years, accommodating between 200 and 1000 persons each. Individual counties took pride in their asylums; some sought out the most renowned architects of the day and the most accomplished landscape gardeners, and the magnificence of some of these buildings prompted one commentator to remark, 'In France, they house their royalty in such buildings, but in England, they are where lunatics reside' (Porter, 1987). Asylums were generally located in the midst of good farming land because keeping residents active and enabling the asylums to be self-sufficient were cornerstones of the new system. Each asylum was managed by an asylum board made up of local people, the majority of whom were either from the landowning or professional classes. It was left to medical superintendents to oversee all that took place in the institution. Few superintendents had any specific training in the management of mentally ill people, and asylum medicine was not highly respected.

At the turn of the twentieth century, psychiatry had no firm scientific basis and was unclear about what it could actually achieve. There were competing models of mental illness: the biological, psychological and social (Pressman,

1998). Superintendents who tried to develop better medical practices embraced a range of interventions with a physical basis, such as deep insulin therapy, malarial therapy, leucotomies and various forms of psychosurgery. Although therapeutic optimism prevailed, few if any successful treatments were recorded.

The First World War and its aftermath had important consequences for mental health services in England. This period saw a rapid increase in the number of patients, a reduction in the number of staff and, due to the economic recession, many of the recommendations suggested for the improvement of mental hospitals were never carried out. An important event was the passing of the Mental Treatment Act (1930), which recognised mental health care in England as a branch of medicine. Asylums were now referred to as 'psychiatric hospitals' and designated not only as places for treating patients but also for training doctors and nurses. By 1955, there were around 150000 patients in institutions built to house 85000, a situation that required urgent attention.

Few asylum doctors had any specific training throughout the late nineteenth and early twentieth centuries, but that did not prevent them from criticising the level of education and functioning of the nurses and the attendants, which led to two outcomes. First, superintendents stated that they would assume responsibility for improving the standards of care within the institutions, and secondly, as a means of achieving this, they would initiate a system of training for the asylum nurses comparable to that devised by Florence Nightingale at St Thomas's Hospital in London.

The development of the psychiatric profession

After 1800, the term widely used to refer to the new breed of doctors who specialised in mental illness was 'alienists', a curious term derived from the belief that 'lunatics' were influenced by the moon just as the seas and tides were. Therefore, those who cared for them became known as alienists. In 1841, Dr Samuel Hitch, Superintendent of the Gloucester Lunatic Asylum, decided to form the Association of Medical Officers of Asylums and Hospitals for the Insane. This association soon changed its name to the Medico-Psychological Association (MPA) just as the term 'psychiatry' started to be used by asylum doctors. In 1853, the MPA published the *Asylum Journal*, which in 1858 became the *Journal of Mental Science*. In 1926, the MPA became the Royal Medico-Psychological Association (RMPA) and in 1971, the Royal College of Psychiatrists was founded and its journal became the *British Journal of Psychiatry*.

Prior to the establishment of the NHS in 1948, psychiatrists tended to be generalists. This situation changed during the second half of the century when many psychiatrists took on specialist roles in child and adolescent psychiatry, eating disorders and forensic care. Revill (2003) argues that the current number of psychiatrists is inadequate to meet the level of need there, and some are leaving the profession because of pressure of work, bureaucracy and the growing culture of litigation and blame. Several posts, she contends, remain unfilled and around one consultant in three plans to retire early, putting even more pressure on those left behind. Gee (2007) points to three main problems that prevail within psychiatry:

- declining popularity as a career
- over-reliance on overseas graduates
- unacceptable variation in quality.

The origins of mental health nursing

Towards the end of 1885, two significant events took place which sought to improve the quality of care within institutions. Both were based on the assumption that the introduction of training schemes could rectify any deficits that had arisen within the institutions. First was the introduction of a diploma course in mental disorders for asylum doctors, and second was the publication of what became known as the 'red handbook', entitled *The Handbook for the Instruction of Attendants on the Insane*. The text was divided into five sections dealing with the body, its general functions and disorders, the nursing of the sick, the mind and its disorders, the care of the insane and the general duties of the attendants. This book formed the national curriculum for the training of asylum nurses, and the first successful candidates qualified in 1891.

Florence Nightingale was stridently opposed to this approach to improving the care of patients by training staff. Asylum nurses, she held, were not real nurses because they were poorly educated, had little sensitivity and were largely unemployable. Furthermore, she asserted that asylums were not hospitals and that asylum doctors that taught the nurses were not real doctors. If asylum nurses needed training, then they would have to be taught by general nurse tutors, work in general hospitals and subject themselves to rigorous examinations by general nurses. This difference of opinion between asylum doctors and general nurses resulted in two schemes being devised for the training of psychiatric nurses: one was run by the Medical Psychological Association (MPA), leading to the qualification of MPA, and the other, which started in 1923, was delivered under the direction of the General Nursing Council (GNC) and conferred the title registered mental nurse (RMN). They both ran alongside each other until the introduction of the NHS in 1948, when the training of all nurses became the responsibility of the GNC.

The two schemes varied in form and content. The MPA scheme focused specifically on the management of patients and the running of the institution, whereas the GNC course was more preoccupied with the care and treatment of patients and laid emphasis on such issues as hygiene, nutrition, wound care and infection control. Nolan (1993) described the people who came forward to become psychiatric nurses in the 1920s and 1930s as males who had spent some time in the forces or farming work, while the females tended to have worked in domestic service. The job was seen as secure, as it provided a uniform, food, excellent sporting facilities, accommodation and a social life. All asylums had at least two wards where those with physical illnesses were cared for, i.e. those with highly infectious diseases, such as tuberculosis, venereal diseases and *Streptococcus* skin infections.

Immediately after the Second World War, three significant developments took place which strengthened the position of psychiatric nurses. First, the use of general nurse tutors in psychiatric hospitals was phased out and they were replaced by psychiatric nurse tutors. Gradually, the role of the psychiatric nurse began to shift from that of managing an organisation and controlling violent patients to that of caring for individuals. More discussion was beginning to take place about *nursing skills* as opposed to *nursing work*. Eysenck (1952) was one of the first to ask nurses to confront what they were doing. He stated that recovery rates among psychiatric patients were unrelated to anything doctors did or to any treatments they prescribed. Nurses were further challenged by the introduction of a new drug in 1952, Largactil. It met with some success, and many previously withdrawn and uncommunicative patients responded by being able to converse, talk about their pasts and take an interest in life around them. The downside, however, was that many also developed side effects, particularly disorders of gait, or the 'Largactil shuffle', as it became known. This caused consternation in the minds of some nurses who felt that whereas before they were being asked to care for people who were mentally ill, now their job was to care for people whose problems were brought about by the treatment they were given.

The third development was the publication of the Salmon Report (Department of Health, 1966), which suggested that nurses should play a much greater part in providing clinical supervision, management of personnel and the transforming of the face of nursing. Thenceforth, nurses ceased to be managed by doctors and were to be no longer seen as adjuncts to doctors, but collaborators in the provision of mental health services.

Deinstitutionalisation

The search for another model of mental health care was formally stated in the policy document *Better Services for the Mentally Ill* (Department of Health, 1975), which stated that admission to a psychiatric hospital had to be a last resort. Despite some innovations, deinstitutionalisation had now become an urgent priority. However, the origins of deinstitutionalisation had begun some years before, with the work of social psychiatrists Rudolf Freudenberg at Netherne Hospital in Surrey and Duncan Macmillan at Mapperly Hospital in Cambridgeshire (Clark, 1996). They found that active rehabilitation coupled with improved patient management brought about reduced hospital stays, a reduction in bed occupancy and closer relationships between patients and their families. This initiative further reduced the number of psychiatric beds while emphasising the importance of integrating physical and mental health.

Preparation by nurses for the new approach to mental health care can be detected within their training schemes. By the mid-1970s, most training courses included psychology, sociology and the theory and practice of community-based interventions. A short experimental course aimed to prepare psychiatric nurses to work in the community was initiated in London in 1970 and became the only formal means by which psychiatric nurses could prepare for the role of community psychiatric nurse (CPN) (White, 2000). Throughout the 1970s and 1980s, courses were developed for nurses on behavioural therapy, family systemic therapy, cognitive behavioural therapy and dynamic therapy, and some nurses began to assume the title of *therapist* or *nurse therapist*. Following a national review of psychiatric nursing in England in 1993, the term *mental health nurse* emerged to represent the ideal that nurses were endeavouring to assist clients to regain mental *health* rather than merely assisting in the treatment of psychiatric *illness*.

White (2000) considered that the move to community-based care caused 'a crisis of occupational identity' for mental health nursing and left it threatened by encroachment from other professions, particularly social workers and psychological therapists. Certainly in community settings, a whole variety of different professions do 'jostle for space, attention and independence' (Coppock and Hopton, 2000). Significantly, many early CPNs were individuals disaffected with the dominance of psychiatrists within hospitals and research suggested that these general developments, together with changes in management arrangements and nurse education, allowed claims to be made that by the 1980s nurses were no longer 'the minions of doctors' (Brimblecombe, 2005). Nurses were instrumental in retreating from becoming too involved in primary care and instead began to refocus their efforts on preventing the severely mentally ill from relapsing and being readmitted.

Attitudes to mental health problems

The Department of Health carried out a national survey of attitudes towards mental illness in 1999, which was repeated in 2009 (Department of Health, 2009a). The overall conclusion was that: 'People are broadly sympathetic towards people with a mental illness'.

However, when comparing the two studies, it was apparent that in some respects, attitudes towards people with mental illness were worse in 2009 although there were some clear improvements:

- There was a clear indication of increasing tolerance on the part of the general public towards people with mental health problems.
- It was strongly felt that integrating people with mental illness into the community was a positive strategy.
- People with mental health problems were considered to be entitled to the same rights to a job as everyone else.
- Responses indicated that those with mental health problems could do more to help themselves.
- Respondents were not in agreement with spending more money on new services.

The changing position of service users

Between the two world wars, such terms as 'asylum', 'mad' and 'lunatic' were replaced by such terms as *psychiatric hospital*, the *mentally ill* or psychiatric *patients*. This reflected the growth of medical influence and the medicalisation of institutional practices. Towards the end of the Second World War, under the influence of Carl Rogers, many psychologists and psychiatrists who aspired to be psychotherapists began to use the term *client* to refer to those whom they treated (Masson, 1990). Rogers had changed *patient* to *client* on the grounds that the people whom he saw chose to visit him, without coercion, and most paid a fee. During the 1980s, the new term *service user* emerged in England, stemming from the service user movements in the US and Australia, which focused on the experience of people using mental health services and embodied the belief that service users could recover and assist each other in the recovery process. Today all mental health providers are charged by the external regulator, the Care Quality Commission, and through contracts with commissioners of services, with gathering 'service user feedback' (see below) and need to be able to indicate how this is used to improve services.

Current mental health care

In 1999, the *National Service Framework for Mental Health* (NSF), a 10-year programme, laid out standards for mental health services in England (Department of Health, 1999). Services were to focus heavily on ensuring that people with severe mental health problems had their needs met and that care should be provided in community rather than hospital settings whenever possible. Standards in the NSF focused on:

i) mental health promotion and overcoming discrimination and social exclusion associated with mental health problems

ii) access to services in primary care for people with mental health problems

iii) effective services for people with severe mental illness
iv) the welfare of carers of people with mental health problems
v) taking action to reduce suicides.

The NSF led to the development of specialist multidisciplinary community services across the country, which have considerably reduced the amount of admissions, including:

- *Community mental health teams:* Community mental health teams typically manage people with long-term, serious and enduring mental health problems. They can provide medication and a range of psychological and social services.
- *Crisis/home treatment teams:* Government policy emphasises that people with mental health problems should be cared for in their own homes. In the event of a crisis, specialist teams provide rapid assessment and can provide intensive care at home as an alternative to hospital admission.
- *Early intervention teams:* These teams aim to detect and treat psychosis as early as possible, with the aim of reducing the number and severity of relapses. Their work is especially directed towards young people.
- *Assertive outreach teams:* These teams work with an identified client group of severely mentally ill adults who do not effectively engage with mental health services. Assertive outreach staff expect to see their clients frequently and to stay in contact, however difficult that may be.

Arguably, such government policies are beginning to change the ethos of mental health care in England and the biomedically based psychiatry of the asylums is being replaced by social psychiatry which is most concerned about the disadvantages of social exclusion (Bracken and Thomas, 2001). A counterview is that the control of psychiatry over people's lives has been extended (from beyond the hospital wards to the community) and that biomedicine has really only changed enough to become more acceptable, but essentially remains unable to respond to people's real needs (Barker, 2003). Micale and Lerner (2001) suggest that even though English psychiatry showed signs of 'beginning to awake from its lethargy' in the twentieth century, it still lacks the cognitive and professional unity enjoyed by general medicine and remains torn between ideological models, therapeutic strategies and organisational theories.

Common treatments

Medication remains a primary intervention for most people receiving mental health services. For example, 95% of working-age inpatients receive psychotropic medication as a part of their treatment (Care Quality Commission, 2009). The National Institute for Health and Clinical Excellence (NICE, 2002), an organisation that sets national and quality standards and seeks to improve people's health and prevent and treat ill health, has increasingly emphasised the potential contribution of psychological interventions for a wide range of conditions. However, it is acknowledged that many services struggle to have sufficient staff able to provide such interventions. The use of electroconvulsive therapy has reduced over past years as national guidance has become more specific and limiting about the range of conditions for which it should be utilised (NICE, 2003).

Quality monitoring and effectiveness of mental health services

England, in common with the rest of the UK, has always had in place systems of monitoring, regulatory agencies and a means of evaluating the quality of mental health services. Many of these regulatory agencies have recently been subsumed into the Care Quality Commission (CQC), which regulates health and adult social care services, whether provided by the NHS, local authorities, private companies or voluntary organisations. Providers of mental health services are required to provide evidence to the CQC that they are compliant with standards relating to diverse issues including patient safety, medication management, meeting physical health care needs, providing suitable support and training for staff, and infection control. Although monitoring is seen as important, Salzer *et al.* (1997) noted that many of the processes and instruments used in monitoring mental health services were poorly designed and unsystematically administered and that few were ever validated. Goldman *et al.* (2009) identified some of the problems associated with poor practice as diagnostic/formulation errors, communication problems, system-based problems and class/culture misunderstandings. Any one of these could result in poor quality care, but when all four were present, care was inevitably of a very low calibre.

In judging the success of the shift from institution-based care to that based in community settings, Leff and Trieman (2000) found that although there was little improvement in clinical state or social functioning, patients did acquire domestic and community living skills. They also acquired friends and enjoyed more freedom in their lives than when they were in hospital. The majority wanted to remain at home. The study concluded that more mental health nurses and psychiatrists should be allocated to community services because:

- people prefer being treated at home, rather than in hospital
- community care reduces the number of suicides
- patients feel that medication management and treatment are better under community care than in hospital.

Service users' experience of services
. . . .

Annual national surveys have taken place for several years of those receiving community services, and in 2009 the first survey took place of inpatient services. This process is seen as key to improving quality by many, although inevitably there are complaints from services that the surveys are not representative (being based on relatively small samples compared to the large numbers receiving services overall).

A recent study of inpatients in 212 NHS and independent sector facilities in England and Wales found that 19% were from black and ethnic minority groups (National Institute for Mental Health in England, 2005). This study found that not only were people from several black and ethnic minority groups disproportion-ately represented in the inpatient population but also that they had longer periods of seclusion once detained. The association between mental health problems and ethnicity has been recognised for some time and would seem to be at least partly related to disadvantage in housing, education, employment and social isolation, which are correlated with mental health problems (Department of Health, 2003).

Staffing

There have been significant increased numbers of clinical staff employed within the NHS in the 10 years since the recommendations of the *National Service Framework for Mental Health* were introduced. There have been 10 000 more nurses, 55% more consultants and 69% more psychologists. There are now 10 451 medical staff in the psychiatry group, of whom 5179 are consultants, 3175 under-taking various training and 998 either retired or working part-time. That means that there are approximately 12.7 psychiatrists per 100 000 of the population, higher than the European average of 8.9, but lower than in some countries such as France and Sweden. Nurse staffing levels in English mental health settings are also higher than average, with 51.9 nurses per 100 000 people, as opposed to the European average of 18.7 (WHO, 2008).

Hospital-based services

Although the numbers of inpatient admissions have reduced slowly over the last few years, this remains a core part of statutory mental health services. The major-ity of wards for working-age adults are defined as 'acute admission wards'. Bed numbers vary in size from low teens to high twenties and are typically found in:
 i) *Adapted Victorian institutions:* Although the number of such wards used to be the majority, they have significantly reduced in the last few years. In some areas, most of the wards on Victorian sites have been replaced with more modern buildings and merge with category iii below.
 ii) *Psychiatric units based on general hospital sites:* This model was popular in the

1960s and 1970s, and significant numbers continue. Problems associated with such wards are lack of outdoor space (being on a busy general hospital site), and wards that are not on the ground floor exacerbate this and add a degree of risk. More generally, tensions can exist between general hospital staff and psychiatric units with anxieties about the potential behaviour of psychiatric patients sometimes leading to restrictive rules.

iii) *Specialist psychiatric facilities:* The size of such facilities can vary from 'psychiatric hospitals with a significant number of wards' to single 'stand alone' units. Isolated units have the advantages of typically being based in the locality of the populations they serve, but have challenges in having sufficient staff to cope with emergencies, which can make them either expensive to run or risky.

Standards of care in inpatient settings have received much criticism in the past few years (Quirk and Lelliott, 2002; Priebe and Turner, 2003), with issues such as low staffing, poor environments, threatening atmosphere and problems of underoccupation and boredom being cited. The Department of Health (2002) has produced guidance, but recent surveys of inpatient service users' views suggest that standards remain highly variable across England (see above).

Mental health law

Historically, distinguishing normality from insanity, and criminality from insanity, has never been thought to require medical expertise. Lawyers relied on friends and family to testify in court. The insanity plea became controversial in England in 1843, when the trial of Daniel McNaghten for the murder of the prime minister's private secretary was stopped on the grounds of insanity (Porter, 2002). During the court hearing, it became apparent that McNaghten could not follow the trial proceedings; he was incoherent when questions were put to him. Almost immediately, the McNaghten Rules were formulated, which became the basis of modern British law and are as follows:

● Was the nature of the offence serious?
● Did the perpetrator intend to commit a crime?
● Was the perpetrator aware at the time of the crime of its seriousness?

Current mental health legislation in England also exists in the context of racial legislation, civil liberties and human rights. Since the Enlightenment, the protection and freedom of the individual has been central to British justice. The main purpose of the legislation is to ensure that people with serious mental disorders which threaten either their own health and safety or the safety of the public can be treated irrespective of their consent. The Mental Health Act of 1983 was amended in 1987 and governs the formal detention and care of mentally disordered people in hospital. The 2007 MHA also governs care of some people in the community with community treatment orders (CTOs), a new development which was extremely controversial in the passage of the act through Parliament, as to how this was going to be implemented.

When detaining a person in hospital, appropriate treatment must be available on site and to the patient. Detention requires the agreement of an approved mental health professional, most of whom are social workers, although the role is now open to other professionals, two doctors, one of whom must be a psychiatrist, and the patient's nearest relative. The right of the nearest relative to block admission can be legally removed if he or she is not seen as acting in the patient's best interests. In the first instance, detention can be for up to 6 months, but this period can be extended. The overall care of the patient falls to the responsible clinician, who used to have to be a senior psychiatrist, but recent changes in the law have opened up this role to other senior professionals.

The act defines mental disorder as 'any disorder or disability of mind'. Drug and alcohol dependence are not considered mental disorders in themselves. Inpatients who are not detained are described as 'informal' patients, but can be detained for up to 72 hours by a doctor, or for up to 6 hours by a nurse, if the patient wishes to leave but the professionals involved think they should be detained until a full assessment can be carried out. Mental health law also allows a police officer the power to remove someone who appears to be suffering from a mental health disorder in a public place (not, for example, in a person's own home) to a place of safety. In the past, in many areas, this place would be a police station, but increasingly this is now most frequently a mental health unit. This is to allow a full assessment to take place under the Mental Health Act. The following people/roles can discharge someone from a section of the MHA:

- the responsible clinician (the professional in overall charge of the detained patient's care)
- the patient's nearest relative (although the responsible clinician has the power to block this)
- a mental health tribunal (an independent panel from an external national body)
- hospital managers.

Current role of nursing in mental health care

Mental health nurses (MHNs) are found in virtually every service area in mental health. This includes inpatient care for adolescents, adults and older people, in community teams for all age groups and in the whole range of specialist teams, such as crisis/home treatment, drug and alcohol, assertive outreach. In many areas, such as in inpatient settings, they form the bulk of the workforce, but they are also found working in speciality areas such as psychotherapy services, where their primary skill would be a specialist one, but they would still retain nursing registration.

Recently a Department of Health-led national review of mental health nursing took place (Department of Health, 2006). The review emphasised the importance of mental health nurses providing 'holistic' care, i.e. that which took into account the psychological, social, physical and spiritual needs of service users. The review supported the continued development of new roles for nurses, particularly those which had previously been the exclusive domain of other professions in the past, for example, prescribing and carrying out various functions under mental health law.

Service users' views of mental health nursing

Gray *et al.* (2006) undertook a literature review of how service users viewed mental health nursing. Their conclusion was that mental health nursing was seen as a multifaceted role that requires both human qualities and specific clinical skills and that mental health nurses were expected to deliver both practical and social support alongside clinical skills and more formal psychological therapies. Relationships between service users and mental health nurses working in community settings generally appeared to be good. In national surveys of the views of service users for the 5 years between 2004 and 2008 inclusive, consistent scores of 80%–81% of those surveyed stated that nurses 'definitely listened carefully to me', with only 3%–4% saying that they did not do so (Care Quality Commission, 2011). However, the picture in acute inpatient care settings is different and more varied, with only 48% of service users stating that nurses always listened carefully to them, 40% stating that they did so sometimes and 12% saying they did not listen carefully most of the time (MIND, 2008; McGeorge and Lelliott, 2006).

Effectiveness of mental health nursing

Gray *et al.* (2006) examined the evidence from 52 randomised controlled trials (mostly based in the UK), where mental health nurses delivered specific clinical intervention. They found that the interventions delivered by mental health nurses had, broadly speaking, a positive effect. Overall, a meta-analysis of the randomised controlled trials demonstrated that nurses made a positive difference clinically. It should be noted that those controlled trials covered only a very narrow aspect of the day-to-day work of mental health nurses.

Relationships with other professions

It is important to understand that historically both nursing and psychiatry have been closely linked. Even when most of psychiatry's formal management responsibility for nursing came to an end, implicit influence over many nursing activities was slow to fade (Brimblecombe, 2005). However, the steady growth of more independent nursing roles outside the hospital setting, the increase in more specialist and senior roles (such as nurse consultants and nurse practitioners) and acquisition of advanced skills (such as psychosocial interventions) has supported the profession in belatedly asserting its independence.

Many MHNs want their profession to become more confident and autonomous, and also to have improved relationships with other professions (Gowodo and Nolan, 2008). Yet recently, mental health nursing has had to challenge threats to its survival as a separate and distinct branch of nursing from its own nursing regulatory body, the Nursing and Midwifery Council. The outcome, following much vigorous lobbying by mental health nurses, was a continued commitment to having separate branches, rather than follow the model of generic nursing as the basic qualification for all areas of practice, as followed in most of the rest of Europe.

Future plans for mental health care

Following the completion of the 10-year plan emerging from the *Mental Health National Service Framework*, the new coalition government has recently released a new strategy – *No Health Without Mental Health: a cross-government mental health outcomes strategy for people of all ages* (HM Government, 2011). There are six main aims:

 i) More people will have good mental health – particularly focusing on strengthening the mental health of young people.
 ii) More people with mental health problems will recover – focusing on improving social inclusion for people with mental health problems, through education, employment and generally strengthening social relationships.
 iii) More people with mental health problems will have good physical health – responding to the evidence of increased morbidity in people with severe mental health problems.
 iv) More people will have a positive experience of care and support – building on previous work done on improving services, providing evidence-based care and ensuring that they are provided in the least restrictive environment.
 v) Fewer people will suffer avoidable harm – ensuring that services are provided in a safe way.

vi) Fewer people will experience stigma and discrimination – negative public attitudes towards mental health will improve.

This strategy document has a number of significant changes from the earlier NSF, not least in that it has no prescriptive emphasis on particular service models. Rather there is a focus on measuring outcomes as opposed to inputs. One criticism of the new strategy approach is that, unlike the earlier NSF, there are no targets that mental health providers and commissioners will be penalised for failing to meet, the argument being that providers should be held accountable primarily for the outcomes of individuals receiving services.

A further important and recently developed strategy, *Living Well with Dementia: a national dementia strategy*, arose from the need to develop and strengthen services for people with dementia, to respond to estimates of massively increased need over the next 50 years (Department of Health, 2009). This strategy focuses on a wide range of activities in both health and social care, including:

- improving access to early diagnosis
- improving support for carers
- utilising technology to improve independence and safety
- improving knowledge and training of health care professionals.

Conclusions

In many ways, England has mental health services that can be seen as exemplary, at least when compared to others. The proportion of health spend that goes to mental health is one of the highest in Europe. Large isolated institutions are rare. There are relatively high numbers of mental health professionals and a range of community services providing input for both those with short-term crises and those with longer-term needs. There has recently been a considerable expansion in the availability of psychological treatments for those with common mental disorders. The level of monitoring of the quality of services is also extensive, compared to most countries in Europe. However, few in England would claim that services are yet uniformly excellent, nor do they meet the whole range of needs of people with mental health problems. There are still challenges from some quarters that the focus of care remains too heavily on the removal of symptoms rather than helping to meet the social inclusion needs of people. Medication is still frequently the main form of treatment, despite guidelines increasingly emphasising the value of psychological interventions. Inpatient care remains problematic in terms of often providing an unsatisfactory experience for service users. People with mental health problems still occasionally kill others, and, more frequently, kill themselves. While many of these issues can be addressed to a degree, it is unclear what a realistic expectation of mental health services actually should be in a world with finite resources and working in a field inevitably filled with risks.

Case scenario

A 23-year-old unemployed man is reported by his landlord as acting increasingly strangely. He has barricaded his room, talking about being spied upon by the CIA. He can be heard shouting within his room in an angry and incoherent way. He has not been seen by a psychiatrist in the past, although his mother has told the landlord that he has been isolating himself and acting increasingly oddly over the last couple of years.

In this scenario, there is little factual information on which to make a clinical decision. Whilst people involved may presuppose that this behaviour denotes a mental illness, there could be other explanations, e.g. an abusive landlord whose sole intent is to increase the rent or a mother who refuses to have him live in her home. In the UK, it would be likely that the man's general practitioner would be contacted if it was known who this was. The GP might try and visit if he or she knew the man. In a situation such as this, the police might also be called if he was seen as being at risk or threatening. If attempts to speak to the man did not gather enough information to reassure the police or GP, then it is likely that an assessment might be carried out under mental health law. This process would be led by an approved mental health professional (normally a social worker). Once contact is made, an assessment will determine what the nature of the problem is. Does it relate to a major mental health problem? If yes, then what level of risk exists, e.g. is the person safe to leave? A range of actions are then available, for example, arranging for one of the community services, such as a crisis and home treatment team (CRHT) to come back and visit again and provide treatment and continued assessment at home. If the person proves to be ill, and a risk to himself or others, and declines to be treated at home or this cannot be done safely, then he may have to be compulsorily admitted to acute inpatient services, with police help if necessary.

If treated at home by a crisis home treatment team, then he could receive visits several times a day. Typical interventions would be continued monitoring of his mental state and any risk, ensuring that his personal care needs, such as eating, were being met, providing support to him and possibly others around him and, if he were diagnosed with a psychotic disorder then he would receive medication, which potentially the CRHT could bring with them on each visit. A CRHT would typically work with someone for a few weeks until he was well enough to be seen less frequently by other services, such as community mental health teams.

If admitted to hospital, there would be further assessments carried out by nursing and medical staff. The care would be under the leadership of a consultant psychiatrist (although other professions can potentially take this role on, but this is rare as yet). The type of treatment given would be similar to that provided by the CRHT. For example, the nursing staff would be expected to monitor the patient's mental state and his response to medication but also provide individual one-to-one sessions. Typically, such sessions would include supportive counselling, but some nurses have basic training in other interventions such as brief solution-focused therapy or cognitive behaviour therapy. Additionally on an inpatient ward, structured activities would be provided, normally in group sessions, and these would commonly be led by occupational therapists or sometimes support workers. The activities provide entertainment in what can be a boring experience on a ward, but also can provide distraction from disturbing thoughts and a means to assess the concentration and skills of individual patients. The other feature of admission to a ward would be the ability of staff to provide very close observation over 24 hours, including one-to-one 'specialing' if risk factors suggested this.

As the man's condition improves, he is likely to be given time off the ward, initially escorted but eventually on his own. Links with community services would be made (normally provided from the same organisation as runs the ward) and a community key worker identified. This person (normally a mental health nurse or social worker) would coordinate follow-up care following discharge form hospital.

Whether treated by a CRHT or on a ward, a formal process for planning future care (the care programme approach) would provide a structure for a full assessment of future need, and should include physical health care and social needs, e.g. housing and employment, although dependent on the area, such things can be slow to find. The man would also see a doctor periodically to have his medication reviewed after discharge (although increasingly, specifically trained nurses are also able to review medication).

References

Appleby L, Butterworth T. Fifty years of endeavour, prevention and health in mental health policy. *J Res Nurs.* 2009; **14**: 489–92.

Barham P, Hayward R. *Relocating Madness.* London: Free Association Books; 1995.

Barker P, editor. *Psychiatric and Mental Health Nursing: the craft of caring.* London: Arnold; 2003.

Bracken P, Thomas P. Post-psychiatry: a new direction for mental health. *BMJ.* 2001; **322**: 724–7.

Brewer M, Muriel A, Phillips D, *et al. Poverty and Inequality in the UK.* London: The Institute for Fiscal Studies; 2008.

Brimblecombe N. The changing relationship between mental health nurses and psychiatrists in the United Kingdom. *J Adv Nurs.* 2005; **49**(4): 344–53.

Care Quality Commission. Community Mental Health Survey 2011. Available at: www.cqc.org.uk/

public/reports-surveys-and-reviews/surveys/community-mental-health-survey-2011 (accessed 20 February 2012).

Chishti DH, Stone P, Corcoran E, *et al.* Suicide mortality in the European Union. *Eur J Public Health.* 2003; **13**: 108–14.

Clark D. *The Story of a Mental Hospital: Fulbourn 1858–1983.* London: Process Press; 1996.

Clarke B. *Mental Disorder in Early Britain.* Cardiff: University of Wales Press; 1975.

Coppock V, Hopton J. *Critical Perspectives on Mental Health.* London: Routledge; 2000.

Department of Health. *The Report of the Committee on Senior Nurse Staffing Structure* (The Salmon Report). London: Her Majesty's Stationery Office; 1966.

Department of Health. *Better Services for the Mentally Ill.* Cmnd. 6233. London: Her Majesty's Stationery Office; 1975.

Department of Health. *Mental Health Nursing: addressing acute concerns.* Report by the Standing Nursing and Midwifery Advisory Committee, London: The Stationery Office; 1999.

Department of Health. *National Service Framework for Mental Health: modern standards and service models.* London: Department of Health; 1999a.

Department of Health. *Mental Health Policy Implementation Guide: adult acute inpatient care provision.* London: The Stationery Office; 2002.

Department of Health. *Mental Health Policy Implementation Guide: national minimum standards for general adult services in psychiatric intensive care units (picu) and low secure environments.* London: The Stationery Office; 2003.

Department of Health. *Personality Disorder: no longer a diagnosis of exclusion – policy implementation guidance for the development of services for people with personality disorder.* London: Department of Health; 2003.

Department of Health. *From Values to Actions: the chief nursing officer's review of mental health nursing.* London: Department of Health; 2006.

Department of Health. *Attitudes to Mental Illness 2009 Research Report.* 2009a. Available at: www.dh.gov.uk/en/Publicationsandstatistics/Publications/PublicationsStatistics/DH_100345 (accessed 20 December 2009).

Department of Health. *Living Well with Dementia: a national dementia strategy.* London: Department of Health; 2009b.

Digby A. *Madness, Morality and Medicine: a study of the York Retreat 1796–1914.* Cambridge: Cambridge University Press; 1985.

Eysenck J. The effects of psychotherapy: an evaluation. *J Consult Psychol.* 1952; **16**: 319–24.

Fazel S, Danesh J. Serious mental health disorder in 23,000 prisoners: a systematic review of 62 surveys. *Lancet.* 2009; **359**: 545–50.

Gee M. New Ways of Working threatens the future of the psychiatric profession. *The Psychiatrist.* 2007; **31**: 315.

Goldman M, David R, Demaso M, *et al.* Psychiatry morbidity and mortality rounds: implementation and impact. *Acad Psychiatry.* 2009; **33**: 383–8.

Gowodo F, Nolan P. Taking stock. *Ment Health Pract.* 2008; **12**(4): 24–8.

Gray R, Barnes P, Bee P, *et al. Mental Health Nursing: literature review synthesis and recommendations.* 2006. Available at: www.nursing.manchester.ac.uk/projects/mentalhealthreview/reviewsynthesisandrecommendations.pdf (accessed 15 April 2011).

Green H, McGinnity A, Meltzer H, *et al. Mental Health in Children and Young People in Great Britain.* London: National Office of Statistics; 2005.

HM Government. *The Case for Change: why England needs a new care and support system.* 2008. Available at: www.dh.gov.uk/en/Publicationsandstatistics/Publications/Publications PolicyAndGuidance/DH_084725 (accessed 5 April 2011).

HM Government. *No Health without Mental Health: a cross-government mental health outcomes strategy for people of all ages.* 2011. Available at: www.dh.gov.uk/prod_consum_dh/groups/dh_digitalassets/documents/digitalasset/dh_124058.pdf (accessed 8 April 2011).

Howarth J, Lees J, Sidebotham P, *et al. Religion, Belief and Parenting Practices.* London: Joseph Rowntree Foundation; 2008.

Hunter R, Macalpine I. *Psychiatry for the Poor: 1851 Colney Hatch Asylum-Friern Hospital.* London: Dawsons of Pall Mall; 1974.

Information Centre for Health and Social Care. *Statistics on Alcohol, England 2010.* 2011a. Available at: www.ic.nhs.uk/pubs/alcohol10 (accessed 7 April 2011).

Information Centre for Health and Social Care. *Statistics on Obesity, Physical Activity and Diet: England, 2011.* 2011b. Available at: www.ic.nhs.uk/statistics-and-data-collections/health-and-lifestyles/obesity (accessed 7 April 2011).

International Monetary Fund. *World Economic Outlook Database: October 2009.* 2009. Available at: www.imf.org/external/pubs/ft/weo/2009/02/weodata/index.aspx (accessed 1 October 2009).

Jones K. The culture of the mental hospital. In: Berrios GE, Freeman H, editors. *150 Years of British Psychiatry 1841–1991.* London: Gaskell; 1991.

Leff J, Trieman N. Long-stay patients discharged from psychiatric hospitals: social and clinical outcomes after five years in the community. The TAPS Project 46. *Br J Psychiatry.* 2000; **176**: 217–23.

McCrone P, Dhanasiri S, Patel A, *et al. Paying the Cost of Mental Health Care in England to 2006.* London: King's Fund; 2008.

McGeorge M, Lelliott P. The national audit of violence: in-patient care for adults of working age. *The Psychiatrist.* 2006; **30**: 444–6.

Masson J. *Against Therapy.* London: Harper Collins; 1990.

Mental Health Network. *Key Facts and Trends in Mental Health.* London: The NHS Confederation; 2009.

Micale M, Lerner P. *Traumatic Pasts: histories, psychiatry and trauma in the modern age, 1870–1930.* Cambridge: Cambridge University Press; 2001.

Micale M, Porter R, editors. *Discovering the History of Psychiatry.* Oxford: Oxford University Press; 1994.

MIND. *The Statistical Aspects of Mental Health Problems. Fact Sheet 5.* London: MIND; 2008.

National Institute for Health and Clinical Excellence. *The Economic Effectiveness and Cost Effectiveness of the Newer Atypical Anti-psychotic Drugs for Schizophrenia: Technology Appraisal 43.* London: NIHCE; 2002.

National Institute for Health and Clinical Excellence. *Electroconvulsive Therapy (ECT): Technology Appraisal 59.* London: NIHCE; 2003. Available at: http://guidance.nice.org.uk/TA59/Guidance/pdf/English (accessed 25 December 2009).

National Institute for Mental Health in England. *Count Me In: result of a national census of inpatients in mental hospitals and facilities in England and Wales.* London: National Institute for Mental Health in England; 2005.

National Mental Health Developmental Unit. *Factfile 2: mental health and housing.* London: National Mental Health Developmental Unit; 2010a.

National Mental Health Developmental Unit. *Factfile 3: the cost of mental ill health.* London: National Mental Health Developmental Unit; 2010b.

National Mental Health Developmental Unit. *Factfile 5: equalities in mental health.* London: National Mental Health Developmental Unit; 2010c.

National Mental Health Developmental Unit. *Factfile 6: Stigma and discrimination in mental health.* London: National Mental Health Developmental Unit; 2010d.

National Statistics. *Mortality Statistics Cause.* London: Office for National Statistics; 2006.

NHS Information Centre. *Adult Psychiatric Morbidity in England, 2007: results of a household survey.* 2009. Available at: www.ic.nhs.uk/pubs/psychiatricmorbidity07 (accessed 22 December 2011.

Nolan P. *A History of Mental Health Nursing.* Cheltenham: Stanley Thornes; 1993.

Office for National Statistics. *Social Trends no. 39.* Basingstoke: Palgrave Macmillan; 2009.

Office of National Statistics. *Social Trends no. 40.* Basingstoke; Palgrave Macmillan; 2010.

Parry-Jones WL. *The Trade in Lunacy: a study of private madhouses in England in the 18th and 19th centuries.* London: Routledge and K Paul; 1971.

Philo C. *A Geographical History of Institutional Provision for the Insane from Mediveal Times to the 1860s in England and Wales.* Lampeter: The Edwin Mellen Press; 2004.

Porter R. *A Social History of Madness: stories of the insane.* London: Weidenfeld and Nicolson; 1987.

Porter R. *The Greatest Benefit to Mankind: a medical history of humanity from antiquity to the present.* London: HarperCollins; 1997.

Porter R. *Madness: a brief history.* Oxford: Oxford University Press; 2002.

Pressman J. *Last Resort: psychosurgery and the limits of medicine.* Cambridge: Cambridge University Press; 1998.

Priebe S, Turner T. Deinstitutionalisation in mental health care: this largely unnoticed process requires further debate and evaluation. *BMJ.* 2003; **326**: 175–6.

Quirk A, Lelliott P. Acute wards: problems and solutions – a participant observation study of life on an acute psychiatric ward. *Psychiatr Bull.* 2002; **26**: 344–5.

Revill J. (2003) Shrinking number of psychiatrists sparks crisis. *The Observer.* 2 March 2003.

Roberts ADL, Coid J. Personality disorder and offending behaviour: findings from the national survey of male prisoners in England and Wales. *J Forens Psychiatry Psychol.* 2010; **21**(2): 221–37.

Sainsbury Centre for Mental Health. *Mental Health at Work: developing the business case.* Policy paper 8. London: Sainsbury Centre for Mental Health; 2007.

Salzer M, Nixon C, James L, *et al.* Validating quality indicators. *Eval Rev.* 1997; **21**(3): 292–309.

Scull A. A quarter of a century of the history of psychiatry. *J Hist Behav Sci.* 1999; **35**: 235–54.

Shorter E. *A History of Psychiatry: from the era of the asylum to the age of Prozac.* New York: Wiley; 1997.

The King's Fund. *Paying the Price: the cost of mental health care to 2026.* London: King's Fund; 2008.

Webster C. *The National Health Service: a political history.* Oxford: Oxford University Press; 2002.

Wenchao J, Joyce R, Phillips D, Sibieta L. *Poverty and Inequality in the UK: 2011.* Available at: www.ifs.org.uk/comms/comm118.pdf (accessed 28 December 2011).

White E. *The Future of Psychiatric Nursing by the Year 2000: a Delphi study.* Manchester: Manchester University, Department of Nursing; 2000.

World Health Organization. *Policies and Practices for Mental Health in Europe: meeting the challenges.* Geneva: World Health Organization; 2008.

www.cqc.org.uk (Care Quality Commission).

11

Conclusions: is there a common European approach to delivering mental health services?

Neil Brimblecombe and Peter Nolan

Introduction

This chapter, in drawing on the contents of the previous chapters, seeks to explore the broad question: Is there a common European approach to what mental health services should be and how they should be implemented? As was alluded to in the introduction to this book, even though EU and WHO mental health policies indicate directions of travel and what the aims of good mental health services should be, no mention is made of the required structures, systems and services that would ensure their full implementation, nor is there any mention of how services should be funded, staffed, measured, monitored or reviewed. It would appear that WHO mental health policy is the result of collating best practice and then recommending it to all. Whereas WHO policy provides a direction or preferred outcomes, it would also appear that the formulation, interpretation and implementation of policies are left to the discretion of each member country, utilising and revising their existing resources, systems and structures as they see fit. In considering the above questions, there are a number of important secondary questions that need to be addressed:

- How similar are mental health services across Europe?
- Have they developed in similar ways and are they likely to continue to do so in the future?

- To what extent have local need or local culture, politics and economics influenced the past and the present, and are hence likely to influence the future?
- What evidence is there that attempts to improve services have been successful?

It cannot be claimed that sufficient information is provided in the previous chapters to answer all of these questions in detail; nevertheless, authors provide sufficient accounts that enable one to see differences and make comparisons between the countries. In addition to describing the structures and systems of health care that exist in the nine countries, the authors also allude to a range of contextual issues. The individual case scenario included in each chapter illustrates how a common mental problem would be dealt with within their respective services. Comparing mental health care in various countries is a difficult enterprise, because of linguistic differences, differences in terminologies, different methods used in collecting and analysing data, and different criteria against which the efficacy of services are judged. Arguably, the greatest difficulty is that mental health care remains a relatively underdeveloped science and improvements may be due as much to the application of particular values or beliefs as opposed to scientific evidence. Whilst the World Health Organization has striven hard to produce accurate data to allow comparisons to be made between countries, for example about the numbers of people accessing services, details of the workforce and the types of treatments and interventions used, there remain concerns about the reliability of the data. As has been seen in the previous pages, not only do some countries simply not hold central data, in others different government departments hold different data sets which are produced depending on which organisation asks to see them. The type of data produced depends not just on the questions asked, but on how the questions are asked and for what purposes.

This book focuses specifically on the nature of mental heatlth services and does not explore in any detail the many factors that may impact directly on the mental health of individuals, e.g. unemployment levels, housing availability, level of familial support and access to community support, which may vary from country to country. These are important and should influence the nature of individual mental health services. Just one example of such a factor is the pressure that exists within families and between family members. In a recent study (Relationships Foundation, 2011) it was found that when both parents go out to work, families sometimes struggle to hold it together. According to the study, the two EU countries in which family pressure was highest were Romania and Malta, closely followed by Slovakia and Latvia.

Population and demographics

The population of the European Union, encompassing 27 countries, is currently over 500 million. Member states have democratic governments, with varying degrees of centralisation, some with strong devolved state structures, while others are strongly centralised. There is great variation in the geographical size of states, their economic status, population and histories. The countries explored in this book range in size from Luxembourg, with a population of 500 000, to Germany, with 80 million.

The political structure of a country can strongly influence the structure, functioning and, sometimes, the legal frameworks in which mental health services have to operate, for example, Germany's state structure with its more localised laws and decision-making. Similarly, national politics have a huge impact on the nature of health services, in terms of the level of investment, the means of funding and, to a lesser degree, the philosophy of health care provision, for example, the degree to which it is state controlled and state delivered. A striking example is provided by Novotná and Petr (Chapter 2), who suggest that the current Czech population's reluctance to adopt models of personal responsibility for health is derived directly from the historical influence of the communist structure wherein the state rather than individuals assumed responsibility for all aspects of individual welfare.

Population size and geography have implications for population densities, for example, ranging from 16 people per square kilometre in Finland to 393 in Holland. Such variation presents challenges for those who plan and deliver mental health services, for example, in terms of the practical difficulties of providing services in rural or thinly populated areas, or, conversely, in cities, with their typically higher levels of social deprivation and psychiatric morbidity. These variations, coupled with the economic status of the country, have a bearing on the need for resources allocated to services.

History also influences population demographics: countries with imperial heritage often have significant immigrant populations from the lands of former empires, such as in the United Kingdom and Holland. In some EU regions, negative natural change in population size has been offset by positive net migration. This is at its most striking in Austria, the United Kingdom, Spain, the northern and central regions of Italy, and in some regions of western Germany, Slovenia, southern Sweden, Portugal and Greece (Eurostat, 2009).

The challenges faced by countries in responding appropriately to the mental health needs of immigrant communities have been seen as particularly challenging in some countries, for example, the United Kingdom and Holland. Some of the challenges relate to different presentations of disorders in different population groups (Jablensky *et al.*, 1994), culture-bound syndromes apparently unique to individual cultures (Jilek and Jilek-Aall, 1985) and the possible negative effects of conscious, or unconscious, racism within mental health services (Sainsbury Centre for Mental Health, 2002).

The development of mental health services

Accepted wisdom is that all mental health services across Europe have followed a common developmental pathway, with the establishment of large institutions in the nineteenth and early twentieth centuries and, towards the end of the twentieth century, these being gradually replaced, at least theoretically, by community-based services (Priebe, 2004). Whereas the structures and systems have similarly evolved, it would appear that the nature of what was provided for people within them varied considerably.

These recent changes have been linked with post-war public rejection of institutional care, with mounting evidence of the potentially harmful effects of such care (Barton, 1959; Goffman, 1961) and following numerous public exposures of poor and abusive practice in asylums in some countries. An important facilitator of change was the introduction of antipsychotic medication from the mid-1950s onward, enabling people with psychosis to be managed and cared for in less restrictive environments. However, it does seem likely that this effect has been overstated, as in some countries, such as the United Kingdom, significant bed reductions had taken place prior to the common use of chlorpromazine.

When trying to compare the historical development of mental health services across countries, an undoubted challenge is the variability in quality and availability of secondary source material (Gijswift-Hoftra and Oosterhuis, 2005). However, the picture that does emerge from the contributors to this volume is remarkably consistent in general features, although greatly variable in terms of exact timing and local circumstance.

Asylums were certainly significantly developed in the nineteenth century in all of the countries contributing to this volume. In some, specific institutions for the mentally ill or 'insane' were available prior to that date, for example, in Portugal there were specialised wards for 'patients who lost their minds' in the sixteenth century, and in Finland institutions specifically for the purpose of housing the mentally ill were available from the late eighteenth century; the Bethlem Hospital ('Bedlam') in London had admitted the insane from the fourteenth century. The church certainly played a role in many countries, with monastic orders providing care framed within a religious understanding of mental illness.

There is evidence of some early attempts to encourage the care of the mentally ill by families and community. In Ireland, the Brehon laws, which originated in pre-Christian Ireland, had effect up to the Elizabethan period and attempted to ensure the provision of care for the insane person by their family or the community, featuring various penalties for failure to care for the insane person. However, most commonly, prior to the establishment of specific asylums, the mentally ill would be likely to wander the country or be contained in other institutions, such as, for example, houses of correction, gaols, houses of industry and workhouses.

The universal growth of asylums in the nineteenth century seems to relate to a number of factors, including:

- the growth of central power in nation states
- the wish for such states to typically both better control and better care for their populations
- evidence produced at the time that seemed to demonstrate the beneficial effects of compassionate care in asylums
- the strengthening of the medical profession and its attempt to take authority over the field of mental illness, which was best done in the controlled environment of the asylum.

Once established, the number of beds in institutions typically rose well beyond initial expectations, limiting the ability of the asylums to provide therapeutic care and consequently resulting in the warehousing of large numbers of people. The latter reframing of asylums as 'hospitals' and the further emphasising of the medical nature of mental illness did little to improve conditions, treatment or outcome, with the exception of such demonstrably biologically based illnesses as general paralysis of the insane, caused by syphilis.

Between the end of the Second World War and the end of the century, countries recognised the need to replace large institutions with other forms of care at varying pace and with varying emphases. The moving of wards to general hospital sites was important symbolically, although it neither significantly reduced the stigma of mental illness nor changed the reliance on hospital admission as the main mode of service intervention.

In Portugal, it was not until the end of 1970 that an attempt was made to regionalise and decentralise mental health services so that a greater emphasis was given to the creation of community-based support structures. Similarly, in Germany, it took until the mid-1970s for the psychiatric landscape to change, when in a general climate of social and political reform, the country turned towards community-based mental health care. The high point for bed numbers in both Ireland and Finland was reached in the 1970s. These were in contrast to England, where bed occupancy was at its highest in the mid-1950s.

The impact of the church on mental health services

Although the role of the church has been referred to in several chapters, in terms of the provision of care by religious orders, less has been reported as to the potential impact of the church's beliefs on attitudes towards mental health problems and treatments. Ann Sheridan (Chapter 6) reports that the Roman Catholic church in Ireland in the 1940s, 1950s and 1960s was hostile to dynamic psychologies which were then being slowly implemented. Church leaders at the time held that the 'psyche' was synonymous with the soul and hence this was the province of the church's jurisdiction. In fact, hypnosis was proscribed in Ireland until 1955, when priestly ministries gave way to therapeutic interventions (Healy, 1996). In the Netherlands, the Catholic community equally viewed therapy as a threat to Roman ethics, and during the 1950s psychotherapy and psychoanalysis became the main areas of conflict between clergy and conservative doctors on the one hand and psychiatrists and psychologists on the other (Oosterhuis, 2005). The rejection of dynamic psychologies by the Roman Catholic church was associated with the focus of therapy on self-directedness, autonomy and self-regulation vis-à-vis sexuality in particular, a position at variance with the church's teaching on obedience and adherence to rules. However, in the Netherlands, Catholic resistance was mitigated by the existence and equal recognition of other Christian groups as well as a strong academic tradition within psychiatry. It would appear that in the Netherlands, when an amiable compromise was reached between Catholic, Protestant and secular mental health service providers, the care and treatment of patients improved, as did the cooperation between the services. Though no mention is made of religion or religious institutions in EU policies, nevertheless it is possible that faith communities have more to offer by way of supporting people with mental health problems than has been the case hitherto, and religious orders are still significant providers of services in some states, e.g. Belgium.

History's legacy

Finnane (2009, p. 6) rightly points out that 'More than other modern medical institutions, mental hospitals labour under the burdens of their histories'. The descriptions from the contributing countries show this to be the case in two key ways. Firstly, and most pervasively, is the burden of stigma attached to the asylums. In Luxembourg (Chapter 7), the modern psychiatric hospital is still associated with the Ettelbruck asylum, seen by the population as 'a dark place to which mad people are sent for lengthy periods of time'. Stigma remains one of the greatest obstacles in all countries to improving community care facilities and continues to be a priority if mental health improvement is to become a reality.

The second major burden is that of resources. Many countries illustrate the struggle to move the proportion of resources that have been bound up in central institutions towards care closer to people's homes or even within the homes of mental health service users.

General health need

Across Europe, as well as in the rest of the 'developed' world, the last 100 years have seen a huge shift from mortality related to infectious diseases and death in childhood, to longer lifespans and mortality largely connected with diseases associated with ageing, for example, cardiac disease and cancer. Such diseases are also heavily linked to lifestyle issues, such as diet, lack of exercise and smoking. Whilst there is an established cultural belief that mental health conditions related to stress have grown (Karpf, 1988), the reality is that the evidence is simply not available to demonstrate this. As diagnostic criteria change over time, access to health services and staff trained in identifying mental health conditions has increased, individuals are more likely to acknowledge that they have a mental health problem and the language of 'stress' has come to cover a wide range of emotions that may formerly have been labelled in other ways (or not expressed at all).

In the previous chapters, contributors cited a range of general health care issues as being significant today and likely to become even more so in the future. Certainly the shift from infectious disease, as the primary killer, to others related to lifestyle and age was clear and consistent. Two factors, commonly cited, are closely linked to mental health issues. Firstly, across Europe the population is ageing, as life expectancy increases. A striking example is provided by Finland (Chapter 3) where life expectancy has increased by 10 years in the last 30 years and over 30 years since the time of Finnish independence in 1917. At the moment, the average life expectancy for children born in 2000 is 83 years for females and 76 years for males (Statistics Finland, 2007). The primary mental health impact of this demographic change has been, and will increasingly be, a rise in the incidence of dementia, although other mental health problems such as depression can increase with age, especially in the presence of physical illness or social isolation (Djernes, 2006). A related challenge to mental health services is the practical one of a typically decreasing demographic pool of people to employ staff from compared to a growing population with high levels of morbidity.

The second commonly cited health challenge that relates directly to mental health need is that of alcohol, or alcohol and drug abuse. Europe has the highest alcohol intake of any region in the world (WHO, 2005a), and alcohol use and abuse is linked with increased risk of suicide, and is related to and can be a causative factor for a number of other mental health problems, as well as a litany of physical diseases. Whilst some countries, such as Portugal (Chapter 9), are claiming some success in pushing back the spread of alcoholism and addiction, others, such as Finland (Chapter 3), see it as continuing to be a serious problem. Ellilä and colleagues point out the rise in alcohol consumption and increasing addiction, cirrhosis and other medical problems linked to alcohol abuse, and that alcohol abuse and its related problems are regarded as the biggest general health problem in Finland today.

Funding health services

The distinguishing feature of the funding of health services is that every country has its own unique arrangements, and most have a number of sources from which services are funded. Generally, it is not clear how well the range of different funding bodies collaborate with each other, how they reach agreement as to the amount of resources required to provide services and whether or not they agree with the outcomes achieved. The most common means of funding are:

- *Central taxation*: being the predominant form in the United Kingdom.
- *Compulsory employee health care insurance*: either payable to the government or to insurance companies, as in Germany, Holland and Luxembourg.
- *Voluntary health care insurance*: an important addition to central national funding in Ireland, and part of a range of payment sources in Greece.
- *Direct patient payments*: found as a 'top up' for specific services in many countries, for example, prescription charges in England, payment for visits to general practitioners in Ireland and a fixed charge for examinations and treatment in the Czech Republic.

Undoubtedly, the commonest picture is one of a mixture of funding sources. In many countries, individuals who are unable to work have access to health care without contributing to the compulsory insurance schemes. However, in those countries that generally rely more on direct payments by patients for treatment, this potentially limits the engagement for treatment by people with mental health problems, although the actual effect is hard to quantify.

Delivering health services

Just as the means of funding health care in EU countries vary, so do the structures and systems that exist for delivering services. These include:

- *Direct employment of health care workers by the government*: as is still the common position in the United Kingdom, although there has been a recent emphasis on more pluralistic provision in the name of competition and based on a view that large governmental organisations may not always be the best or the cheapest. Other countries also have most services provided through state-provided services, for example, in Portugal, the public sector represents about 70% of total health care.
- *Funding of non-governmental organisations to provide health care*: in Germany, many services are provided by non-governmental organisations. Similarly, in the Czech Republic, most services are non-governmental; they have been established by regional governments, municipalities, churches and

individuals. Governmental health care facilities make up less than 1% of all the health care facilities.

- A *mixed economy of health care provision*: in fact, all countries appear to have some element of mixed provision. Even in the UK, there is, for example, major provision of forensic inpatient services by the private sector, and community drug and alcohol services are often provided by government-funded charities. Ireland also has provision from a mix of state employees, the charity sector and private (profit-making) organisations.

All of these models have potential benefits and drawbacks. Certainly the provision of complex mental health care pathways by utilising several different organisations that may need to be involved in separate or overlapping stages of an individual service user/patient's care can lead to significant challenges in terms of having joined-up processes and good communication. In Germany (Chapter 4), this issue contributes to the problem referred to as the 'German disease', the fragmented system of mental health care provision and mental health care funding with its 'potential to hamper mental health care planning and cause under- and oversupply.'

Policy and structure

The WHO (2001) reported that, at that time, one third of European countries did not have specific mental health policies, suggesting that policies were a major driver of change and improvement. However, as Machiavelli rightly pointed out several centuries ago, drawing up laws and policies without having the means of enforcing them is futile (Fischer, 2000). Of the nine countries reported on in this book, only the Czech Republic seems not to have a national policy of some kind, apart from having the current intention to devise a strategy for dementia. Several other countries appear to have had a whole series of policy initiatives over the years, which have contributed disappointingly little to the overall improvement of services or meeting stated goals in the planned timescales. This was so in Ireland, Germany, Portugal and Greece. Santos and colleagues (Chapter 9) comment that 'Portugal considers the production of policies, guidelines and directives to be important, but by themselves, they are insufficient'. The relationship between the production of policies, no matter how relevant they are, and the production of change is often not strongly correlated. Schulz takes a more forgiving view when commenting on the slow progress made in Germany to creating change (Chapter 4): 'progress in German mental health services is slow and deliberate, and perhaps attempting to speed up the process might result in confusion and failure'.

Most national plans/strategies in the recent past have tended to place most emphasis on planning the move from large psychiatric hospitals to general hospitals and on increasing community-based services. Little prominence appears to have been attached to increasing mental health promotion activities or devising methods of preventing mental health problems (WHO, 2005a). Even where the need for such action is specifically cited, such as in the English *National Service Framework for Mental Health* (Department of Health, 1999), the reality is that this particular objective has not been realised. This is largely due to the fact that resources would have to be diverted from services that currently provide treatment to those that deliver health promotion, always a challenging prospect politically.

Whilst national governments have taken on the task of planning the future of mental health care services, the degree to which their strategies actually come to fruition varies depending on a number of issues, the most important of which are outlined below:

The degree to which governments are prepared to develop detailed plans

Possibly the most detailed example of mental health policy that has actually been enforced is in England, where the *National Service Framework for Mental Health* (Department of Health, 1999) laid out detailed structures for services, down to the level of skill mix, type of team design and number of expected patients per area. This level of detail, which was subsequently enforced by measuring local health organisations' performance against some of these criteria, is rare. Conversely, the Czech Republic has had a dearth of central planning for mental health services, although recently a plan has specifically been developed to tackle the challenge of dementia (Chapter 2).

Generally, detailed planning is preferable to sweeping strategic generalities, and Petrea (Chapter 1) notes that national documents frequently tend to set ambitious goals and cover a wide range of areas, from mental health promotion to deinstitutionalisation and human rights. What they often miss, however, are specific targets to be achieved within a determined time frame, the means by which any progress towards these targets will be measured, and clearly established funding mechanisms and funding sources for the implementation of policy and achievement targets. In their absence, the goals set remain aspirational.

The degree to which plans are then implemented

The principal division in the planning of health care lies between national and local governments, while the degree to which the responsibility is divided varies from country to country. As discussed above, the English National Service Framework provided governmentally devised detailed plans to be applied locally, whilst in Finland the Ministry for Social Affairs and Health administers the overall functioning of health and social care services, but the municipalities are responsible for the local organisation and planning of health services.

One of the major problems relating to planning as seen in the previous accounts is that the allocation of resources seems to be targeted on existing services and often not on the locations where need is greatest. The challenge of uneven distribution of resources is found in Portugal (Chapter 9) and Greece (Chapter 5), where although all residents are entitled to health services, the availability is often limited in some areas, especially on the many Greek islands. In the Czech Republic, there is also an unbalanced distribution of resources, with inadequacies outside of large cities (Chapter 2),

The degree to which plans are supported

An important consideration in attempting to implement policies that aim at the provision of more care away from institutional settings and in the community is the willingness or otherwise of the community itself and health and social care professionals, not specifically working in the mental health field, to accept that and share some of the responsibility for at least tolerating people with evident mental health problems being in their midst (see 'Attitudes to mental health problems', p. 310). Where this does not happen, incidents that inevitably occur from time to time can be framed as demonstrating a failed system and can attract disproportionate media interest, creating further barriers to the care of people and reinforcing stigma. Not only does the risk to the development of community-based care come from those who, arguably, may simply be influenced by the weight of historical and cultural stigma, but, as Porritt (2005) notes, some of the most vociferous opponents of community care are actually mental health professionals who fail to see any therapeutic advantages.

Mental health need

Mental health is essential to enable human beings to live happy, fulfilled and productive lives (Knapp et al., 2007). However, trying to identify the level and nature of mental health need in a particular country is a challenge everywhere. There are issues concerning:

- the availability of data
- the reliability and comparability of that data
- the 'meaning of data', i.e. how it should be interpreted.

Petrea (Chapter 1) points out that 'Ideally, policy-makers would have access to adequate information on the scale and nature of mental health problems, to ensure that the representation of mental health on the political agenda is commensurate with its magnitude, and to promote sufficient investment in strategies and interventions to address mental ill health.' She also takes a view that in terms of epidemiological data available to policy-makers, the situation in which European countries find themselves today is far from ideal. Muijen (2008) concurs by adding that he believes reforms across Europe are hampered by a lack of reliable comparable information and research.

Consistently, both national and international studies of mental health need suggest very high levels of untreated morbidity. For example, preliminary data from a study recently conducted by the WHO and Harvard University, coordinated in Portugal by Almeida (2010), indicates that, in the last year, more than one in five Portuguese citizens were suffering from a psychiatric illness (23%) at any given time. Elsewhere, it is estimated that 27% of the adult population (aged 18–65) in the EU, Iceland, Norway and Switzerland have experienced at least one mental disorder within a 12-month period, ranging from somatoform disorders, depression, anxiety and psychosis to substance use or eating disorders (Wittchen and Jacobi, 2005). What particularly produces concern is that many fewer people are accessing mental health services than are estimated actually to be experiencing mental health problems (Kohn *et al.*, 2004). The results of such a treatment gap can be serious. For example, failure to identify and treat people with psychosis at the earliest opportunity can result in prolonged individual suffering or prolonged expensive hospital stays (Marshall and Rathbone, 2006).

Major concerns raised by recent research findings

Should these figures be taken at face value – that is, that around a quarter of the population at any one time has a mental health problem? Of course, mental health problems cover a wide range of conditions, some debilitating, others less so. An important critique of the prevalence of mental health problems within various societies is that this calculation reflects the medicalisation of the normal range of human experience and the confusion of common unhappiness with pathological conditions. Wootton (2007) contests that data concerning the prevalence of mental health problems is often exaggerated and methodologies deployed in gathering it lack rigour; whilst Richter *et al.* (2008) raise the challenge that high rates of mental health problems may be due to the diagnostic practices deployed.

If such high figures are accepted as reflections of a reality and that all such cases needed treatment, then the implications would make the design and provision of services simply impossible, in terms of sheer size, cost and manpower. It is estimated that only 10% of people with alcohol problems currently receive effective treatment for alcohol problems (Kohn *et al.*, 2004). Does this suggest that we need 10 times the volume of capacity to treat alcohol problems in the future? Such figures are clearly alarming when taken to their logical conclusion.

However, one thing that such figures do achieve is to apply pressure to fund mental health services, even though they could never seriously attempt to respond to such levels of possible need. The WHO tends to adopt the more reassuring statistic that 20% of health need relates to mental health (WHO, 2005a), a figure that argues for a larger proportion of the cake rather than describing a level of need that no government could reasonably be expected to meet.

There have been claims that psychiatric diagnostic reliability – that is, the ability of clinicians to diagnose a similar presentation with the same diagnosis – has improved with newer iterations of diagnostic systems (e.g. Spitzer *et al.*, 1979; Jakobsen *et al.*, 2005), although reliability still varies between diagnostic categories (Cheniaux *et al.*, 2009). There has also been a great deal of debate as to how valid diagnoses are across cultures (Alarcon, 2009; Canino and Alegría, 2008). It is, as yet, unclear as to whether 'cultural differences' between individual countries (or regions within countries) may affect demographic estimates of mental health problems. Despite the increasing number of cross-country studies and increasingly standardised approaches to diagnoses over the last few years, there appears to still be a deal of scepticism when studies show apparent differences in the epidemiology of mental health problems in different countries. For example, Ellilä and colleagues (Chapter 3) contend that although the lifetime prevalence of all psychoses in Finland is estimated to be higher than other comparable countries, this may simply be due to data collection bias.

One area where reasonably reliable data is available is suicide. Petrea (Chapter 1) describes the very wide variation in prevalence across Europe, with the highest levels being found in the former Soviet countries. Suicide rates may relate to many issues, from the degree of personal psychopathology in a population to the elusive concept of 'culture'. The rates certainly do not appear to be directly correlated with investment in mental health services. For example, Greece has one of the lowest rates of suicide and self-inflicted injuries in all ages, at 2.85 per 100 000, one of the lowest in the European Union, despite having a relatively low spend on mental health services. The low suicide rate in Greece has been attributed to cultural and social factors. Koukia (Chapter 5) suggests the importance of the role of families in Greece who 'stick together' and support each other, especially during times of crisis. This kind of social and psychological support by family and friends plays a protective role in diminishing the effects of social isolation and feelings of loneliness that may eventually lead to suicidal behaviour. One factor that does seem universal across Europe is the high proportion of male compared to female suicides, for which although there is variation between countries, this is small compared to variation between numbers of suicides in countries.

Attitudes to mental health problems

For people with severe mental health problems, one of the most important problems they face is the stigma they encounter, contributing to lowered self-esteem, disrupted family relationships, and their ability to socialise, obtain housing and become employed (Wahl, 1999). The Helsinki Agreement (WHO, 2005a) made a specific pledge to tackle stigma, discrimination and social exclusion. All three of these issues are significant problems right across Europe. Negative attitudes and stereotypes have been well documented through studies of public attitudes and media portrayals. A smaller number of large-scale studies have documented massive social exclusion (e.g. Social Exclusion Unit, 2004).

Whilst all countries included in this book have some evidence of negative attitudes in their populations towards people with mental health problems, the nature and focus of that evidence varies widely. Angermeyer and Dietrich (2006) note that although attitude research in psychiatry has made considerable progress in recent years, there is still much to be done to provide an empirical basis for evidence-based interventions to reduce stigma.

A major negative consequence of the stigmatisation of both mental health problems and mental health services is the decreased likelihood that those with mental health needs will come forward voluntarily for treatment. In Portugal, evidence from a study of 843 people led the authors (Loureiro *et al.*, 2008) to conclude that negative beliefs are still deeply rooted in the social and cultural context, especially views about dangerousness and incurability. However, on the positive side, they found that people with mental health problems were prepared to seek professional help and comply with prescribed treatments, suggesting some success in destigmatising services. Conversely, in a study of 300 patients and relatives and 330 psychiatrists and psychologists in Finland (Finnish Central Association for Mental Health, 2010), 70% of those under 25 stated that they (including mental health professionals) would not mention their own mental health problem to their fellow workers and 45% would not tell their superior.

A positive note is provided by some limited evidence that attitudes can change to become more positive over time. In Greece, Madianos *et al.* (1987) sought to discover the attitudes of 1574 adult members of the public towards people with mental health problems, and after 10 years they undertook a follow-up study in which they compared the attitudes towards mental illness of the general public and those personnel who worked in the same community mental health centre (Madianos *et al.*, 1999). Both groups expressed more positive attitudes towards the mentally ill than had been the case previously. Both groups were more favourably disposed towards social integration than had previously been the case, they held less authoritarian attitudes to social restriction and they possessed a good level of knowledge about the aetiology of mental illnesses. In the UK, a public survey carried out in 1999 was repeated in 2009, and the results indicated increasing tolerance on the part of the general public towards people with mental health problems (Department of Health, 2009).

Despite the bold objective in the Helsinki Accord to reduce stigma across Europe, there is little evidence of systematic national approaches to achieve this aim. Where action has been taken, a common feature has been engaging with the media to reduce sensationalist reporting of incidents possibly involving people with mental health problems. One approach taken is that services invite journalists to see what is being done and the difficulties that those with mental health problems have to endure.

Various specific schemes exist across Europe to tackle stigma and discrimination. For example, in the Czech Republic, a Week of Mental Health is held, with musical and theatre festivals in psychiatric sanatoria, online consultancy services, education programmes and debates at schools or publication of magazines. In Nuremberg, Germany, the Alliance Against Depression carries out intervention on four levels: co-operation with GPs, an information and awareness campaign for the general public, educational training for people, such as teachers, priests, nurses and other caregivers for older people, as well as the support of self help activities.

Public attitudes cannot be changed overnight, but strategies can be put in place to start the process – by campaigns to raise awareness of mental health issues, publishing literature, highlighting good practice and encouraging those who suffer with mental health problems to speak out about their needs and experiences. An enormous amount was achieved in Norway when Prime Minister Kjell Magne Bondevik acknowledged that he had a mental illness which had required him to take time off work (Knapp et al., 2007). He spoke openly about his condition, how it disabled him and what he needed in order to recuperate. In doing so, he evoked a sympathetic reaction from the public, the media and his colleagues to such an extent that recommended improvements in mental health services met with little resistance.

Arguably, the changes most likely to have a major cumulative impact over time are the changing structure and focus of mental health services. As discussed above, the shifting from large institutionally based care is the stated intent in most countries, although the reality of the extent of that shift varies enormously. The original development of institutions for, undoubtedly, mixed reasons of humanitarianism and benevolent paternalism, together with the perceived need for greater social control, created closed environments, largely away from population centres, where fears and fantasies could be projected into the symbol of the asylum and the 'mad' who inhabited it. The creation of community-based services stands a better chance of being effective in assisting individuals and reducing stigma if local people are consulted, involved and invited to participate.

Expenditure on mental health

Estimating whether the expenditure on mental health services in any country is 'sufficient' requires having the answers to a number of questions including:

- What is the level of mental health need?
- The potential effectiveness of such services – is it money that could be/is being well spent?
- Does the structure, focus and skills of staff employed in mental health services allows maximum effectiveness to be attained?
- What can be afforded?

These are questions that are all very difficult to answer. As indicated above, estimating mental health need is challenging, and can produce such high potential levels of need that no amount of investment could realistically 'treat' all conditions. If tighter criteria are applied, for example, by focusing on 'severe mental illness', then estimates produce small numbers, but there is still some doubt as to whether identified differences in national illness demographics are real or the results of sampling bias or methodological flaws.

There is undoubtedly a burgeoning literature that looks at the effectiveness of specific interventions, although the 'halo' effect of new interventions seems as significant in mental health as other areas of medical endeavour, with an overestimate of value before robust data becomes available, e.g. for antidepressant medication (American Psychiatric Association, 2006) and atypical antipsychotic medication (Bagnall *et al.*, 2003); as is the difficulty in transferring findings from clinical trials, with tight exclusion criteria to real-world practice where people often need to receive a service regardless of whether they neatly fit specific parameters.

Trying to understand whether *services* are well designed to work effectively is more difficult. Two measures provide information on spend: firstly, spend per head of the population, which provides a raw figure; and secondly, how much is spent proportionately as compared to other forms of health spend, which allows a sense of comparative priority. These interlinking issues also need to be contextualised by the fact, as discussed in the introduction of this book, that *mental health services* are not the same thing as *mental health care* in its totality, as this tends to exclude many other relevant activities in social care, primary care and within families. So actually measuring spend is difficult in the first place, as many services provide elements of mental health care but no estimate of cost can be placed against this, for example, general practice.

Even with these caveats, it seems unarguable that across Europe, funding for mental health typically remains small relative to the burden of disease (WHO, 2005a). As indicated above, the data suggests very high levels of mental health need across all countries, with depression and alcohol abuse, in particular, being predicted to continue to grow. The variation between countries in their spend on mental health, as a proportion of their total budget, is between 2% and 14%, a huge range.

There is a general correlation between affluence and mental health spend. Petrea (Chapter 1) also, interestingly, suggests a link between countries with 'higher achievements in different areas of human development' and higher spend on mental health. The implicit suggestion that mental health spend may somehow reflect an interest by governments in the value of people, more generally, is provocative and challenging, although unevidenced at this point (and possibly hard to evidence in the absence of a clear definition of words such as 'achievement').

Although a philosophical leaning towards developing people may play a part in governmental decisions on prioritising spend, a factor that may be playing an increasingly important role is the increasing recognition, at least in some countries, of the cost to the nation of mental health problems themselves. In Finland, sickness allowance due to mental health problems increased by 93% between 1990 and 2003. Mental health problems are currently the most common reason for receiving a disability pension (Järvisalo et al., 2005). In the UK, a report has estimated that impaired work efficiency associated with mental health problems costs the country approximately €15.6 billion a year (Sainsbury Centre for Mental Health, 2007). In Germany, Schulz (Chapter 4) points out that the numbers of days and cases of sick leave due to mental disorders have increased by about 80%, according to health insurers' statistics. Mental disorders have become the single most frequent cause of early pensions, and the numbers of inpatient cases due to mental disorders have been rising, in contrast to a general trend towards a constant number of somatic hospital cases. Whilst these costs may be a result of an increase in mental health problems, they may also be the result of an increased recognition or acceptance of mental health problems and a greater willingness to receive such a diagnosis.

If a government believes that mental health problems can be effectively treated, then spending on mental health can be seen, in part, as an investment to reduce costs in the future. Interestingly, in the Czech Republic, a country with a relatively low proportional health budget spend on mental health, the levels of pensions related to mental ill health remain relatively small, with 14.2% of newly granted full disability pensions being granted for a mental illness and 9.5% of partial disability pensions being granted for psychiatric reasons (Dlouhý, 2009). Cause and effect may become inextricably linked in such a case, where a low understanding of and low tolerance for mental health problems, combined with low levels of diagnostic identification, may lead to underreporting and hence less pressure to invest in services.

So if there is significant evidence that 'Effective solutions for mental disorders are available' (WHO, 2001, p. 109), then what other reasons may result in countries not investing more in mental health care? In some European countries, this question has to be preceded by the larger question: Why do countries not spend more on health care generally? The answer to this first question tends to be tied up with the overall wealth of a country, although this is certainly not always the case; for example, until relatively recently the United Kingdom spent less of its GDP on health care than many other nations with comparable GDP. Political will and political prioritisation are always important mediators.

The answer to the more specific question – why is more not spent (proportionally) on mental health services? – can produce a range of answers. Undoubtedly the influence of history is important. Where historically relative underspending has taken place, it is harder to reach a desired current position, as investment would need to be relatively large, and also, expectations of professionals, patients and society may be lower and thus there will be less internal drive for change in the system. Such a conclusion is not without potential challenge, however, as it is clear that shocking failures within mental health systems (linked directly or indirectly with funding) have driven change in many countries. Examples can be found in the United Kingdom, with various scandals in psychiatric hospitals in the 1960s and more recently homicides carried out by individuals with severe mental health problems that had demonstrated flaws in community care (Coid, 1994), which have led to governmental reviews, and in Greece, where the appalling treatment of people on Leros led to international concern and subsequent major change (Chapter 5). Certainly, the impact of medical politics is likely to be important where the issue is the proportion of total spend. The most powerful and influential grouping within medicine remains strongly linked to the more invasive specialities. The impact of stigma and the fact that mental health issues do not win votes is also a significant factor influencing spending decisions. Additionally, the argument that effective solutions for mental disorders are available is often not enough to convince governments of the need for more investment, as the translation of that promise into effective action is more complex than simply increasing the spend on mental health. Where the majority of spend remains tied into inpatient resources, the degree of planning and investment to move to more community-focused models is potentially very large. Knapp *et al.* (2011) reviewed European experiences of deinstitutionalisation and concluded that community-based models are not inherently more costly than institutions, once account is taken of individuals' needs and the quality of care. The highly important caveat is that community-based models could be more expensive, but more *cost-effective*, when properly set up and managed, because they could deliver better outcomes. For a country with limited financial resources, there are a number of 'ifs' in this equation.

A final, and important, contextual point relates to the reality that even where mental health need is evidenced, it appears that services frequently prove unable to engage with those with that need, as discussed above. European research reveals that more than half the population of people with mental health problems do not wish to engage with mental health services (Codony *et al.*, 2009). Therefore, even where extra investment is available, simply increasing the size and quality of current services without changing the model of engagement may, frankly, be missing the point.

Current mental health care

All countries with mental health policies, including those of central and Eastern Europe, have planned reforms that embrace deinstitutionalisation and a greater role for community mental health services (Becker and Kilian, 2006; Becker and Vazquez-Barquero, 2001; Thornicroft and Rose, 2005). However, there are still many countries with very limited community resources (WHO, 2005a). Even a country such as Finland, which invests relatively heavily in mental health services, has suffered criticism for having a lack of diverse and flexible community care services (NOMESCO, 2007).

The Helsinki Agreement stated that subject to national constitutional structures and responsibilities, signatories would commit themselves to:

> Recognising the need for comprehensive evidence-based mental health policies and to considering ways and means of developing, implementing and reinforcing such policies.

Furthermore the agreement aimed to pursue:
- promoting mental well-being
- tackling stigma, discrimination and social exclusion
- preventing mental health problems
- providing comprehensive and effective interventions for people with mental health problems whilst offering involvement and choice
- rehabilitating and including in society people who have experienced serious mental health problems.

The role of the WHO was relatively limited with respect to mental health as compared with other public health issues, such as alcohol consumption, obesity and smoking, until the late 1990s. Still, over the last 10 years it has adopted a number of influential policy documents, as noted above, that have steered policy-making on mental health in European countries. Although none of these documents are legally binding, they typically include a requirement on member states that the WHO monitors their implementation.

The agreement recognised that mental health is crucial to the quality of life of individuals, families and communities, and to the prosperity and well-being of nations. Homogeneity across services was not advocated, and the structure, resourcing and monitoring of services was to be determined by the individual nations for whose peoples services were provided.

The European Union has provided funding to support the development of mental health services, although Parker (2010) raises concerns about how EU structural funds have been used to assist Central and Eastern European (CEE) member states. These funds were intended for EU countries where mental health has been severely neglected to help services move from an institutional base into the community, and thereby reduce disparities between different regions of Europe. The funding comes from the European Social Fund (ESF) and the European Regional Development Fund (ERDF). Although some countries have applied for and received additional funding to help protect the rights of disabled people and promote their social inclusion, many people with disabilities continue to be segregated in large, remote, residential institutions where their exclusion from society is virtually absolute. Resources allocated to Hungary and Romania have, for example, been used to provide additional *institutional* care. Structural monies, which were meant to accelerate provision of community services have, in these instances, Parker argues, actually hindered progress. Other countries that have been successful in obtaining funding have found that they do not have the administrative infrastructure to deliver the services required. Good intentions are clearly not enough.

In reality, all countries struggle to deliver the mental health services that governments espouse and users of services and professionals request. The Merano Declaration on Mental Health in CIS countries (WHO Regional Office for Europe, 2005b) identified a number of common challenges to developing services. These challenges are related to implementation of national policies and legislation, availability of mental health care in primary care settings, poor conditions in mental health institutions, which remain the main provider of mental health services in these countries, limited availability of specialist mental health staff, and poor funding. Although these related to CIS countries at the time, the individual stories told in this book suggest that these factors can be applied to all countries to a greater or lesser extent. Even in countries with (until recently) highly successful economies, such as Ireland, there has been a significant lag between the development of government policy and its delivery.

In reality, a fundamental challenge underpins the development of extensive mental health services. Whilst services in the UK may be extensive and the proportion of health spend is relatively high compared to most other countries, what is lacking is convincing empirical evidence that the extent and/or nature of mental health service predicts better outcomes for individuals or, indeed, a country. Unlike other health areas, in which improvements can be linked to, for example, acquisition of high-quality equipment, linear correlations cannot be simplistically drawn in relation to improvements in mental health.

Despite these challenges, the vast majority of countries have made significant progress over recent years (Petrea and Muijen, 2008). Whether the current Europe-wide financial downturn will allow further gains to be made (or even to maintain those already made) is unclear. The rapid growth in investment that has taken place in countries such as the UK has ceased, and even relatively wealthy states, such as Luxembourg, are having to take control of expenditure much more tightly. It is likely to be those countries who have suffered most from the economic downturn, such as Ireland, where this is likely to have the most impact, and this will be doubly felt in those where the economic impact is on top of a relatively low spend even prior to that, such as in Greece.

Where community resources do exist, they vary in scope, constitution and aims. In several countries, they are provided by a range of organisations. An area where services are rarely available are those for specific mental health crises, i.e. those that are able to respond rapidly and see individuals in their own homes, particularly out of office hours. The most extensively resourced example of such services is in England, where crisis resolution/home treatment teams are available in all areas and are expected to be able to carry out emergency assessments within a few hours and can then offer intensive home treatment as an alternative to hospital admission where this appears clinically safe to do so. Many other countries struggle with provision of expert emergency assessments. For example, in Germany a mental health crisis in the home is likely to be initially approached by health technicians (without any specific training in mental health) from the national emergency department. Many other countries have little or no resources to assess a person in their own home, with all assessments taking place in offices or health facilities.

There is also considerable variability as to the extent of services available to offer treatment in a home setting. Whilst all countries have an element of 'psychiatric outpatients' available, typically provided by psychiatrists in office settings, a number of countries, such as Luxembourg, have recently increased their ability to provide a level of home-based care primarily utilising nurses. Psychiatric day hospitals are key features of the community services found in Portugal and Ireland. England, Holland and Ireland all have assertive outreach services focusing on the needs of people with severe mental health problems.

Whilst the number of psychiatric beds has been significantly reduced in many states, paradoxically, Priebe *et al.* (2005) argue that reinstitutionalisation is actually taking place in some European countries with different traditions of health care, although with significant variation between the six countries they studied. While stating that the precise reasons for the phenomenon remain unclear, they suggest that general attitudes to risk containment in a society may be significant.

So is the apparent move away from institutional care across Europe a mirage? Certainly if true deinstitutionalisation was reliant on positive attitudes of the public towards people with mental health problems, then it is certainly unlikely that this has happened. However, much depends on definition. The UK has demonstrated one of the most radical approaches to bed closure in Europe, yet this has gone alongside the significant growth in forensic beds (Priebe *et al.*, 2005). The detail behind this is complex. At one end of the spectrum, the most secure and restrictive environments, the 'special hospitals', have drastically reduced bed numbers over many years, whilst there has been a major rise in medium secure facilities. More recently, there has been increasing recognition that many people in medium secure facilities could be adequately cared for in 'low secure' environments (still locked but with less elaborate security). Thus there has been, somewhat paradoxically, a rise in those in secure facilities but a gradual overall reduction in the average level of security in which they are held.

Still in the UK, in terms of community provision, there has been a large scale move from long-term hospital care to a range of other alternatives, including nursing homes, group homes, accommodation supported by housing workers (either living on or off site) and then a range of community-based health and social care teams. A particularly significant development in this regard has been the governmental mandating of the creation of assertive outreach teams (Department of Health, 1999) derived from American models, and focusing on ensuring that individuals diagnosed with severe mental health problems and a tendency to drift away from services are not able to do so by means of 'assertive' follow-up. It is fairly clear that such models do contain elements of the control traditionally associated with large-scale institutions, albeit in a milder way and allowing a larger degree of privacy and choice than would ever have been possible in the past.

Over the past four decades in Ireland (Chapter 6), the number of patients residing in psychiatric hospitals has decreased from 19 801 in 1963 to 3389 in 2006. A key part of this change has been the development of community residences with a spectrum of 'support' graduating from higher to lower levels of support. In line with this policy priority, the number and composition of community residences have grown considerably over the past 25 years. In 1984, there were 121 community residences, with 900 places; 20 years later in 2004, the number of people living in community residences exceeded 3000 (Mental Health Commission, 2006). So, certainly, by one definition, there has been a degree of reinstitutionalisation, but if the aim is to increase the level of independence from institutions, rather than have a simplistic aim of always seeking total freedom from institutional forms of care, then this can be seen as a success.

Mental health law

All European Union countries have means by which individuals can be detained in psychiatric facilities against their will if they meet certain criteria and certain procedures are followed. This suggests a universal acknowledgement that people with mental health problems may, at times, need to be compulsorily treated because of the level of risk they pose to themselves or others or the severity of their mental health problem. The WHO rightly points out, however, that the existence of a mental health law (or other laws that perform that function) is not in itself a guarantee against human rights violations (WHO, 2005a).

The majority of countries have specific legislation regarding the processes and safeguards concerning the detention of individuals with mental health problems where they do not consent, although this may be divided into a number of different laws. For example, in Germany the relevant legal framework comprises 'police laws' to maintain public safety and order and the law on tutelage (or guardianship), which gives powers to intervene with people who apparently need treatment, but are not (yet) in a situation requiring them to be hospitalised right away. An interesting exception to the general clarity of legal frameworks is found in the Czech Republic (Chapter 2), where there is no specific law, but rather a number of different statutes work together to provide a practical approach to such detention.

The need to prevent detention being used as a purely social control, as opposed to an intervention for specific mental illness, is often reflected by exclusion criteria that cannot be held as a reason for compulsory admission. For example, in Luxembourg a 'lack of congruity with moral, social, political or other societal values cannot be considered, per se, as a mental disorder' (Chapter 7).

Finland's law regarding the detention of patients against their will carries many of the typical features found elsewhere. Thus, according to the Finnish Mental Health Act 1116/1990, a person can be ordered to have treatment in a psychiatric hospital against his/her will only if:

- the person has been found to be suffering from a severe mental illness, or
- they are in need of psychiatric care, without which the mental illness will get worse, or
- it could seriously threaten their own or other people's health or safety; and
- no other form of mental health service is available or the service is deemed to be insufficient.

The most significant variation between countries relates to the involvement of the courts early in the process for involuntary detention. Some countries are characterised by having no judicial involvement early in the assessment and detention process, for example, in England, Finland and Ireland. However, judges or their equivalent are typically involved in these countries at later stages through processes of review or appeal. Other countries have more active court/judicial involvement at early stages of detention processes, although exactly when and how varies. In Greece, an initial police-led process can lead to detention to enable the person to be examined by two psychiatrists in the emergency department of a mental or general hospital rather then in his or her home; whilst in Holland an initial application for admission by a psychiatrist must be supported by the mayor and then, and within no more than 3 days, a judge will visit the person and conduct a face-to-face interview in the hospital to validate the compulsory admission or release the person from involuntary stay in the hospital.

A common feature in all systems appears to be the right of appeal, for example, in Ireland and England, to specific mental health tribunals. Once detained, there is a range of legal approaches to the enforcement of treatment, in particular the giving of medication against the will of the patient. In Germany, medication can only be prescribed against the patient's will if there is immediate danger of aggression or violence. In Holland, similarly, the implications of the law are that even if a person were suffering from a severe psychosis, a depot medication would not be able to be given against the patient's will. By contrast, in England medication is frequently given against the will of a detained patient as part of 'treatment'.

Some countries have a system of limited continued compulsion after discharge, although this does not allow for the physical administration of medication against the patient's will outside of hospital. For example, in Luxembourg, if the patient fails to comply with conditions set at the point of hospital discharge, the person who had requested the admission may readmit the person to the institution on request, without producing a new medical certificate. In England, a community treatment order can be imposed on individuals who have had a period of detention in hospital. Similarly, conditions are placed which, if broken, can lead to a return to hospital.

Mental health law across the EU therefore has certain commonalities, mostly in the principles relating to proportionality of detention (i.e. relating to a serious condition), processes involving either expert (medical) or legal (i.e. judges) officials, fixed maximum terms of detention and the right of appeal. Differences are to be found in the nature of processes (who is involved and when) and significant differences in the right of individuals to decline certain treatments.

The mental health professions

Petrea (Chapter 1) describes the enormous variation across Europe in staffing levels. For instance, there are 30 times more psychiatrists per 100 000 population in Switzerland than in Turkey. This intercountry gap is even greater for nurses working in mental health. Finland has 163 nurses per 100 000 population, while Greece has only three nurses per 100 000. There is no clear evidence of a direct relationship between recovery rates from severe mental health problems and the number of staff available; in fact, some evidence exists of the opposite being the case when comparing the Western and developing worlds (Warner, 2009). However, what is clear is that the 'treatment gap', i.e. the proportion of people with mental health problems who do not receive treatment, will typically be higher where there are less professionals available.

There are differences in numerical availability, but also some differences in the training and roles of key mental health staff. Nursing staff are the largest profession within mental health services. Significant differences exist across Europe in terms of whether they train specifically to practice solely in mental health settings, as in the United Kingdom, Ireland and Malta, or they are generally trained nurses who then just choose to work in mental health settings (Nolan and Brimblecombe, 2007). Even where postgraduate specialist mental health training for general nurses is 'expected', the reality is that it is often only a small proportion of nurses working in the mental health field who achieve this. For example, Schulz comments that in Germany it is not uncommon to have a psychiatric ward where there are two qualified psychiatric nurses and 10 general nurses (Chapter 4).

Across Europe, the majority of mental health services are led by psychiatrists. In some states, this is actually embedded in legislation. For example, in Ireland mental health services are defined as 'services which provide care and treatment to persons suffering from mental illness or a mental disorder under the clinical direction of a consultant psychiatrist'. Whilst other disciplines have grown in numbers and academic strength, and exist in what is normally termed the 'multidisciplinary team', this is contextualised by the reality of the current power structure. This is particularly clearly illustrated by the relationship between nursing and psychiatry. The historical context of this relationship across Europe is that psychiatric nursing was born in a managerially subservient position to the fledgling psychiatric profession in the asylums of the nineteenth century (Brimblecomb, 2005), and although nursing has increasingly professionalised and is typically a graduate profession, in most countries psychiatrists still define the work that nurses can do with individual patients.

Whilst nurses may be theoretically responsible for any decisions that they take in all countries, it is clear that the range of decisions that they are permitted to make independently varies greatly from country to country. A frequent position is that nursing actions need to be 'prescribed' by medical staff, as in Germany where nurses are expected, by law, to carry out the prescribed care of medical staff, even where working in community settings.

There are exceptions to this situation. The nurses' role in Finland is seen as independent, and nurses are responsible for the decisions they make in daily nursing care. In the UK, psychiatrists are typically the clinical lead for the care in inpatient settings, but nurses must make decisions based on their view of what is in the patient's best interests, and the instructions of a psychiatrist cannot make them act in a way that they believe is not in such interests. Interestingly, a recent change in mental health law in England theoretically allows nurses (following recognition as having the right experience and abilities) to become the lead clinician in multidisciplinary teams for individual inpatients. It is even more interesting that this opportunity has, as yet, been rarely taken up, suggesting that 150 years of tradition is hard to change.

Future mental health services

The majority of European states have comprehensive plans for the future development of mental health services. These all focus on the provision of community-focused services. The reality, as described above, is that such policies typically deliver slow change and change that does not fully meet the stated goals. Some states have revisited former strategies which have not delivered their promise and have restated them. The major concern about these is that the current economic climate across Europe is likely to make further successful development less of a priority, despite the growing economic arguments that evidence-based mental health interventions have potential significant financial benefits attached, particularly in terms of savings on incapacity/invalid benefits, at least in the commoner mental health disorders, such as anxiety and depression.

The role of the WHO and the European Union is important in continuing to highlight the issue. The most important WHO European policy documents are the *Mental Health Declaration* and the *Action Plan for Europe* (WHO Regional Office for Europe, 2005a,b). Both of these instruments were endorsed by European health ministers in January 2005, at the first ministerial conference on mental health in Europe. The action plan set out in detail the responsibilities of both member states and the WHO. These include reductions in stigma and discrimination, access to good primary health care, effective care in the community, partnerships across sectors, a competent workforce and adequate and fair funding. Whilst the determination of individual states to meet all these requirements may sometimes be somewhat lacking, the fact that they officially aligned themselves with the EU and WHO agendas make them easier to be held to account for failing to do so. However, some commentators (Dowding, 1995; Marmot, 2005) are critical of adopting a policy-first approach, which they consider naïve in that it fails to take account of the different health infrastructures of

EU countries. There is no recognition of the circumstances – political, economic and social – that have given rise to gross health inequalities within and between European countries. Without an understanding of these, health care policy may be little more than a cosmetic exercise.

At the level of individual professions, there is huge scope for change. Cox (2007) foresees future psychiatrists as requiring the ability to work as partners in multidisciplinary teams, a significant change from the current position where other professions are frequently seen as subordinate to psychiatrists. Conversely, the potential for developing the role of nursing, by far the largest profession working in mental health, to become more independent and to utilise new skills is currently a vastly untapped resource across much of Europe, despite growing evidence that extended roles can be effective and safe (Gray *et al.*, 2006; Dobel-Ober *et al.*, 2010).

Case scenarios

In each of the chapters describing the mental health services of individual countries, the authors were invited to respond to a common mental health case scenario (see below) and to discuss how the person in question would be likely to be treated and cared for in their respective country. This was to try and illustrate important features of their country's system; in particular, the availability of community-based resources, the process of mental health law in relation to involuntary detention, the nature of inpatient care and the resources and processes used to provide post-hospital care.

A 23-year-old unemployed man is reported by his landlord as acting increasingly strangely. He has barricaded his room, talking about being spied upon by the CIA. He can be heard shouting within his room in an angry and incoherent way. He has not been seen by a psychiatrist in the past, although his mother has told the landlord that he has been isolating himself and acting increasingly oddly over the last couple of years.

In asking this question, there are certain caveats that need to be attached to all responses. In particular, the view received may be individualistic, based on a particular experience of the author's mental health system, and it may describe what is supposed to happen, as opposed to what typically does happen (although authors were asked to be aware of this tendency).

A great deal was found to be in common across the nine countries. The majority of respondents appeared to immediately assume that the nature of the problem was a severe psychiatric one that was likely to require psychiatric treatment. Only two contributors, England and Holland, raised caution about this, querying whether there may be potential non-psychiatric causes for such 'disturbed' behaviour, although in a book about psychiatric services, it would not be unreasonable to assume that the case study was to be about a psychiatric problem.

The question of who or what type of service would be available to see the man initially revealed significant differences between countries, with a general dearth of emergency psychiatric services, with the exception of England and Holland, to offer assessment and a possible alternative to hospital admission. In some countries, e.g. the Czech Republic, a community-based psychiatrist would be able to see the person in his home, however in some countries, such as Germany, this is often not available because of the office-based nature of the practice of psychiatrists. More frequently, a general practitioner would make an assessment and start proceedings for compulsory detention in hospital, e.g. in Ireland.

Once admitted to hospital, the main intervention was seen as being through medication. As described above, the legal right of services in different countries to administer medication against an individual's will varies. The role of nurses in inpatient care was also highlighted, in particular the providing of support, ensuring the patient's safety and providing help in meeting basic needs, such as nutrition and hygiene. More advanced technical skills were said to be available in some countries, social skill training and psycho-education interventions in Holland, and in Germany adherence therapy would be delivered by nurses in some institutions.

As described above, the availability of community-based care varies markedly form country to country, although most provide 'outpatient clinics' of some description, whilst, more rarely, others have specialist assertive outreach teams for people with severe mental health problems.

Conclusions

This chapter set out to explore the question: Is there a common European idea about what mental health services should be like, and has it been implemented? Based on the information considered here, the answer seems to be a very cautious 'yes, but . . .'; the 'but' relating to the myriad of differences between countries in context and the degree to which the idea had been turned into reality. Sometimes differences exist because decisions are made that the particular difference is actually a preferred one; for example, different ways of funding services or different models of multidisciplinary working or different approaches to mental health law. Other differences arise more from the constraint of circumstances, or probably almost as often, because of the *apparent* constraint of circumstances. The clearest example is of the level of spend on mental health services, where less affluent countries clearly have less to spend; however, some more affluent countries 'choose' to spend a smaller proportion of their health budget on mental health and others arguably do not spend what they do allocate in an efficient way. Luxembourg is extremely affluent relatively, yet is constrained in its service models by a focus on medically led provision that limits the comprehensiveness and increases the costs of services.

The detailed responses from the nine countries who contributed to this book suggest a number of other common features:

- Mental health services are typically and essentially *psychiatric services*, led (clinically, if not managerially) by psychiatrists and with a largely medicalised model of care. Little mention was made of the contribution of social care, despite the evidence of social factors contributing to both the genesis and recovery from mental health problems. This may, of course, be an artefact of asking for descriptions of mental health services which may have narrow meanings and does not rule out the possibility of social care services working alongside but not in an integrated manner.

- The stated intention to deliver services from an increasingly community-based service, as opposed to an inpatient-based service, is universal. However, the degree to which this has been attained varies markedly. The factors in some countries that have caused slow or minimal change are powerful and would require a radical change to bring about a shift to community-based services. These include: organisational structures that make change complex; employment and payment structures that, if changed, may alter the favourable position of powerful professional groups; lack of finances; lack of political will; and antipathy from the public and media. The reality is that few countries in Europe have comprehensive community-based mental health services, even for people with severe mental health problems. In particular, there is a lack of crisis services, and those that offer any realistic alternative to hospital admission for those with acute or severe presentations of mental health problems. When more common mental health problems, such as anxiety or depression, are considered, then the position is even more limited, with immense amount of potential need but very little in the way of comprehensive planned provision, despite a clear evidence base demonstrating high rates of recovery.

- With no external, i.e. non-European models, being held up in comparison in the analyses presented here, it is hard to gauge whether European states have more in common with each other than with other non-European systems. Whilst it is clear that some European countries have adopted aspects of psychiatric processes from North American models, for example, the concept of 'assertive community outreach', they have done so in somewhat different ways and often in very different systems of delivery. For example, the service developed in Wisconsin (Stein and Test, 1980) has certainly been cited as influencing service design in the UK, but the original model has changed significantly to separate, specific, specialist teams delivering long-term assertive care and short-term crisis care, and all within a largely nationally funded and provided system, unlike the multiple providers in the US working in a mix of insurance, charitable, state and nationally funded systems.

- What this chapter also has not been able to address is to gather information about how the people who use mental health services experience those services, and even less of those who have no access to suitable services. In terms of the participation of people with mental health problems in the planning and evaluation of services, this is a largely undeveloped area. Nor has it been possible to describe the reality of probably the vast majority of the provision of care for people with mental health problems, i.e. the care provided within families and social networks that is typically neither recognised, supported or rewarded.

- At the moment, a European idea of what constitutes good mental health services may exist, but the reality lags well behind this. However, this should not prevent recognition of the fact that most countries have made significant changes in their services, in particular in beginning the movement towards more community-based services, with a consequent reduction in the most negative aspects of institutional care. To progress further will require each country to reflect on the structural issues that may have hindered progress to date. As the World Health Organization rightly points out, 'Society cannot afford not to invest in mental health' (WHO, 2005a, p. 127), and investment includes both money and the investment in supporting changes even when it goes against vested interests or prejudice.

References

Alarcon RD. Culture, cultural factors and psychiatric diagnosis: review and projections. *World Psychiatry.* 2009; **8**(3): 131–9.

Almeida C. *Portugal é o país da Europa com mais doenças mentais.* Lisboa: Entrevista conduzida por Rute Araújo; 2010.

American Psychiatric Association. *Practice Guidelines for the Treatment of Psychiatric Disorders: compendium 2006.* Arlington, VA: American Psychiatric Association; 2006.

Angermeyer MC, Dietrich S. Public beliefs and attitudes towards people with mental illness: a review of population studies. *Acta Psychiatr Scand.* 2006; **113**(3): 163–79.

Bagnall AM, Jones L, Ginnelly L, *et al.* A systematic review of atypical antipsychotic drugs in schizophrenia. *Health Technol Assess.* 2003; **7**(13): 1–193.

Barton R. *Institutional Neurosis.* Bristol: J Wright & Son; 1959.

Becker T, Kilian R. Psychiatric services for people with severe mental illness across Western Europe: what can be generalized from current knowledge about differences in provision, costs, and outcomes of mental health care? *Acta Psychiatr Scand.* 2006; **113**(Suppl 429): 9–16.

Becker T, Vazquez-Barquero JL. The European perspective of psychiatric reform. *Acta Psychiatr Scand.* 2001; **104**(Suppl 410): 8–14.

Brimblecombe N. The changing relationship between mental health nurses and psychiatrists in the United Kingdom. *J Adv Nurs*. 2005; **49**(4): 344–53.

Canino G, Alegría M. Psychiatric diagnosis – is it universal or relative to culture? *J Child Psychol Psychiatry*. 2008; **49**: 237–50.

Cheniaux E, Landeira-Fernandez J, Versiani M. The diagnoses of schizophrenia, schizoaffective disorder, bipolar disorder and unipolar depression: interrater reliability and congruence between DSM-IV and ICD-10. *Psychopathology*. 2009; **42**: 293–8.

Codony M, Alonso J, Almansa J, *et al.* Perceived need for mental health care and service use among adults in Western Europe: results of the ESEMeD project. *Psychiatr Serv*. 2009; **60**: 1051–8.

Coid J. The Christopher Clunis enquiry. *Psychiatr Bull*. 1994; **18**: 449–52.

Cox JL. European psychiatry: moving towards integration and harmony. *World Psychiatry*. 2007; **6**(1): 54–6.

Department of Health. *National Service Framework for Mental Health: modern standards and service models*. London: Department of Health; 1999.

Department of Health. *National Service Framework for Mental Health: modern standards and service models*. London: Department of Health; 2009a.

Department of Health. *Attitudes to Mental Illness 2009 Research Report*. 2009b. Available at: www.dh.gov.uk/en/Publicationsandstatistics/Publications/PublicationsStatistics/DH_100345 (accessed 20 December 2009).

Djernes JK. Prevalence and predictors of depression in populations of elderly: a review. *Acta Psychiatr Scand*. 2006; **113**(5): 372–87.

Dlouhý M. [Economics of mental health care in the Czech Republic] [Czech]. *Political Economy*. 2009; **6**: 797.

Dobel-Ober D, Brimblecombe N, Bradle E. Nurse prescribing in mental health: national survey. *J Psychiatr Ment Health Nurs*. 2010; **17**: 487–93.

Dowding K. *The Civil Service*. London: Routledge; 1995.

Eurostat. *Population Change at Regional Level*. 2009. Available at: epp.eurostat.ec.europa.eu (accessed 15 March 2011).

Finnane M. Australian asylums and their histories. introduction. *Health and History*. 2009; **11**: 6–8.

Finnish Central Association for Mental Health (2010) Mielenterveysbarometri. Available at: www.mtkl.fi/?x752385=1230924 (accessed 13 June 2010).

Fischer M. *Well-Ordered License: on the unity of Machiavelli's thought*. New York: Lexington; 2000.

Goffman E. *Asylums: essays on the social situation of mental patients and other inmates*. New York: Doubleday Anchor; 1961.

Gijswift-Hoftra M, Oosterhuis H. Introduction: comparing national cultures of psychiatry. In: Gijswift-Hoftra M, Oosterhuis H, Vijselaar J, *et al.*, editors. *Psychiatric Cultures Compared*. Amsterdam: Amsterdam University Press; 2005. pp. 9–28.

Gray R, Barnes P, Bee P, *et al. Mental Health Nursing: literature review synthesis and recommendations*. 2006. Available at: www.nursing.manchester.ac.uk/projects/mentalhealthreview/reviewsynthesisandrecommendations.pdf (accessed 21 December 2010).

Healy D. Irish psychiatry in the twentieth century. In: Freeman H, Berrios G, editors. *150 Years of British Psychiatry Volume II: the aftermath*. London: Athlone Press; 1996. pp. 268–91.

Hyun J, Nawka P, Hang SH, *et al.* Recovery- and community-based mental health services in the Slovak Republic: a pilot study on the implications for hospitalization and inpatient length-of-stay for individuals with severe and persistent mental illness. *Int J Psychosoc Rehab*. 2008; **13**(1): 67–80.

Jablensky A, Sartorius N, Cooper JE, *et al.* Culture and schizophrenia. *Br J Psychiatry*. 1994; **165**: 434–6.

Jakobsen KD, Frederiksen JN, Hansen T, *et al.* Reliability of clinical ICD-10 schizophrenia diagnoses. *Nord J Psychiatry*. 2005; **59**(3): 209–12.

Järvisalo J, Andersson B, Boedeker W, *et al. Mental Disorders as a Major Challenge in Prevention of Work Disability: experiences in Finland, Germany, the Netherlands and Sweden.* Helsinki: Kela; 2005.

Jilek WG, Jilek-Aall L. The metamorphosis of 'culture-bound' syndromes. *Soc Sci Medicine.* 1985; **21**: 205–10.

Karpf A. *Doctoring the Media.* London: Routledge; 1988.

Knapp M, Beecham J, McDaid D, *et al.* The economic consequences of deinstitutionalisation of mental health services: lessons from a systematic review of European experience. *Health Soc Care Comm.* 2011; **19**(2): 113–25.

Knapp M, McDaid D, Mossialos E, *et al. Mental Health Policy and Practice across Europe.* Milton Keynes: Open University Press; 2007.

Kohn R, Saxena S, Levav I, *et al.* The treatment gap in mental health care. *B World Health Organ.* 2004; **82**: 858–66.

Loureiro L, Dias C, Aragão R. Crenças e Atitudes acerca das doenças e dos doentes mentais – Contributos para o estudo das representações sociais da loucura. *Referência.* 2008; **2**(8): 33–44.

Madianos MG, Economou M, Hatjiandreou M, *et al.* Changes in public attitudes towards mental illness in the Athens area 1979/1980–1994. *Acta Psychiatr Scand.* 1999; **99**(1): 73–8.

Madianos MG, Madianou D, Vlachonikolis J, *et al.* Attitudes towards mental illness in the Athens area: implications for community mental health intervention. *Acta Psychiatr Scand.* 1987; **75**(2): 158–65.

Marmot M. Social determinants of health inequalities. *The Lancet.* 2005; **365**: 1099–104.

Marshall M, Rathbone J. Early intervention for psychosis. *Cochrane Database Syst Rev.* 2006; 18(4): CD004718.

Mental Health Commission. Community *Mental Health Services in Ireland: activity and catchment area characteristics 2004.* Dublin: Mental Health Commission; 2006.

Muijen M. Focus on mental health care reforms in Europe: mental health services in Europe – an overview. *Psychiatr Serv.* 2008; **59**(5): 479–82.

Nolan P, Brimblecombe N. A survey of the education of nurses working in mental health settings in 12 European countries. *Int J Nurs Stud.* 2007; 44(3): 407–14.

NOMESCO. *Health Statistics in the Nordic Countries 2005. Theme section: mental health.* Copenhagen: Nordic Medico Statistical committee 80; 2007.

Oosterhuis H. Insanity and other discomforts: a century of outpatient psychiatry and mental health care in the Netherlands 1900–2000. In: Gijswijt-Hofstra M, Oosterhuis H, Vijselaar J, *et al.,* editors. *Psychiatric Cultures Compared: psychiatry and mental health care in the twentieth century.* Amsterdam: Amsterdam University Press; 2005. pp. 72–80.

Parker C. Wasted time, wasted money, wasted lives . . . a wasted opportunity. *Tizard Learning Disability Review.* 2010; **15**: 7–14.

Petrea I, Muijen M. *Policies and Practices for Mental Health in Europe: meeting the challenges.* Copenhagen: WHO Regional Office for Europe; 2008.

Porritt J. *Capitalism, as if the World Matters.* London: Earthscan; 2005.

Priebe S. Psychiatry in the future. Where is mental health care going? A European perspective. *Psychiatr Bull.* 2004; **28**: 315–16.

Priebe S, Badesconyi A, Fioritti A, *et al.* Reinstitutionalisation in mental health care: comparison of data on service provision from six European countries. *BMJ.* 2005; **330**: 123–6.

Relationships Foundation. *The Family Pressure Gauge.* 2011. Available at: www.relationship foundation.org (accessed 10 July 2011).

Richter D, Berger K, Reker T. Are mental disorders on the increase? A systematic review. *Psychiatr Prax.* 2008; **35**(7): 321–30.

Sainsbury Centre for Mental Health. *Breaking the Circles of Fear.* London: Sainsbury Centre for Mental Health; 2002.

Sainsbury Centre for Mental Health. *Mental Health at Work: developing the business case*. Policy paper 8. London: Sainsbury Centre for Mental Health; 2007.

Social Exclusion Unit. *Mental Health and Social Exclusion: social exclusion unit report*. London, DHSS; 2004.

Spitzer RL, Forman JB, Nee J. DSM-III field trials: I. Initial interrater diagnostic reliability. *Am J Psychiatry*. 1979; **136**: 815–17.

Statistics Finland. *Life Expectancy of Newborn babies in Finland 1751–2006*. [Information brochure] 10 October 2007.

Stein LI, Test MA. Alternative to mental hospital treatment: I. Conceptual model, treatment program, and clinical evaluation. *Arch Gen Psychiatry*. 1980; **37**(4): 392–7.

Thornicroft G, Rose D. Mental health in Europe. *BMJ*. 2005; **330**(7492): 613–14.

Wahl OF. Mental health consumers' experience of stigma. *Schizophr Bull*. 1999; **25**: 467–78.

Warner R. Recovery from schizophrenia and the recovery model. *Curr Opin Psychiatry*. 2009; 22(4): 374–80.

WHO. *The World Health Report 2001. Mental Health: new understanding, new hope*. Geneva: World Health Organization; 2001. Available at: www.who.int/whr/2001/en/whr01_en.pdf (accessed 20 June 2010).

WHO Regional Office for Europe. *Mental Health Action Plan for Europe: facing the challenges, building solutions*. Copenhagen: WHO Regional Office for Europe; 2005a.

WHO Regional Office for Europe. *Mental Health Declaration for Europe: facing the challenges, building solutions*. Copenhagen: WHO Regional Office for Europe; 2005b.

Wittchen H, Jacobi F. Size and burden of mental disorders in Europe: a critical review and appraisal of 27 studies. *Eur Neuropsychopharmacol*. 2005; **15**(4): 357–76.

Wootton D. *Bad Medicine: doctors doing harm since Hippocrates*. Oxford: Oxford University Press; 2007.

12

Epilogue

Peter Nolan and Neil Brimblecombe

Reducing the implications of this book to a few salient points is to do a disservice to the myriad accounts and insights that have been presented here. There are so many areas of interest and concern that potentially merit further detailed discussion and examination, but space does not permit this. However, we have decided to highlight those points that we consider particularly important and which, we believe, should be given stronger consideration when seeking to improve mental health services in the future. We anticipate that many readers will not find them new, but we earnestly invite them to contemplate them with renewed vigour. In the first instance, we want to acknowledge the honesty and integrity which the authors who have contributed to this book have demonstrated in writing about mental health services in their respective countries; each one has portrayed their national situation as they have experienced it and believe it to be.

Of course, by the time this book is published, services may have altered beyond recognition to when the chapters were written. In reality, what ultimately gets implemented is highly dependent on the economic conditions, the political will and the abilities of service providers. A very real obstacle to change is the economic crisis which is enveloping the whole world, and it is conceivable that mental health policies, strategies and plans may have to be curtailed or put on hold. If this turns out to be the case, the efforts and enthusiasm of countless people in the EU who are eager to improve the care and treatment of people with mental health problems may be thwarted. Ironically, during times of economic recessions, the mental well-being of certain sections of society deteriorates; these include the poor, the unemployed, single-parent families, children and the old. The challenge to all governments is that mental health services can become so disadvantaged that they revert to being what they were over half a century ago. While governments do have a part to play in avoiding such an occurence, service users, families, the professions and the general public have an even more important part to play in not allowing this to happen. The voices of concern of these groups should reverberate through the corridors of power in every land, alerting leaders of the dire consequences of ignoring the general well-being of countless thousands of people. Not only do unrecognised and untreated mental health problems cause untold suffering to individuals and their familes, they can also affect members of extended families, communities and society at large.

It has been remarked on throughout this book that the quality of mental health policies is not solely dependent on their content. Equally important is the organisational climate in which they are implemented and the quality of support and supervision available to mental health professionals and carers. The outcome for individuals receiving services is closely correlated with the quality of care provided, and this particularly, but not solely, depends upon honest relationships, up-to-date information, affording choices to people, recognising the context of people's lives and being willing to assist people to shape the lives they wish to live.

As has been alluded to throughout this book, policies are no more than a set of propositions agreed on by ministers of state, stating how they would like things to be. Rarely do policy statements define what good mental health is; instead they point to what it should be, sometimes in utopian terms. In referring to scientific evidence, policy-makers attempt to strengthen their chances of certain policies being accepted, funded and implemented. Such policies inevitably need to be politically palatable, publicly acceptable and achievable within existing resources. In order for policies to be implemented, much needs to be known about human organisations, the values that people hold, the meanings they attach to actions and what they expect change to bring about. Policies can sometimes overstate what can realistically be achieved, and can be couched in terms that are difficult to discern. Policies often appear to be an extension of the philosophies of central government, with little or no input from professional staff, consumers of services or the general public. However, while central government gives direction, it is generally left to local government, local health services, individual health and social care managers to oversee what can realistically be implemented. It is now obvious that the future of mental health care is not about building more hospitals, extending existing services and employing more health professionals; instead it is about keeping people healthy. Health services that are government dependent are in a precarious position because governments change, priorities change and there will always be competing demands on existing services. So creating services which are independent of government should be an aim of all service providers.

In order to avoid the situation of staff feeling that they are constantly on a merry-go-round of being asked to provide more than their competence and resources permit, it is important to ask them what can be achieved, what obstacles exist and what help is required to overcome them. Where policy demands outweigh what can reasonably be delivered, it is frequently the case that patients are not well served by staff who themselves feel pressurised, bullied or lacking in competence and confidence.

The slow and sometimes disturbing evolution of mental health care has been illustrated in the chapters of this book. Now is the time when critical decisions need to be made about future direction. If bold decisions are not taken, mental health services could stagnate, frustrated by a situation in which policy states the desired direction of travel but where there is neither the political nor the professional will to provide the means of travel, nor insist that the means be found. Improvement in the well-being of people with mental illness in the future can no longer just be left to policy-makers, politicians and service providers; whole societies must be educated and encouraged to take more responsibility for decision-making. As part of this change, there is an urgent need to move away from the concept of mental *illness* services, as referred to in the introduction and which the Helsinki Agreement (WHO, 2005), the Foresight Project (2009) and WHO (2010) have strongly advocated. What is required now is a mixed economy of care where packages can be devised that meet the specific needs of individuals. For this to happen, boundaries between services need to be broken down and, in some cases, disappear. Alternatively, it will need to be much more explicit that *mental health services* will, in the future, only be one component of meeting *mental health need*, and other contributors will be as important. Those most at risk of developing mental health problems – the poor, uneducated, unemployed and socially excluded – are helped not just by individual therapies, but by the integration of services that allow them opportunities to become self-determining. Budgetary and conceptual divisions remain important barriers in this endeavour.

Considerable agreement has been reached on the factors that help people who are recovering from mental health problems; however, knowing what helps is not the same as acting on that knowledge. Providing restorative care makes demands on individuals, families, communities and on society. Improving mental health care cannot only be done by mental health personnel; mental health needs to be 'everyone's responsibility'. It is apparent from preceding chapters that mental health personnel who focus exclusively on expanding their own services or their professional sphere of influence either don't understand the 'bigger social picture' or feel they are unable to influence it. Increasing the number of inpatient beds and the number of outpatient appointments and providing more higher-education programmes for professionals may be helpful, but will have minimum impact on increasing social cohesion within a community, building social capital and removing the stigma that lead to inequality and oppression.

In the pages of this book, we have seen that it used to be customary to isolate the mentally ill from their families and communities and confine them in institutions; this approach, at the time, was seen as both humane and beneficial. Scientific thinking held that mental illness could be located, described and treated, thereby ultimately eradicating it from the human condition. This belief was enthusiastically embraced by those who were charged with caring for the mentally ill. Today, we have reached a point where it is considered that the best therapeutic environment is one in which the person is living their life, the best buffer against mental ill-health to be a life that is satisfying, and the best support an individual can receive to be provided by those who freely offer it as an expression of shared humanity. This is not to say that well-planned, well-delivered and well-evidenced clinical interventions are not valuable, or, indeed, essential. However, most aspects of clinical care remain largely unevidenced, or where evidence exists, history has often shown research evidence to be less robust than initially imagined.

It has been noted in this book that some of those who have lived under communist regimes may find it hard to take responsibility for their own health, having grown up in an environment where the state knows best. Nor is a feeling of powerlessness confined to people from countries of the former Soviet bloc. Indeed, there are many who have lived all their lives in democratic states who share this feeling, including people with mental illness. While their sense of powerlessness may stem from the debilitating effects of long-term mental health problems, it may also be due to experiences they have had of restrictive psychiatric practices and of living in communities where the toxic effect of stigma has contributed to a downward spiral of disability. Therefore, it cannot be assumed that the panacea for mental health problems is to return people to their communities and treat them there. The communities themselves must first be addressed, and then early intervention, accurate assessment, information and education can play their rightful part in preventing long-term incapacity. Whilst we are advocating the concept of mental health as 'everybody's business', we recognise that the reality is that, currently, much of the European population does not share this view and still holds negative views about those with mental illness.

Our aim in producing this book was not to provide another 'official' account of mental health services in the EU, but to explore the perspectives of those closely involved in delivering and managing services. In doing so, we hope that we are adding a new dimension to the current literature. While health policy-makers aim to improve services for patients and service users, it is left to others to decide how to implement their ideas. Policy-makers tend to assume that there are adequate resources (financial and human) to implement what their policy directs, that staff are willing and able to embrace change, and that management and information systems are supportive and flexible. However, if the vision is poorly communicated, or is itself insufficiently clear, and if there is not wholehearted cooperation from those who must realise it, there will inevitably be a disjuncture between aspiration and reality.

Although the creation of the EU was inspired by an urgent and heartfelt desire to prevent another war, such as those that traumatised Europe in the first half of the twentieth century, it was never the intention to impose administrative homogeneity on member countries. In fact, from the earliest days, it was recognised that the strength of the EU lay in its cultural diversity and its rich and turbulent history. Its success would depend on an increased level of cooperation between member states and a rejection of what some see as authoritarian ideologies such as fascism, communism and, indeed, in some historical contexts, Catholicism, which most countries had at some time been associated with. These ideologies had often stifled independent thought and creativity, originality and enterprise in those holding public office. It was not the intention of the EU founders to impose conformity, and indeed, today there are considerable differences of opinion on issues such as the war in Afghanistan, political turbulence in the Arab world and the management of the current economic crisis.

When analysing the relevance of mental health policies, it is important to recognise that they are not value-free and that they make demands on the existing status quo by challenging vested interests and professional securities. They involve speculating about what could be achieved if social structures and health care systems were sufficiently accommodating. This is totally contrary to the nature of modern mental health services, which are awash with treatment ideologies, therapeutic approaches and tightly defined professional boundaries and which demonstrate extreme caution when engaging with communities. Mental health professionals, constrained by the requirements of their professional codes, traditions and roles can often become defensive and change-resistant. However well-reasoned and reasonable, however persuasive and evidence-based, policy still relies totally on the good will of service providers and their commitment to what is being proposed. Health policies may also be presented in 'policy-speak' language which deliberately or unintentionally obscures the detail of how they are to be implemented, or falsely suggests that implementation is easily achievable or can occur with little extra effort.

As the chapters of this book have shown, policies and their implementation take many forms and one policy does not fit all occasions and circumstances. Mental health service improvement is 'work in progress' and requires regular monitoring and constant vigilance if it is to be sustained. It is a sad fact that if human services are capable of changing, they are also capable of reverting to what they once were. The overutilisation of change rhetoric can lead to the belief in providers that change is actually happening and all that requires to be done is being done. The creation of this belief is dangerous and can result in instances where mental health care staff 'hit the target but missed the point'. In England, similar to what occurred in other countries; targets were introduced by the Blair government in the early 2000s on the assumption that improvement could be driven by shortage of funding (Bevan and Robinson, 2006). When Blair came to power in 1997, there were 5 million people employed in the NHS, and when he left, that figure had risen to 6 million, and many of these new staff were employed in managing services, not providing them. His intention was to empower health care managers so as to contest the traditional power of doctors and nurses. Even though the English health care system groaned under regulation and audit, the data on which performances were based was often both fragmentary and episodic. This resulted in what a number of commentators referred to as 'gaming'; that is, where staff report what their managers or auditors wish to hear, rather than what is actually happening. 'Gaming' can become so endemic that it thwarts any or all attempts at changing or improving a culture or a health care system. The danger of this occurring within mental health services is very real, especially if staff are being asked to do more in the absence of adequate support, sufficient resources and appropriate training, and it must be resisted at all costs, as failure to do so could result in even further degeneration of the availability and quality of services.

Bearing the above commentary in mind, we now invite readers to reflect on the contribution from the nine countries represented in the preceding chapters. The key points have been stated before, but we feel it is useful to restate them, the most self-evident truths often being overlooked.

Creating services that are *not* mental illness-focused

Often, mental health providers and managers interpret mental health policy with a mindset that can imagine only more of what already exists. Modern mental health services require thinking that is creative and imaginative and outside institutional and biomedical parameters. The challenge now is to assist people without removing them from the context of their daily lives and without manipulating their identities. This demands that mental health personnel demonstrate far greater insight into social structures and collaborate with those who are best placed to ensure that all people are treated fairly according to their need.

Strengthening leadership

The chasm that has existed and currently exists between policies and their implementation should be a priority for the next generation of change agents. Some recent policies do not specify whose responsibility it is to initiate change; some call for a new type of leadership that transcends professional, service and agency boundaries. This threatens professional securities and may result in confusion on the part of those seeking help. Leaders are therefore needed who can support multidisciplinary and multiagency team functioning whilst managing the insecurities of mental health professionals and engaging with service users and their carers.

Supporting greater public involvement

Professionals may fear community action on the grounds that the community may insist on accountability; they may prefer to keep service users in a position of deference and compliance, rather than dealing with citizens who demand value for money and demonstrable results. However, it is likely to be in community contexts that the quality of mental health care will, in future, be assessed. The terms of reference will be the efficacy of individual care packages and the quality of support people are able to find for themselves. In such an environment, it will be less possible to remove people from their normal social environment and treat the condition, rather than the individual. In the same way that professionals will need training in their new roles, the public will also need education as to what is required of them.

Fighting stigma

The effects of stigmatisation would appear to be one of the biggest problems facing people with mental health issues, and mental health services, across the EU. Fear and distrust of those with mental illnesses remains as prevalent as ever, and it constitutes an obstacle to the treatment and recovery of people with mental health problems. Stigma affects those who suffer with poor mental health, those who provide services for them and the families of those in treatment. Fear of stigmatisation may deter families and individuals from seeking help. A much greater effort to destigmatise mental health is required both from the EU and individual governments if existing policies are to have the impact which they are intended to have. Without addressing this, it is possible that existing and future policies will always meet resistance and indifference and desired aims will become illusions.

Increasing social equality

Where social inequality exists, there is attendant marginalisation, low aspiration, material and spiritual poverty, poor health and a lack of personal resources to overcome deficits. Countries which are unable to address inequalities witness an intergenerational recycling of poor physical and mental health coupled with a poverty of ambition. Mental health personnel, who know the consequences of cutting services for lower-income people during times of recession, should feel able to speak out about the long-term damage that is being done to those who are vulnerable and dependent. Those with a voice or who have access to a means of expressing their feelings should assume a position where they make public the consequences of political, economic and social activities that further disadvantage the weak and disabled.

Strengthening interprofessional and interagency education

The mental health care agenda requires a strong emphasis on educational pro-grammes that bring together different disciplines and services. Enabling people to study and learn alongside each other is an important step towards assisting them to work more closely together. Knowing the roles of others gives a better understanding of their own. For services to progress, critical and self-assured people are needed who can see the rationale for improvement and create the conditions in which it can be achieved. Improvement is thwarted when staff withdraw into their respective disciplines and refuse to cooperate through fear of being seen as less competent than others and of not being able to function in a multidisciplinary setting.

Strengthening quality measurement

Regardless of the type of mental health service provided, continuous evaluation of those services is essential. The need to be able to evaluate clinical effective-ness, impact on quality of life and, equally importantly, acceptability to those people who use services is often missing currently. The manner in which serv-ices measure and judge themselves (or fail to do so) speaks loudly of the culture within those organisations. The absence of evaluation suggests a lack of healthy self-criticism, and a focus on purely clinical measures illustrates a narrow view of the needs of service users.

Listening to the user voice

Service users in all countries have been historically deprived of a voice, and defined as being passive recipients of institutional management and biomedical control. By definition, they have not had a view that should be taken seriously or given moral authority to influence professional concepts of success, failure and quality. A fundamental change is still required, so that the experiences of people with mental health problems are sought out and listened to, so that they become true partners in defining need, deciding on action and evaluating outcomes. This transformation is at very early stages in most countries.

Moving away from reactive services

Mental health services in the past were only available to people once they became ill. In countries where access to care is problematic or delayed, people can be considerably worse by the time they get seen, thus reducing their chances of full recovery. The direction of travel now should be towards minimising the threats to adult mental health which present in the formative years of life. There has been insufficient attention paid to the clear link between maternal mental health and the physical, social and cognitive development of babies. Could monies directed at addressing behavioural problems in school-age children be redirected towards the implementation of programmes for promoting optimum parenting and nurturing parental relationships in the first year of a baby's life, when infant brain plasticity is at its maximum? Of course, the challenging question is always 'money redirected from where?' The issue of prioritisation is one that requires a fresh look. It would be a major change for most mental health services to think outside their current remit and creatively engage with proactive measures to prevent ill health from occurring in infancy.

This book has identified many challenges to delivering high-quality mental health services and, more generally, improving the well-being of people with mental health problems. However, whilst it is important to studiously avoid any 'evolutionary' historical viewpoint which celebrates all change as 'progress', changes have happened that are likely to have improved the lives of many. Whilst the World Health Organization can certainly be criticised for some details of its approach to change, undoubtedly it has had some success at raising the profile of mental health issues, and beginning to change the focus of the debate from *mental illness* to *mental health*. Increasingly, countries have closed their large asylums which, although originally constructed for the best of motives, had typically become warehouses for the sick and socially inappropriate. Most countries now have, at least, embryonic community services and have officially 'signed up' to WHO-influenced models of service delivery. This alignment may not always affect major change, but it certainly makes it easier to hold individual governments to account for their failure to do so.

The future of mental health services and mental health care across Europe is in the balance at the moment, with key issues about resources and focus at a critical point. Only with a positive belief as to the possibility of change, amongst health professionals, service users and the public at large, can positive change be brought about and the required policies finally be translated into reality.

References

Bevan G, Hood C. What's measured in that which matters: targets and gaming in the English public health care system. *Public Admin*. 2006; **84**: 517–38.

Foresight Project on Mental Capital and Well-Being. *Mental Capital and Well-Being: making the most of ourselves in the 21st century – final project report*. London: Government Office for Science; 2009.

World Health Organization. *Report on the European Ministerial Conference on Mental Health*. Helsinki: WHO; 2005.

World Health Organization. *Mental Health: strengthening our response. Fact sheet no. 220*. 2010. Available at: www.who.int/mediacentre/factsheets/fs220/en (accessed 10 April 2011).

Index

Index

Index

Printed and bound by CPI Group (UK) Ltd, Croydon, CR0 4YY

23/10/2024

01777678-0010